H. Menge M. Gregor G. N. J. Tytgat
B. J. Marshall C. A. M. McNulty (Eds.)

Helicobacter pylori 1990

Proceedings of the Second International Symposium on Helicobacter pylori
Bad Nauheim, August 25–26th, 1989

With 55 Figures and 52 Tables

Springer-Verlag
Berlin Heidelberg New York London
Paris Tokyo Hong Kong Barcelona

Professor Dr. H. Menge
Medizinische Klinik II, Krankenanstalten der Stadt Remscheid,
Akademisches Lehrkrankenhaus der Universität Bonn,
Hans-Potyka-Str. 28, 5630 Remscheid, FRG

Professor Dr. M. Gregor
Abteilung für Innere Medizin mit Schwerpunkt Gastroenterologie,
Klinikum Steglitz der Freien Universität Berlin,
Hindenburgdamm 30, 1000 Berlin 45, FRG

Professor Dr. G.N.J. Tytgat
Department of Gastroentero-Hepatology, Academisch Ziekenhuis
bij de Universiteit van Amsterdam, Academisch Medisch Centrum,
Meibergdreef 9, 1105 AZ Amsterdam Zuidoost, The Netherlands

Dr. B.J. Marshall
Division of Gastroenterology, Department of Internal Medicine,
University of Virginia, Charlottesville,
Virginia 22908, USA

Dr. C.A.M. McNulty
Public Health Laboratory, Gloucestershire Royal Hospital,
Great Western Road, Gloucestershire GL1 3NN, United Kingdom

ISBN-13:978-3-642-75728-0 e-ISBN-13:978-3-642-75726-6
DOI: 10.1007/978-3-642-75726-6

2127/3140/543210 – Printed on acid-free paper

Preface

In 1987, we organized the First International Symposium on *Campylobacter pylori* in order to evaluate the information accumulated since the first description of *Helicobacter pylori* in 1983, and to discuss the questions that should be answered in the near future. Since then substantial progress has been made in *Helicobacter pylori* research and it is obvious that the classical concepts of the pathogenesis of chronic gastritis and peptic ulcer disease must be revised to integrate this organism. At this exciting moment it seemed worthwhile to us to have a Second International Symposium on *Helicobacter pylori* in order to discuss its role in diseases of the upper gastrointestinal tract.

Since it is hardly possible to cover all facets of *Helicobacter pylori* research during one symposium, we have focused our interest on five topics of major clinical importance. The first topic includes the virulence factors of *Helicobacter pylori*. The second section deals with the epidemiology of *Helicobacter pylori*, chronic gastritis, and peptic ulcer disease. Thereafter, theoretical and clinical aspects of different regimens for treating *Helicobacter pylori* – associated diseases are considered. The last session is dedicated to a discussion about the optimal design of clinical studies for the treatment of diseases of the upper gastrointestinal tract. The organizers hope to have covered with these topics some of the most interesting clinical aspects of *Helicobacter pylori* infection.

The conference would not have been possible without the extraordinary generosity of Röhm Pharma and the organizational talent of Mrs. C. J. Klein and her staff, whose help and innovating spirit is highly appreciated by the organizers of this symposium. We also thank all those behind the scenes for having created a pleasant atmosphere for this gathering. Finally, we wish to express our appreciation to all the speakers and the moderators who with their high-standard presentations and enthusiastic discussions greatly contributed to the success of the meeting.

H. Menge M. Gregor G. N. J. Tytgat B. J. Marshall C. A. M. McNulty

Table of Contents

Section 4 Clinical Trials for *Helicobacter pylori* Treatment

Section 5 Optimal Design of Clinical Trials

Chairmen and Senior Authors

Börsch, G.
Medizinische Klinik, Elisabeth-Krankenhaus, Akademisches Lehrkrankenhaus der Universität Essen, Moltkestr. 61, 4300 Essen, FRG

Classen, M.
II. Medizinische Klinik und Poliklinik rechts der Isar der TU München, Ismaninger Str. 22, 8000 München 80, FRG

Colin-Jones, D. G.
Queen Alexandra Hospital, Cosham, Portsmouth PO6 3LY, United Kingdom

Glupczynski, Y. G.
Department of Microbiology, Brugmann University Hospital, 4, Place Van Gehuchten, 1020 Brussels, Belgium

Graham, D. Y.
Digestive Disease Division, Baylor College of Medicine, VA Medical Center (111D), 2002 Holcombe Blvd., Houston, Texas 77030, USA

Gregor, M.
Abteilung für Innere Medizin mit Schwerpunkt Gastroenterology, Klinikum Steglitz, Freie Universität Berlin, Hindenburgdamm 30, 1000 Berlin 45, FRG

Hazell, S. L.
School of Microbiology, University of New South Wales, P.O. Box 1, Kensington, NSW 2033, Australia

Heilmann, K. L.
Pathologisches Institut, Städtisches Krankenhaus, Robert-Koch-Str. 1, 8300 Landshut, FRG

De Koster, E.
Department of Gastroenterology, Brugmann University Hospital, 4, Place Van Gehuchten, 1020 Brussels, Belgium

Krakowka, S.
Department of Veterinary Pathobiology, College of Veterinary Medicine,
Ohio State University, 1925 Coffey Road, Columbus, Ohio 43210-1093, USA

Lee, A.
School of Microbiology, University of New South Wales,
P.O. Box 1, Kensington, Sydney, NSW 2033, Australia

Mai, U.E.H.
Department of Microbiology, University of Maryland, College Park,
Maryland 20742, USA

Marshall, B.J.
Division of Gastroenterology, Department of Internal Medicine,
University of Virginia, Charlottesville, Virginia 22908, USA

McNulty, C.A.M.
Public Health Laboratory, Gloucestershire Royal Hospital,
Great Western Road, Gloucester, GL1 3NN, United Kingdom

Mégraud, F.
Laboratoire de Bactériologie, Hôpital des Enfants,
168 Cours de L'Argonne, 33077 Bordeaux, France

Menge, H.
Medizinische Klinik II, Krankenanstalten der Stadt Remscheid,
Akademisches Lehrkrankenhaus der Universität Bonn,
Hans-Potyka-Str. 28, 5630 Remscheid, FRG

Newell, D.G.
Division of Pathology, Centre for Applied Microbiology and Research,
Public Health Laboratory, Porton Down, Salisbury,
Wiltshire SP4 OJG, United Kingdom

Nwckolo, C.U.
Academic Department of Medicine, Royal Free Hospital School of Medicine,
London NW3 2QG, United Kingdom

Petersen, H.
Section of Gastroenterology, Faculty of Medicine, Trondheim Regional Hospital,
University of Trondheim, 7000 Trondheim, Norway

Rauws, E.A.J.
Department of Gastroentero-Hepatology, Academisch Medisch Centrum,
Academisch Ziekenhuis bij de Universiteit van Amsterdam,
Meibergdreef 9, 1105 AZ Amsterdam Zuidoost, The Netherlands

RAEDSCH, R.
Klinikum der Universität Heidelberg, Med. Klinik,
Bergheimer Straße 58, 6900 Heidelberg, FRG

SIPPONEN, P.
Department of Pathology, Jorvi Hospital, 02740 Espoo, Finland

SLIKKERVEER, A.
Toxicology Laboratory, University Hospital,
P.O. Box 9600, 2300 RA Leiden, The Netherlands

SLOMIANY, B. L.
Dental Research Center, University of Medicine and Dentistry,
110 Bergen Street, Newark, New Jersey 07103-2425, USA

STOLTE, M.
Institut für Pathologie, Klinikum Bayreuth,
Preuschwitzer Str. 101, 8580 Bayreuth, FRG

TALLEY, N. J.
Gastroenterology Unit, Mayo Clinic, 3rd St. and 4th Avenue SW, Rochester,
Minnesota 55902, USA

TYTGAT, G. N. J.
Department of Gastroentero-Hepatology, Academisch Medisch Centrum,
Academisch Ziekenhuis bij de Universiteit van Amsterdam,
Meibergdreef 9, 1105 AZ Amsterdam Zuidoost, The Netherlands

VAIRA, D.
Via S. Petronio Vecchio, 18, 40125 Bologna, Italy

VELDHUYZEN VAN ZANTEN, S. J. O.
Division of Gastroenterology, Department of Medicine, McMaster University,
1200 Main Street West, Hamilton, Ontario L8N 3Z5, Canada

WADSTRÖM, T.
Department of Medical Microbiology, University of Lund,
Sölvegatan 23, 22362 Lund, Sweden

WESTBLOM, T. U.
Division of Infectious Diseases, St. Louis University School of Medicine,
1402 S. Grand Blvd., St. Louis, Missouri 63104, USA

WYATT, J. I.
Department of Pathology, St. James's University Hospital,
Beckett Street, Leeds LS9 7TF, United Kingdom

Section 1

Virulence Factors and Pathogenicity of *Helicobacter pylori*

Urease and Catalase as Virulence Factors of *Helicobacter pylori**

S. L. HAZELL

Introduction

Since the first report of the urease activity of *Helicobacter pylori* [1], this enzyme has captured a large amount of attention from researchers interested in the detection and pathogenicity of this gastric bacterium. This interest is in part aroused by the extraordinary urease activity seen in *H. pylori* [2–5]. Another enzyme of *H. pylori* noted for its vigor is catalase [6]. While not the subject of intense investigation to date, this latter enzyme may be as important to *H. pylori* as urease with respect to virulence and pathogenicity.

In reviewing urease and catalase as virulence factors we venture into an area where ideas are more abundant than data. However, as part of the rationale of this symposium is to discuss the questions that should be answered in the future, I do not hesitate in addressing these ideas. To discuss this issue thoroughly a definition of virulence factors is required. I will define virulence factors as those attributes that allow the pathogen to establish and induce disease in the host; this definition excludes core biological functions that may be classed as basic to the growth and viability of the microbe. Building on this definition, virulence factors may be classed as either primary, those permitting the establishment of the agent in the host, or secondary, those promoting or inducing pathology.

Urease

While *H. pylori* urease (Table 1) has received much attention because of its utility as a diagnostic marker – starting with the biopsy urease tests [9–11], followed by urea

Table 1. Characteristics of *Helicobacter pylori* urease [4, 5, 7, 8]

Property	Value
Molecular weight	300 K (625 K)
p*I*	5.9
pH optima	5.8–8.2
K_m	0.8 ± 0.1 m*M* urea
Isoenzymes	2?

* Stuart Hazell is a H.J. Martin Fellow supported by the National Health and Medical Research Council of Australia. This work was supported in part by Veterans Affairs and in part by grant DK-39919 from the National Institute of Digestive and Kidney Diseases

H. Menge et al. (Eds.)
Helicobacter pylori 1990

breath tests [12, 13] and of late as a specific antigen for the detection of antibodies to *H. pylori* [5, 14, 15] – the focus of this commentary will be on urease as a virulence factor.

Urease as a Core Biological Function

The function of urease in a diverse range of eukaryotic and prokaryotic organisms has recently been reviewed [16]. This article reaffirms that the major function of urease is to release nitrogen, in the form of ammonia, from urea,, thus making it available to the cell. Indeed ammonia is the common linkin the assimilation of inorganic nitrogen (Fig. 1). Based on this principle, it has been argued that the urease of *H. pylori* fulfills the role of a core biological function, in that it makes urea nitrogen available to the bacterium [3, 5]. The pronounced urease activity of *H. pylori* may facilitate the flux of urea from the blood and across the gastric mucosa by the generation of a urea gradient [3, 5; Fig. 2]. This principle has previously been established for the bacteria that colonize the wall of the rumen in animals to obtain their nitrogen from blood urea [17, 18]. The apparent localization of *H. pylori* urease in the outer membrane of the bacterium and the unheeded access of the enzyme to urea is consistent with the above function [4, 14, 19].

Where urease exerts a known pathological effect, e.g., in struvite nephrolithiasis, the effect is precipitated by an alteration in pH [20, 21]. For those bacteria that induce kidney stone formation the essential function of urease remains unaltered: the provision of urea nitrogen to the microbe. The pathological effect of urease looks to be essentially a manifestation of the environment in which the organism is found [22].

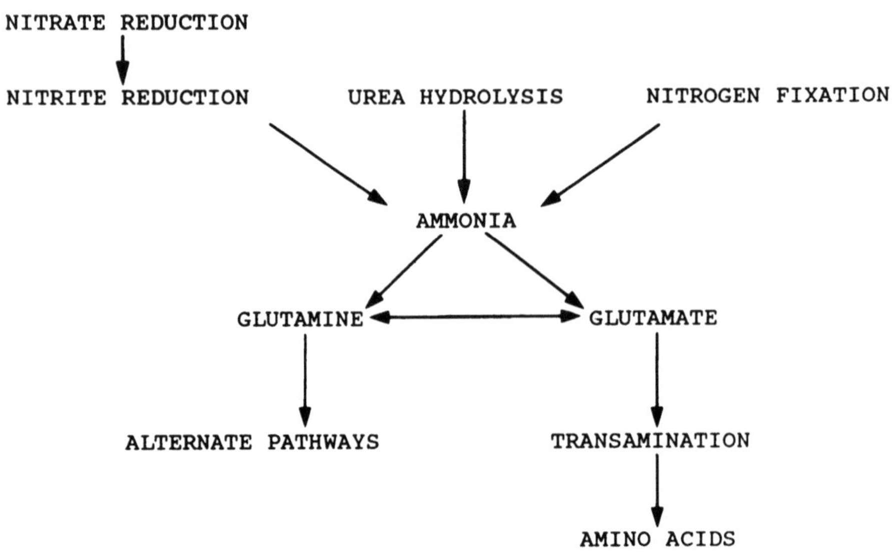

Fig. 1. Ammonia holds a key position in the assimilation of nitrogen by bacteria, be that nitrogen derived from the reduction of nitrate and nitrite, nitrogen fixation, or urea hydrolysis

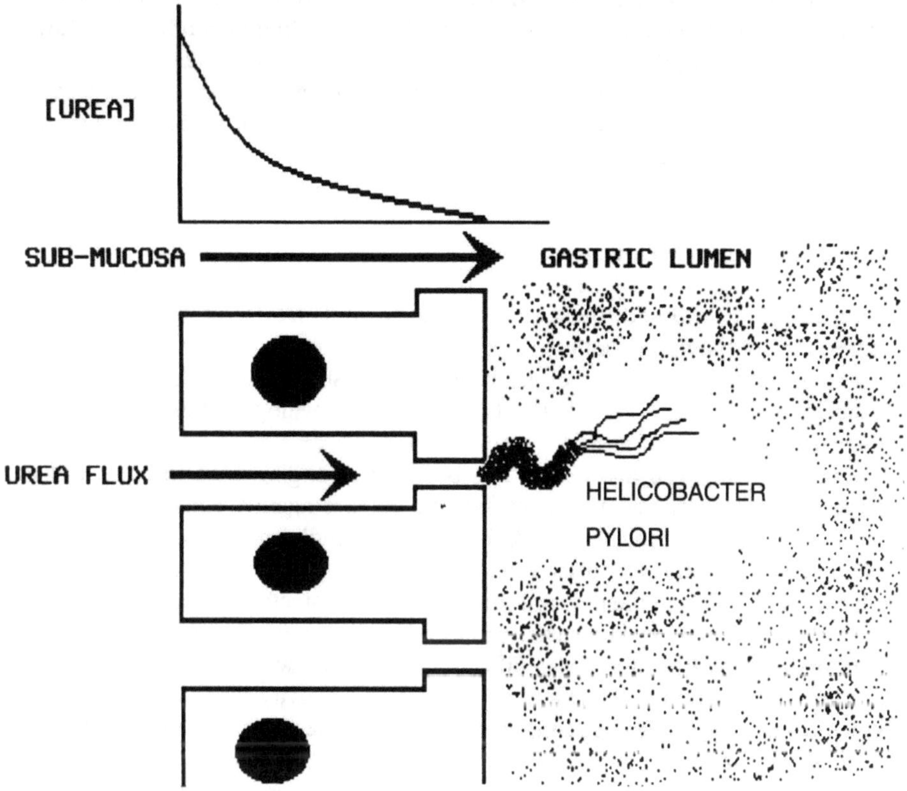

Fig. 2. Rapid urea hydrolysis by *Helicobacter pylori* produces a urea concentration gradient across the mucosa which increases the flux of urea from the submucosa toward the gastric lumen

Urease as a Primary Virulence Factor

Urease has been proposed to protect *H. pylori* from the damaging effects of gastric acidity by providing a buffering "cloud of ammonia" [23]. This hypothesis is both simple and appealing, and has gained some credence in the literature. The ability to evade the damaging effects of gastric acidity by the production of a buffering "cloud of ammonia" would rank *H. pylori* urease as a primary virulence factor (i.e., permitting the establishment of the agent in the host).

In contemplation of this view, the chance that *H. pylori* urease protects from gastric acidity should not be considered in isolation. An important question remains: Is protection from acid the foremost activity of *H. pylori* urease or is this property subordinate to an existent role of the enzyme? Based on the studies involving *H. pylori* and non-*H. pylori* gastric spiral bacteria, the presence of urease undoubtedly endows some advantage to these organisms and may contribute in part to their organ tropism [24–28]. A recent report on the urease activity of *H. pylori* compared the enzyme activity of the latter with that of an apparently related organism isolated from rodents [5]. The rodent bacterium colonizes the mucus-filled crypts of large bowel [29] yet has urease activity comparable to that of *H. pylori* [5]. Further, acidophilic and acid-tolerant bacteria have adapted to such extreme environments by the regulation of their cytoplasmic pH and the development of acid-resistant membrane structures and enzyme systems [30–36]. In this way urease-negative organisms, such as the lactobacilli and yeasts, are able to colonize a diverse range of acidic environments. Thus the argument may be advanced that protection from gastric acidity is a subordinate function or urease.

Urease as a Secondary Virulence Factor

Urease has been proposed to act as a secondary virulence factor by a number of avenues. One of the first hypotheses implicating a role for the urease of *H. pylori* in the pathogenesis of peptic ulcer disease was the "urease-induced hydrogen ion back diffusion hypothesis" [37; Fig. 3]. This hypothesis was developed after consideration of the early literature on "gastric urease" [38–41].

Before it was realized that urease was bacterial in origin, it was presumed that "gastric urease" functioned as part of mucosal defense against acid. Although this latter hypothesis was wrong, it was, like others, both simple and appealing. Yet given a role for acid in peptic ulcer disease, reconciliation of why the "cloud of ammonia" produced by *H. pylori* at the mucosal surface was not protective appeared necessary. Therefore, based on many known and proposed properties of the gastric mucosa, the "urease-induced hydrogen ion back diffusion hypothesis" was developed.

The concept inherent in the hypothesis, that urease activity contributes to the loss of mucosal integrity, has gained some support from studies in rats. In these animals it was found that urea plus urease induces a decrease in the transmucosal potential difference and microscopic damage [42]. These mucosal alterations were found to be mediated by ammonia.

Although the "hypothesis" related primarily to gastric ulcers, its utility in explaining part of the duodenal ulcer story required further development. Some of the remaining questions have been answered by the finding that *H. pylori* colonizes areas of gastric metaplasia in the duodenal bulb and the suggestion that, where duodenal ulcers form, functional heterotopic gastric mucosa may be present [43–46].

A section of the paper dealing with the "urease-induced hydrogen ion back diffusion hypothesis" also discussed the potential for ammonia to be directly toxic to cells by mechanisms such as interference with the Na^+/K^+-ATPase [37]. Others have reported results indicating that *H. pylori* urease produces a cytopathic effect in Vero cells, this effect being attributed to ammonia [47]. As yet no mechanism has been established for this effect. In consideration of ammonia as a toxin for the gastric epithelium a number of factors must be kept in mind. First, cells vary in their susceptibility to ammonia in a concentration-dependent manner [48–51], with some being unaffected by extremely high concentrations of ammonia. Second, it is ammonia (NH_3) and not the ammonium ion (NH_4^+) that is the toxic species [52]; thus the pH of both the extra- and intracellular environment will mediate the apparent toxicity off amonia. Thus, although it is possible in vitro to acidify cells by first loading them with NH_4^+ followed by washing in an ammonium-free solution [53] without apparent toxic effects, this should not be interpreted to mean that ammonia is nontoxic. In the stomach the urease activity of *H. pylori* could result in chronic,

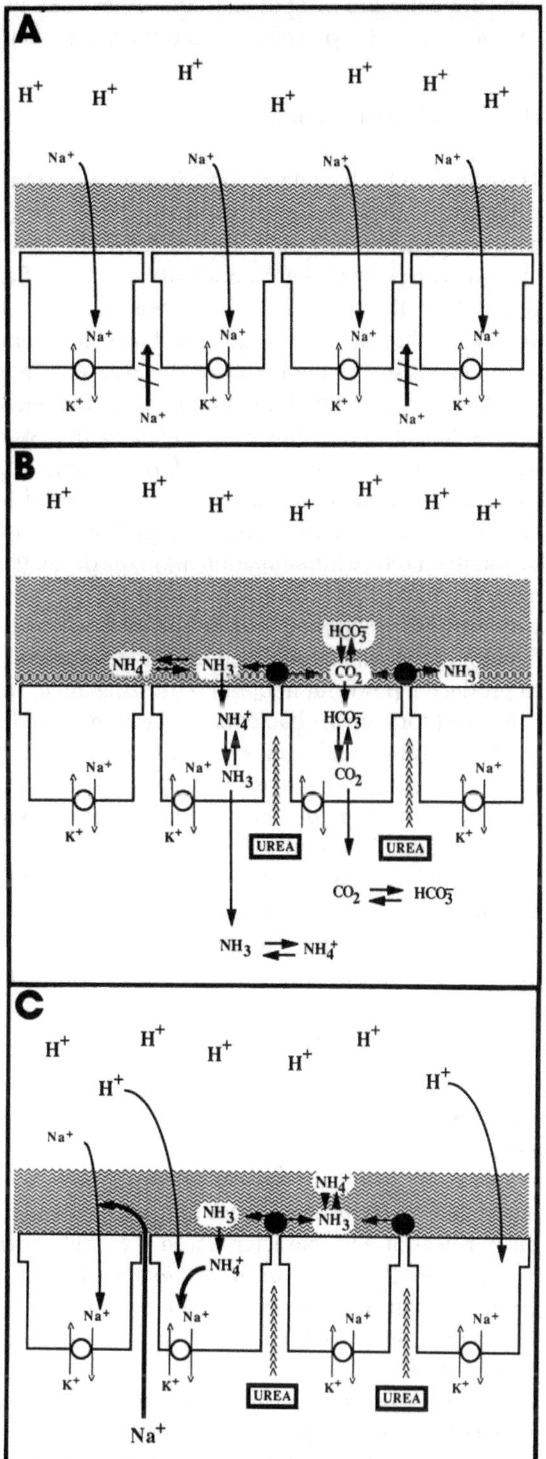

Fig. 3A–C. In the normal stomach the mucus layer has been proposed to act as a one-way barrier for H^+ [69]. The proposed mechanism for this one-way barrier is a combination of ion-exchange characteristics of the mucus gel and the generation of a positive charge on the epithelial surface. This mechanism involves the formation of an Na^+ gradient through the mucus which is maintained by (**a**) a Na^+/K^+-ATPase-dependent unidirectional flow of Na^+ and (**b**) the pH-dependent anionic selective nature of the intercellular space which blocks the passage of Na^+ from the submucosa to the gastric lumen (**A**). When gastric epithelium is colonized by *Helicobacter pylori* (**B**) the urease activity of the bacterium will induce a flux of urea across the mucosa, increase the local pH, and significantly increase the concentration of ammonia/ammonium at the epithelial surface. These alterations bring about urease-dependent hydrogen ion back diffusion (**C**). Where (a) the increase in local pH alters the anionic selective nature of the intercellular spaces and allows Na^+ to pass across the mucosa which destroys the Na^+-dependent surface charge, (b) the NH_4^+ impedes the ion-exchange properties of the mucus gel, and (c) NH_4^+/NH_3 uncouples the Na^+/K^+-ATPase. All of this facilitates the back diffusion of H^+

subacute exposure of epithelial and other cells to ammonia. Potentially this could contribute to cell hyperplasia and tumorogenesis [54–56].

Urease and Inflammation

The claim has been made by some investigators that either the lack of inflammation in animals colonized by urease-positive bacteria or the purported lack of a correlation between gastritis and gastric ammonia invalidates the above hypotheses; even though there was no claim that urease activity was pro-inflammatory [57, 58]. This conclusion is based on the tenet that if an agent is producing an effect, be it cytopathic or otherwise, then this must be manifest in an inflammatory response. This notion is not valid. To illustrate, the toxins of the enterotoxigenic *Escherichia coli* have a major effect on the gut epithelium but are not inflammatory [59].

This concern does, however, highlight the issue of the differences in pathology between humans infected by *H. pylori* and animals colonized by other urease-positive bacteria. Inflammation may represent a crucial factor in events leading to peptic ulceration. Here urease-generated ammonia/ammonium in conjunction with independently induced inflammation may contribute to mucosal damage. In polymorphonuclear leukocytes (PMNs), myeloperoxidase-generated hypochlorous acid will react with nitrogen compounds to produce mono-*N*-chloramine compounds. These mono-*N*-chloramines can be released from PMNs and will react with ammonia/ammonium to produce a powerful lipophilic oxidizing agent monochloramine [60].

Monochloramine is bactericidal, cytotoxic, and cytolytic. Its formation is favored by elevated ammonia/ammonium concentrations. We may ask the question, does part of the duodenal ulcer disease cycle consist of repeated events of colonization of gastric metaplasia by *H. pylori,* induction of inflammation, formation of monochloramine, cell lysis, and ulceration?

As with the discussion of urease as a primary virulence factor, the role of urease as a secondary virulence factor should be considered subordinate to the core biological function of the enzyme. The potential pathological effects of urease outlined above, if proven, will be only a function of the environment in which the organism is found. Urease of comparable activity from another source, delivered to the same site, would be expected to produce the same effects.

Catalase

Whereas *H. pylori* urease has been adopted as a topic of research by numerous investigators, *H. pylori* catalase has, until recently, remained an orphan. A paper on the purification and characterization of *H. pylori* catalase has recently been submitted to the *Journal of General Microbiology* (Hazell, S.L., D.J. Evans Jr., and D.Y. Graham. "Purification and characterization of catalase from *Helicobacter pylori*"). This paper, apart from characterizing the enzyme (Table 2), queried the benefit of catalase to *H. pylori.*

Catalase acts to protect against the damaging effects of oxygen metabolites, specifically H_2O_2, and is potentially important to some bacteria in resistance to killing by polymorphonuclear leukocytes [61–63]. It is now established that *H. pylori* is a major

Table 2. Characteristics of *Helicobacter pylori* catalase. (Hazell, S.L., D.J. Evans Jr., and D.Y. Graham. Purification and characterization of catalase from *Helicobacter pylori*. Submitted to *Journal of General Microbiology)*

Property	Value
Molecular weight	200 K
p*I*	9–9.3
pH optima	Broad
K_m	45 ± 2 m*M* H_2O_2

etiological agent of human active chronic gastritis. Thus the catalase activity of *H. pylori* may protect this bacterium from H_2O_2 released either intra- or extracellularly by polymorphonuclear leukocytes.

Preliminary data suggest that *H. pylori* may be resistant to relatively high concentrations of exogenous H_2O_2 (unreported data). Interestingly, a recent study of ours suggests that *H. pylori* is susceptible in vitro to the toxic effects of peroxidated long-chain fatty acids and that, in the absence of blood or serum, exogenous catalase is required in the medium [64]. While there appears to be no correlation between the ability of peroxidated long-chain fatty acids to damage cells and susceptibility to H_2O_2, the former study indicates that *H. pylori* catalase is not secreted into the environment and hence may only provide a specific local defense against damage by H_2O_2.

While the catalase of some bacteria appears to protect the cells from damage by exogenous H_2O_2 (e.g., from PMNs), in others the enzyme acts to "mop up" endogenously generated H_2O_2 [65, 66]. If *H. pylori* catalase proves to be important in protection from exogenous H_2O_2, this enzyme may represent another primary virulence factor in that it allows the bacterium to survive on the surface of inflamed gastric mucosa. Three factors lend weight to this hypothesis:

a) The relatively high catalase activity of *H. pylori* compared with *C. jejuni;*
b) the apparent lack of enzyme inhibition by high concentrations of H_2O_2, unlike the catalase from a range of other bacteria [66, 67], a notable exception being the mycobacteria [68]; and
c) the spontaneous mutation of *H. pylori* to a catalase-negative phenotype upon repeated culture in vitro (unpublished data).

This latter information suggests that catalase is not required by the bacterium to break down endogenous H_2O_2.

Conclusion

The considerable urease activity of *H. pylori* marks this enzyme as a significant factor in the life of the bacterium. Whereas urease has been a "hot" topic of research in the field of diagnostics, the available data on urease as a virulence factor remain scant. It is hoped that the information and ideas presented here will stimulate both discussion and activity. A full understanding of the value of urease in the colonization of the gastric mucosa by *H. pylori* and other gastric bacteria has yet to be attained. In the investigation of the effect of urease activity on the gastric mucosa, the development and use of cell models that are truly gastric in nature should be a prime consideration.

While urease may be a virulence factor by virtue of the environment into which it is delivered, catalase potentially represents a primary virulence factor in its own right. Further studies of the effect catalase has on the ability of *H. pylori* to withstand H_2O_2-mediated damage are warranted. Such studies, in conjunction with studies that advance our understanding of how *H. pylori* persists in the face of other components of the immune system, may permit novel therapeutic approaches to the *H. pylori* problem to be developed.

References

1. Langenberg ML, Tytgat GN, Schipper MEI, Rietra PJGM, Zanen HC (1984) *Campylobacter*-like organisms in the stomach of patients and healthy individuals. Lancet I:1348
2. Owen RJ, Martin SR, Borman P (1985) Rapid urea hydrolysis by gastric *Campylobacters*. Lancet I:111
3. Hazell SL, Lee A, Brady L, Hennessy W (1986) *Campylobacter pyloridis* and gastritis: association with intercellular spaces and adaption to an environment of mucus as important factors in colonization of the gastric epithelium. J Infect Dis 153:658–663
4. Mobley HLT, Cortesia MJ, Rosenthal LE, Jones BD (1988) Characterization of urease from *Campylobacter pylori*. J Clin Microbiol 26:831–836
5. Ferrero RL, Hazell SL, Lee A (1988) The urease enzymes of *Campylobacter pylori* and a related bacterium. J Med Microbiol 27:33–40
6. Marshall BJ, Royce H, Annear DI, Goodwin CS, Pearman JW, Warren JR, Armstrong JA (1984) Original isolation of *Campylobacter pyloridis* from human gastric mucosa. FEMS Microbios Lett 25:83–88
7. Taylor MB, Goodwin CS, Karim QN (1988) Two urease activities with different pH optima in *Campylobacter pylori* and similar organisms. FEMS Microbiol Lett 55:259–262
8. Taylor MB, Karim QN (1988) Urease activity of *Campylobacter pylori*. J Clin Pathol 41:112
9. McNulty CAM, Wise R (1985) Rapid diagnosis of *Campylobacter*-associated gastritis. Lancet I:1443–1444
10. Marshall BJ, Warren JR, Francis GJ, Langton SR, Goodwin CS, Blincow ED (1987) Rapid urease test in the management of *Campylobacter pyloridis*-associated gastritis. Am J Gastroenterol 82:200–210
11. Hazell SL, Borody TJ, Gal A, Lee A (1987) *Campylobacter pyloridis* gastritis I: detection of urease as a marker of bacterial colonization and gastritis. Am J Gastroenterol 82:292–296
12. Graham DY, Klein PD, Evans DJ, Evans DG, Alpert LC, Opekun AR, Boutton TW (1987) *Campylobacter pyloridis* detected noninvasively by the 13C-urea breath test. Lancet I:1174–1177
13. Marshall BJ, Surveyor I (1988) Carbon-14 urea breath test for the diagnosis of *Campylobacter pylori* associated gastritis. J Nucl Med 29:11–16
14. Evans DJ Jr, Evans DG, Graham DY, Klein PD (1989) A sensitive and specific serologic test for detection of *Campylobacter pylori* infection. Gastroenterology 96:1004–1008
15. Dent JC, McNulty CAM, Uff JS, Gear MWL, Wilkinson SP (1988) *Campylobacter pylori* urease: a new serological test. Lancet I:1002
16. Mobley HLT, Haussinger RP (1989) Microbial ureases: significance, regulation, and molecular characterization. Microbiol Rev 53:85–108
17. Wallace RJ, Cheng K-J, Dinsdale D, Orskov ER (1979) An independent microbial flora of the epithelium and its role in the ecomicrobiology of the rumen. Nature 279:424–426
18. Javorsky P, Rybosova E, Havassy I, Horsky K, Kmet V (1987) Urease activity of adherent bacteria and rumen fluid bacteria. Physiol Bohemoslov 36:75–81
19. Bode G, Malfertheiner P, Nilius M, Lehnhardt G, Ditschuneit H (1989) Ultrastructural localisation of urease in outer membrane and periplasm of *Campylobacter pylori*. J Clin Pathol 42:778–779

20. Gatermann S, John J, Marre R (1989) *Staphylococcus saprophyticus* urease: characterization and contribution to uropathogenicity in unobstructed urinary tract infection of rats. Infect Immun 57:110–116
21. Nickel JC, Olson M, McLean RJ, Grant SK, Costerton JW (1987) An ecological study of infected urinary stone genesis in an animal model. Br J Urol 59:21–30
22. McLean RJ, Nickel JC, Cheng KJ, Costerton JW (1988) The ecology and pathogenicity of urease producing bacteria in the urinary tract. CRC Crit Rev Microbiol 16:37–79
23. Goodwin CS, Armstrong JA, Marshall BJ (1986) *Campylobacter pyloridis,* gastritis, and peptic ulceration. J Clin Pathol 39:353–365
24. Korff RW, Glick D (1951) Role of urease in the gastric mucosa II: in vitro studies with isotopic urea on frog mucosa. Am J Physiol 165:688–694
25. Bronsdon MA, Schoenknecht FD (1988) *Campylobacter pylori* isolated from the stomach of the monkey, *Macaca nemestrina.* J Clin Microbiol 26:1725–1728
26. Baskerville A, Newell DG (1988) Naturally occurring chronic gastritis and *H. pylori* infection in the rhesus monkey: a potential model for gastritis in man. Gut 29:465–472
27. Lee A, Hazell SL, O'Rourke J, Kouprach S (1988) Isolation of a spiral-shaped bacterium from the cat stomach. Infect Immun 56:2843–2850
28. Lee A, Hazell SL (1988) *Campylobacter pylori* in health and disease: an ecological perspective. Microb Ecology Health Dis 1:1–16
29. Phillips MW, Lee A, Leach WD (1978) The mucosa associated microflora of the rat intestine: a study of normal distribution and magnesium sulphate induced diarrhoea. Aust J Exp Biol Med Sci 56:649–662
30. Casiano-Colon A, Marquis RE (1988) Role of the arginine deiminase system in protecting oral bacteria and an enzymatic basis for acid tolerance. Appl Environ Microbiol 54:1318–1324
31. MacNab RM, Castle AM (1987) A variable stoichiometry model for pH homeostasis in bacteria. Biophys J 52:637–647
32. Marquis RE, Bender GR, Murray DR, Wong A (1987) Arginine deiminase system and bacterial adaptation to acid environments. Appl Environ Microbiol 53:198–200
33. Melin AM, Carbonneau MA, Rebeyrotte N (1986) Fatty acids and carbohydrate-containing lipids in four Micrococcaceae strains. Biochimie 68:1201–1209
34. Bender GR, Sutton SV, Marquis RE (1986) Acid tolerance, proton permeabilities, and membrane ATPases of oral streptococci. Infect Immun 53:331–338
35. Harper DS, Loesche WJ (1984) Growth and acid tolerance of human dental plaque bacteria. Arch Oral Biol 29:843–848
36. Costerton JW, Rozee KR, Cheng KJ (1983) Colonization of particulates, mucus, and intestinal tissue. Prog Food Nutr Sci 7:91–105
37. Hazell SL, Lee A (1986) *Campylobacter pyloridis,* urease, hydrogen ion back diffusion, and gastric ulcers. Lancet II:15–17
38. Luck JM, Seth TN (1923) Gastric urease. Biochem J 18:1227–1231
39. Fitzgerald O, Murphy P (1950) Studies on the physiological chemistry and clinical significance of urease and urea with special reference to the stomach. Ir J Med Sci 292:97–159
40. Kornberg HL, Davies RE (1955) Gastric urease. Physiol Rev 35:169–177
41. Fleshler B, Gabuzda G (1965) Effect of ammonium chloride and urea infusions on ammonium levels and acidity of gastric juice. Gut 6:349–356
42. Murakami M, Yoo JK, Inada M, Miyake T (1988) Effect of ammonia on the gastric mucosa in rats: pathophysiological importance of urease in gastric ulcer disease. Jpn J Pharmacol 47:330–332
43. Steer HW (1985) The gastro-duodenal epithelium in peptic ulceration. J Pathol 146:355–362
44. Wyatt JI, Rathbone BJ, Dixon MF, Heatley RV (1987) *Campylobacter pylori* and acid induced gastric metaplasia in the pathogenesis of duodenitis. J Clin Pathol 40:841–848
45. Caselli M, Bovolenta MR, Aleotti A, Trevisani L, Stabellini G, Ricci N (1988) Epithelial morphology of duodenal bulb and *Campylobacter*-like organisms. J Submicrosc Cytol 20:237–242
46. Carrick J, Lee A, Hazell S, Ralston M, Daskalopoulos G (1989) *Campylobacter pylori,* duodenal ulcer, and gastric metaplasia: possible role of functional heterotopic tissue in ulcerogenesis. Gut 30:790–797

47. Barer MR, Elliott TS, Berkeley D, Thomas JE, Eastham EJ (1988) Cytopathic effects of *Campylobacter pylori* urease. J Clin Pathol 41:597
48. Burns TR, Mace ML, Greenberg SD, Jachimczyk JA (1985) Ultrastructure of acute ammonia toxicity in the human lung. Am J Forensic Med Pathol 6:204–210
49. Gregorios JB, Mozes LW, Norenberg LO, Norenberg MD (1986) Effect of cyclic AMP on ammonia-induced alterations in primary astrocyte cultures. J Neuropathol Exp Neurol 45:396–407
50. Renau-Piqueras J, O'Connor JE, Baguena-Cervellera R, Grisolia S (1986) Ammonium chloride-induced alterations in growth kinetics and ultrastructure of murine neuroblastoma cells. A flow cytometric and stereologic study. Virchows Arch [B] 50:271–283
51. Klucinski W, Targowski SP (1984) Ammonia toxicity for mammalian and avian lymphocytes from blood. Immunopharmacology 8:47–52
52. Visek WJ (1984) Ammonia: its effects on biological systems, metabolic hormones, and reproduction. J Dairy Sci 67:481–498
53. Olender EJ, Woods D, Kozol R, Fromm D (1986) Salicylate effects on proton gradient dissipation by isolated gastric mucosal surface cells. Proc Soc Exp Biol Med 183:177–185
54. Perona R, Serrano R (1988) Increased pH and tumorigenicity of fibroblasts expressing a yeast proton pump. Nature 334:438–440
55. de Groot AP, Feron VJ, Immel HR (1988) Induction of hyperplasia in the bladder epithelium of rats by a dietary excess of acid or base: implications for toxicity/carcinogenicity testing. Food Chem Toxicol 26:425–434
56. Smith CE (1984) Hyperplastic lesions of the primitive meninx of fathead minnows, *Pimephales promelas,* induced by ammonia: species potential for carcinogen testing. Natl Cancer Inst Monogr 65:119–125
57. Rathbone BJ, West AP, Wyatt JI, Johnson AW, Tompkins DS (1986) *Campylobacter pyloridis,* urease, and gastric ulcers. Lancet II:400–401
58. Fauchere JL, Rosenau A, Bonneville F (1989) Virulence factors of *Campylobacter pylori.* Gastroenterol Clin Biol 13:59B–64B
59. Richardson SE, Karmali MA, Becker LE, Smith CR (1988) The histopathology of the hemolytic uremic syndrome associated with verocytotoxin producing *Escherichia coli* infections. Hum Pathol 19:1102–1108
60. Grisham MB, Jefferson MM, Melton DF, Thomas EL (1984) Chlorination of endogenous amines by isolated neutrophils. Ammonia-dependent bactericidal, cytotoxic, and cytolytic activities of the chloramines. J Biol Chem 259:10404–10413
61. Wilson CB, Weaver WM (1985) Comparative susceptibility of group B streptococci and *Staphylococcus aureus* to killing by oxygen metabolites. J Infect Dis 152:323–329
62. Beaman BL, Black CM, Doughty F, Beaman L (1985) Role of superoxide dismutase and catalase as determinants of pathogenicity of *Nocardia asteroides:* importance in resistance to microbicidal activity of human polymorphonuclear neutrophils. Infect Immun 47:135–141
63. Schwartz CE, Krall J, Norton L, McKay K, Kay D, Lynch RE (1983) Catalase and superoxide dismutase in *Escherichia coli.* J Biol Chem 258:6277–6281
64. Hazell SL, Markesich DC, Evans DJ, Evans DG, Graham DY (1989) Influence of media supplements on the growth and survival of *Campylobacter pylori.* Eur J Clin Microbiol Infect Dis 8:597–602
65. Hochman A, Shemesh A (1987) Purification and characterization of a catalase-peroxidase from the photosynthetic bacterium *Rhodopseudomonas capsulata.* J Biol Chem 262:6871–6876
66. Meir E, Yagil E (1985) Further characterization of the two catalases in *Escherichia coli.* Curr Microbiol 12:315–320
67. Goldberg I, Hochman A (1989) Three different types of catalase in *Klebsiella pneumoniae.* Arch Biochem Biophys 268:124–128
68. Wayne LG, Diaz GA (1982) Serological, taxonomic, and kinetic studies of the T and M classes of mycobacterial catalase. Int J Syst Bacteriol 32:296–304
69. Smith GW, Tasman-Jones C, Wiggins PM, Lee SP (1985) Pig gastric mucus: a one-way barrier for H^+. Gastroenterology 89:1313–1318

Discussion

Marshall: I am not sure that I disagree with you, Stuart, but let me ask you a question. If urease is a means of providing nitrogen for cell division, you must agree that *H. pylori* grows very well without urea in the environment. Secondly, many species of plants have high levels of urease, particularly the jack bean, and these plants have never been found to contain urea. Thus urease in these species is not used to provide a nitrogen source. Is it perhaps primarily a toxin?

Hazell: With the plant situation, you have to consider the entire ecosystem, for the plants may have urease activity to maintain a microbial environment around their root system. Urease is a fairly ubiquitous enzyme. If you take a nasal swab and test it with your CLO test, you will find plenty of urease activity. You can find urease-positive bacteria in the urinary tract and in the bowel. I think the notion that the *principal* function of the enzyme is protection from acid is not necessarily valid. Again, it is a difficult argument; it does not say that urease does not play a role in protection from acid. However, if you take rats and look at their stomachs, they are colonized by lactobacilli and yeasts. These organisms are urease negative but tolerate the acidic environment quite well. So it is not essential to a microbe to have urease activity to be protected from gastric acid. I like to think of it in terms of air conditioning: you can keep a house cool by air conditioning the inside, or you can turn the air conditioning to the outside and try to cool the whole environment – an inefficient system. If the principal function of urease is protection from acid, it is really doing it the hard way. I think there is enough evidence to show that protection from acid may be a factor, but I believe the urease provides some other function initially.

Talley: Stuart, I have a question on urease inhibitors in man, as this may be relevant clinically. Are there any data on the use of urease inhibitors in *H. pylori* gastritis, and are they of any benefit in gastritis? Also, do heavy metals have any effect on urease or catalase?

Hazell: I will take the last question first. Bismuth inhibits the formation of porphyrins in certain cell lines, so bismuth could potentially inhibit part of the mechanism of the formation of catalase. There are no data to support this, but it is another one of the areas where these metal salts may be important. In terms of urease inhibitors, a few years ago I tried to interest people in urease inhibitors but did not get much of a response. We have a problem; probably the best choice would be acetohydroxamate, which is currently licensed in the United States to treat renal stones. However, this particular drug is a teratogen and a potential carcinogen; so whether it would ever be licensed for use in a treatment trial for gastritis, because of the poor risk-benefit ratio,

I am not sure. You would have to talk to people with more information about this. Thus I am not aware of any data regarding urease inhibitors in gastritis.

Malfertheiner: Stuart, I would like to ask you about the role of vitamin C and copper ions in respect to their inhibiting properties on urease activity. Do you have personal experience with these substances? We did some in vitro experiments inhibiting urease using vitamin C, and its effect was even stronger when copper ions were added.

Hazell: No data.

Megraud: You mentioned that there are differences between cells. What would be, for you, the best cell model to study urease?

Hazell: Some sort of an Ussing chamber type of set-up, if you could actually set up a cell culture on a membrane, but this is very difficult. What I know is that human gastric cells will grow, but they grow in a suspension culture and need to form a monolayer that can then be tested for mucosal integrity. The other possibility is an Ussing chamber type of set-up with explant tissue.

Adhesion Properties of *Helicobacter pylori*

E. De Koster, J. P. M. van Putten, E. A. J. Rauws, and G. N. J. Tytgat

Why Study Adhesion of *H. pylori*?

Adherence of pathogenic bacteria to their target cells is a key event in the pathogenesis of bacterial infection (Beachey 1981). Reasons for studying *H. pylori* adhesion are enumerated in the following:

1. Organ specificity of *H. pylori,* which infects only gastric-type cells in the stomach, gastric metaplasia areas in the bulb, in Barrett's esophagus, in Meckel's diverticula, and in gastric metaplasia in the rectum.
2. Cytopathic effect. Only gastric cells to which *H. pylori* adheres in great numbers show cytopathic changes.
3. Morphologically, adhesion of *H. pylori* to gastric cells involves filamentous structures (pili or fimbriae? Caselli et al. 1989) and adhesion pedestals, i.e., local thickening of the gastric cell membrane in areas of contact with the bacteria (Bode et al. 1988).
4. It must be investigated whether adhesion properties of *H. pylori* are a virulence factor.

What is Bacterial Adhesion?

Specific adhesion of a bacterium to its target cell involves the interaction of an adhesin, a specialized bacterial structure, that is often a protein and is often found on a specialized structure (pili or fibrillae), and the target cell receptor, which is often a sugar (mono- or oligosaccharide). On observing adhesion in vitro, the experimenter should test whether the adhesion is specific, by specifically inhibiting it, using the following methods:

1. Adding a specific sugar to saturate the bacterial adhesin
2. Treating the target cells with a specific saccharidase to destroy the host cell receptors
3. Adding a specific lectin to mask the sugars on the host cell receptors from the adhesin
4. Denaturating the bacterial adhesin by treatment with protease
5. Blocking the bacterial adhesin with a specific antibody
6. Finding another target cell, lacking the specific receptor, which bacteria will not adhere to

The final goal of adhesion studies is the complete characterization of the adhesin and its receptor.

H. Menge et al. (Eds.)
Helicobacter pylori 1990 .

Adhesion of *H. pylori* in Vivo

Hessey et al. (1988) found a relationship between the fraction of the total number of microorganisms which adhered and the activity of underlying gastritis. The relationship they found was rather peculiar and nonlinear; there were, however, two important findings:

1. There is a threshold for epithelial cell degeneration (at least 20% of bacteria visible in the field must adhere to the cells for cytopathic changes to occur).
2. Above this threshold, there is an inverse correlation between the fraction of the total number of adhering microorganisms and the severity of cell degeneration.

It is rather unclear why this correlation is inverse, but its mere existence indicates that the adhesion properties of *H. pylori* might be important for the activity of disease.

Adhesion in Vitro: Models

Two models have been used for studying adhesion of *H. pylori* in vitro: adhesion on cell lines, and hemagglutination. Using cell lines to study adhesion, the investigator hopes that the cell line will have the same or a similar receptor for the adhesin under investigation as in the in vivo situation. Different cell lines are screened for adhesion, and if adhesion is found, its basic properties can be easily studied by adding sugars, lectins, proteases, etc. to the experimental model in order to inhibit adhesion.

Hemagglutination occurs if adhesins (hemagglutinins) on the bacteria bind to receptors on the erythrocytes (RBCs), causing the RBCs to stick together and thus to agglutinate. The same inhibition experiments can be performed as with cell lines. After characterizing the receptor-adhesin interaction in vitro, whether by using cell lines or RBCs, it is necessary to go back to the in vivo situation and check the relevance of the observations in vitro.

Adhesion in Vitro: Adhesion on Cell Lines

H. pylori appears to adhere to a large variety of cell lines (Table 1). Rather unexpectedly, *H. pylori* adheres quite well to intestinal cell lines and less well to gastric cancer cell lines, which may have lost the *H. pylori* receptor during transformation. These observations are thus insufficient to explain the cell specificity of *H. pylori*.

In our own experiments with Chang cells, we consistently observed major differences in adhesion properties of different strains, roughly 40% showing strong adhesion, 40% weak adhesion, and 20% intermediate adhesion (De Koster et al. 1989). Only Graham's group (Evans 1989b) succeeded in determining the characteristic receptor sugar moiety, which they showed to be the same as in their hemagglutination experiments, i.e., *N*-acetylneuraminyllactose.

Table 1. Adherence of *H. pylori* to cell lines

Level of adherence	Cell lines	Reference
Strong	human gastric cells primary culture	(Dunn and Altman 1988)
	buccal epithelial cells	(Dunn and Altman 1988)
	epithelial cells	
	Chang cells	(De Koster et al. 1989)
	HEp-2	(Neman-Simha and Megrand 1988)
	intestinal cells Int 407	(De Koster et al. 1989), Neman-Simha and Megrand 1988; Dunn and Altman 1988)
	HeLa cells, Vero cells	(Rosenau et al. 1988)
	Y-1 mouse adrenal cells	(D. G. Evans et al. 1989)
Moderate	gastric carcinoma	Neman-Simha and Megrand 1988, Dunn and Altman 1988)
Weak	cornea fibroblasts	(De Koster et al. 1989)
	embryonal carcinoma EC	(Dunn and Altman 1988)
	melanoma B16	(Dunn and Altman 1988)
	CHO cells	(Rosenau et al. 1988)

Adhesion in Vitro: Hemagglutination

Hemagglutination will be covered extensively in the chapter by Wadström in this book; we will only treat some relevant points. Wadström's team (Emody et al. 1988) were the first to report that *H. pylori* expresses sialic acid specific hemagglutinin(s). They also found marked heterogeneity of hemagglutination, suggesting the existence of more than one type of hemagglutinin.

Graham's team did a major job in characterizing an *N*-acetylneuraminyllactose-binding fibrillar hemagglutinin (NLBH) (D. G. Evans et al. 1988), to which 75% of *H. pylori* infected individuals make antibodies (D. J. Evans et al. 1989), and which is also involved in the adherence of *H. pylori* to Y-1 mouse adrenal cells (D. G. Evans et al. 1989).

Adhesion in Vitro: The Receptor

Lingwood et al. (1989) from Toronto purified a single *H. pylori*-binding glycolipid fraction, possibly corresponding to the receptor for adhesion. This glycolipid fraction was common to RBCs, human and pig stomach, and HEp-2 cells. It was more prevalent in the mucosa of the stomach antrum than in the mucosa of the fundus, and more prevalent in adults than in children.

Conclusions and Future Research

In the last few years, much has been learned about the adhesion properties of *H. pylori*.

We know *H. pylori* adheres to many different cell types in vitro. The *N*-acetylneuraminyllactose-binding fibrillar hemagglutinin, isolated by Graham's team, seems to be a major adhesin, and the Toronto glycolipid receptor is promising.

There is heterogeneity of adhesion to RBCs and to Chang cells, suggesting *H. pylori* probably carries more than one adhesin. The actual relevance of these observations for the in vivo situation is unclear; the Toronto results are encouraging, suggesting that the human stomach *H. pylori* receptor may be the same as the RBC receptor and the HEp-2 cell line receptor, implicating that in vitro adhesion experiments do have relevance for the in vivo situation.

Many questions are unanswered yet, for instance: Does *H. pylori* carry one or more adhesin(s)? Are the adhesins variants of the NLBH or are they truly different structures? Can one *H. pylori* carry more than one adhesin type? Are these adhesins clinically important primary or secondary virulence factors? What is the influence of drugs or bile on adhesion? What happens in animal models? Can interference with adhesion help to cure or protect against *H. pylori* infection? Is the organ specificity of *H. pylori* the consequence of a peculiar distribution of its receptor in the digestive tract? Future research will have to address these questions.

References

Beachey EH (1981) Bacterial adherence: adhesion-receptor interactions mediating the attachment of bacteria to mucosal surfaces. J Infect Dis 143:325–345

Bode G, Malfertheiner P, Ditschuneit H (1988) Pathogenetic implications of ultrastructural findings in Campylobacter pylori related gastroduodenal disease. Scand J Gastroenterol 23 [Suppl 142]: 25–39

Caselli M, Figura N, Trevisani L, Pazzi P, Guglielmetti P, Bovolenta MR, Stabellini G (1989) Patterns of Physical Modes of contact between Campylobacter pylori and gastric epithelium: implications about the bacterial pathogenicity. Am J Gastroenterol 84:511–513

De Koster E, van Putten JPM, Langenberg W, Rauws EAJ, Tytgat GNJ (1989) Pathogenetic mechanisms of Campylobacter pylori infection: in vitro adhesion characteristics of Campylobacter pylori. Gastroenterology 96:A116

Dunn BE, Altman M (1988) Adherence of Campylobacter pylori to epithelial cells. In: Megraud F, Lamouliatte H (eds) Workshop Gastroduodenal Pathology and Campylobacter Pylori, 7–8 Oct 1988, Bordeaux

Emody L, Carlsson A, Ljungh A, Wadstrom T (1988) Mannoseresistant hemagglutination by Campylobacter pylori. Scand J Infect Dis 20:353–354

Evans DG, Evans DJ Jr., Moulds JJ, Graham DY (1988) N-Acetylneuraminyllactose-binding fibrillar hemagglutinin of Campylobacter pylori: a putative colonization factor antigen. Infect Immun 56:2896–2906

Evans DG, Evans DJ, Graham DY (1989) Receptor-mediated adherence of Campylobacter pylori to mouse Y-1 adrenal cell monolayers. Infect Immun 57:2272–2278

Evans DJ, Evans DG, Smith KE, Graham DY (1989) Serum antibody responses to the N-Acetylneuraminyllactose-binding hemagglutinin of Campylobacter pylori. Infect Immun 57:664–667

Hessey SJ, Wyatt JI, Sobala G, Rathbone BJ, Dixon MF (1988) The relationship between adhesion sites and disease activity in C. pylori – associated gastritis. In: Megraud F, Lamouliatte H (eds) Workshop Gastroduodenal Pathology and Campylobacter pylori, Bordeaux 7–8 Oct 1988

Lingwood CA, Law H, Pellizzari A, Sherman P, Drumm B (1989) Gastric glycerolipid as a receptor for Campylobacter pylori. Lancet II:238–241

Neman-Simha V, Megraud F (1988) In vitro model for Campylobacter pylori adherence properties. Infect Immun 56:3329–3333

Rosenau A, Moyen EN, Bonneville F, Fauchere JL (1988) In vitro study of the association of Campylobacter pylori to epithelial cells. In: Megraud F, Lamouliatte H (eds) Workshop Gastroduodenal Pathology and Campylobacter Pylori, Bordeaux 7–8 Oct 1988

Helicobacter pylori Hemagglutinins*

T. Wadström

Introduction

Studies in the past decade on a number of mucosal surface microbial pathogens have shown that they usually colonize mucosal surfaces by binding to glycoconjugate receptors in the mucin layer of epithelial cells (Wadström et al. 1985). Different bacterial surface proteins (adhesins) or hair-like surface appendages (fimbriae or pili) as well as nonfimbrial adhesins have been reported to be involved in such colonization processes. Pioneering studies by Duguid and Old (1980) showed that many fimbriae of enteric pathogens hemagglutinate erythrocytes of various animal species and can be classified as bacterial surface hemagglutinins or bacterial surface lectins (Wadström and Trust 1984). Despite the great interest in how *Helicobacter pylori* specifically colonizes human gastric epithelium, very few studies have dealt with how this pathogen penetrates the gastric mucus layer, and penetrates into this epithelium to get access to submucosal tissues. Emödy et al. (1988), Evans et al. (1988) and recently also Nakazawa et al. (1989) have reported on the hemagglutination properties of *H. pylori*. We have also recently characterized a sialic-acid-specific hemagglutinin of *H. pylori* (Carlsson et al. 1989), and our data on hemagglutination profiles suggest the presence of two more hemagglutinins in *H. pylori*.

Materials and Methods

Bacterial strains of *H. pylori* were isolated in several Swedish hospitals as described elsewhere (Emödy et al. 1988; Carlsson et al. 1989). Strains were usually stored in 15% (vol/vol) glycerol in calf serum at −70°C and subcultured regularly on chocolate agar or blood agar with 5% (vol/vol) washed horse erythrocytes. All cultures were performed at 37°C under microaerophilic conditions.

Hemagglutination and Hemagglutination Inhibition Assays

Bacterial cells were washed and resuspended in sodium phosphate-buffered saline (PBS; 0.15 *M* NaCl in 0.02 sodium phosphate buffer, pH 7.2) to a density of 3×10^8 cells/ml; Emödy et al. 1988). Venous human, sheep, rabbit, chicken (or cock), dove,

* This study was supported by a grant from the Swedish Medical Research Council (16 x-04723) to T. W. and a visiting scientist fellowship to T. W. and T. J. Trust.

H. Menge et al. (Eds.)
Helicobacter pylori 1990

horse, rat, mouse, bovine, guinea pig, and monkey (African green) erythrocytes were washed once and resuspended in PBS to 4% (vol/vol) cell suspensions. Hemagglutination (HA) and hemagglutination inhibition (HAI) assays were performed on glass slides by mixing equal volumes (20 µl) of bacterial and erythrocyte suspensions. Minimal bacterial hemagglutinating concentrations were determined by titrating bacteria against these erythrocyte suspensions, and HAI experiments were carried out with such titrated bacterial suspensions after preincubation with various potential monosaccharides and other carbohydrate polymer inhibitors for 5 min at 20°C before a red blood cell suspension was added.

Erythrocytes and bacterial cells were treated with various proteases such as trypsin, pronase, proteinase K or *Clostridium perfringens, Vibrio cholerae,* and *Arthrobacter ureafaciens* neuraminidase (Sjöberg et al. 1988a, b).

Other Assays

Cell surface hydrophobicity was assayed by
a) the salt aggregation test (SAT) (Lindahl et al. 1981),
b) by phase partitioning in dextran polyethylene glycerol (Albertsson 1978), and
c) by hydrophobic interaction chromatography (HIC) on Octyl Sepharose equilibrated with 1 *M* NaCl (Wadström et al. 1984).

Heat stability of bacterial hemagglutinins and surface hydrophobicity was determined on bacterial suspensions (5×10^9 cells/ml heated in PBS at 60°C for 15 and 60 min).

Extraction of Cell Surface Hemagglutinins

Various methods have been tried for mild extraction of cell surface hemagglutinins of strains with various hemagglutination profiles such as extractions with different concentrations of urea (2–6 *M*), guanidinium chloride (0.5–5 *M*), Triton X100 (0.1% and 1% vol/vol), lithium chloride (1–2 *M*), and sodium chloride (1 *M*) in 0.02 *M* sodium phosphate buffer, pH 7.0 (Table 1). Acid glycine buffer (pH 2.2) was also used in some extraction experiments (T.J. Trust, J. Guruge, S. Whei, Å. Ljungh, T. Wadström, unpublished work).

Table 1. Patterns of hemagglutinations of *Helicobacter pylori*

Pattern	Strain	Horse	Rabbit	Human	Bovine	Guinea pig	Pig	Sheep	Green monkey	Dove
		Erythrocyte species								
I	33, 66, 32, 73, 19106	–	–	–	–	–	–	–	–	NT
II	71, CCUG17874, 1067, 72, 1139	+/–	+/–	+	+	+	+/–	+	+/–	+
III	915, 5155517	–	+	–	–	–	–	–	–	–
IV	593, 99	–	–	+	+	+	–	+/–	–	+
V	165	–	–	(+)	–	(+)	(+)	+	–	(+)
VI	95	–	(+)	(+)	–	+	–	–	–	+

NT, not tested; +/–, repeated experiments gave varying results; (+), weak hemagglutination

Chemicals

All chemicals used were of analytical grade. Various sialoglycoconjugates were obtained from R. Brossmer. Institute of Biochemistry, University of Heidelberg, Federal Republic of Germany.

Results and Discussion

Screening of *H. pylori* Strains for Surface Hemagglutinins

More than 150 strains isolated from Swedish patients with gastritis were screened for hemagglutination profiles on human, sheep, and rabbit erythrocyte suspensions as described previously (Emödy et al. 1988). Only a few percent of all strains were negative in this screening process. However, since some strains hemagglutinated only rabbit or sheep but not human erythrocytes, a greater selection of erythrocyte species were included in a screening process for 40 strains. Data from this HA profile screening are presented in Table 1 together with data for two culture collection strains (NCTC 11637 and NCTC 11638). These findings suggest that at least *three* major HA patterns can be distinguished:

1. Strains causing HA of human red blood cells (RBCs) and a great variety of RBCs of various species *(pattern I)*
2. Strains causing HA of only sheep erythrocytes (and sometimes one or two other species) *(pattern II)*
3. Strains causing HA of "rabbit erythrocytes only" or two or more RBC species (weak hemagglutination) *(pattern III)*

Addition of D-mannose and other monosaccharides such as sucrose, galactose, and *N*-acetylglucose-amine did not affect hemagglutination of selected strains of patterns I–III, while disialogangliosides type II (Sigma, 2.5 mg/ml) and bovine submandibular mucins (Sigma, 1 mg/ml) and orosomucoid (i.e., serum α-acid glycoprotein) and fetuin caused inhibition of strains of pattern I such as strain 915 (Table 2).

Table 2. Hemagglutination assay of different extracts of *H. pylori* 915

Extracts[a]	Protein concentration[b] (μg/ml)	A280/A260	HA[c] titer	HAI
Glycine HCl	126	0.89	2^{-2}	–
LiCl	680	0.65	2^{-7}	–[d]
5 *M* guanidine HCl	1960	0.69	2^{-2}	–
8 *M* urea	1760	0.55	2^{-6}	–

[a] Extraction solution 0.5 ml was added to 0.1 g cells (wet weight) for each extraction; (1) intramuscular glycine HCl, pH 2.2, RT 2 h; (2) intramuscular LiCl 45°C, 2 h; (3) 5 *M* guanidine HCl, RT 10 min; (4) 8 *M* urea, RT 10 min

[b] Determined with Bio-Rad kit

[c] With rabbit RBCs

[d] Enhancing HA

Neuraminyl-lactose (2.5 mg/ml) and human glycophorin but not asialo-fetuin or asialoglycophorin caused HAI of strains of pattern II we tested for HAI with various sialoglyco-conjugates. Pretreatment of human, sheep, and rabbit RBCs abolished hemagglutination of all three species; one *H. pylori* hemagglutinin can be classified as a sialic-acid-specific hemagglutinin as a number of other bacterial hemagglutinins-fimbrial lectins of enterotoxigenic *Escherichia coli* (ETEC) (Lindahl et al. 1987; Sjöberg et al. 1988; Wadström and Aleljung 1989) and nonfimbrial lectins of *Mycoplasma pneumoniae* and *Plasmodium falciparum* (Wadström and Trust 1984).

Since sialic-acid-specific surface hemagglutinins of ETEC and other enteropathogens commonly express high surface hydrophobicity (Wadström and Baloda 1986; Wadström et al. 1984), we have selected strains I–IV for screening of surface hydrophobicity by SAT. Preliminary studies indicate that strains fall into two major groups;

a) strains expressing high surface hydrophobicity (SAT value < 0.1 *M* ammonium sulfate) and
b) strains expressing low cell surface hydrophobicity (SAT > 1 *M* ammonium sulfate).

Preliminary studies by HIC on Octyl Sepharose and in phase partitioning also indicate that *H. pylori,* unlike fimbriated ETEC strains, is heterogeneous with respect to expression of surface hydrophobicity when grown on various conditions. Preliminary ongoing studies also indicate that growth on agar media and in liquid cultures affects expression of cell surface hydrophobicity and hemagglutinin(s).

Since the sialic-acid-specific hemagglutinin was better expressed in agar-grown cells than in cells grown in various liquid media, various extraction methods were tried to solubilize hemagglutinins of strain 915 (pattern I) and strain 300^6 (pattern III).

Extraction of suspended agar grown cells (approx. 5×10^{10} cells/ml) with urease, guanidinium hydrochloride, and lithium chloride (but not sodium chloride) in equal concentration and glycine buffer (pH 2.2) and by extraction of 1% Triton X100, caused release of cell surface proteins including hemagglutinins without causing much cell lysis (as determined by measuring spectrophotometrically the ratio of absorbance of extracts at 260 and 280 nm). Cell extracts containing 50–200 μg/ml where then titrated in the standard HA assay. Somewhat disappointingly, usually only nondiluted extracts caused hemagglutination (sometimes also extracts diluted tenfold in PBS). More systematic studies are now underway to define optimal conditions for *H. pylori* strains of various HA profiles which promote expression of high HA titers as measured on standard urea cell extracts. Similar systematic extraction studies will probably also define strategies for extracting other cell surface proteins such as surface-located urease, protease(s), and mucinase. This seems likely to be important in the penetration of the gastric mucus layer and epithelium (Hazell et al. 1986). We have recently reported on low surface hydrophobicity of *H. pylori* strains expressing sialic-acid-specific lectin (SAL) (Carlsson et al. 1989). More recent data suggest that maybe coexpression of other surface proteins or other macromolecules contribute to high cell hydrophobicity of certain strains of various HA profiles (pattern I–III). This has possibly to be further explored as well as determining the hydrophobicity of hemagglutinins in cell extracts. In fact, various surface charge and hydrophobic properties can probably be exploited in purification of *H. pylori* surface hemagglutinins and other surface macromolecules.

These studies are now under way and will be reported elsewhere. Serological studies using various cell extracts for immunoassays in patients with gastritis and stomach ulcer disease [enzyme-linked immunoadsorbent assay (ELISA) and immunoblotting] suggest that the sialic-acid-specific lectin is a poor antigen compared with other antigens in these extracts such as urease and flagellar antigens. Evans et al. (1988) recently described a fimbrial sialic-acid-specific hemagglutinin in *H. pylori* and that patients commonly responded with antibody formation to this structure. We have not been able to visualize fimbriae-like surface appendages on SAL-producing *H. pylori,* strain 915, by electron microscopy (Carlsson et al. 1989). Interestingly, Nakazawa et al. (1989) showed that 43 Japanese strains of *H. pylori* tested showed strong HA with human erythrocytes while only 9 out of 18 *C. jejuni* strains caused positive HA. On the contrary, screening of *C. jejuni* strains for HA and cell surface hydrophobicity upon growth in different media did not reveal hydrophobic surface hemagglutinins in analogy with enteric pathogens such as ETEC, various *Salmonellae* and *Shigella species* (Quadri et al. 1988; Wadström 1988). The Japanese investigators found that D-mannose but not L-fucose caused HAI of certain strains but were unable to detect surface filamentous structures such as fimbriae. In conclusion, *H. pylori* strains of various geographic origin produce surface hemagglutinins. However, since Evans et al. (1988) reported that all United States strains tested produced a sialic-acid-specific hemagglutinin, it is possible that *H. pylori* as enterotoxigenic and enteropathogenic *E. coli* (ETEC and EPEC) strains produce both fimbrial and nonfimbrial hemagglutinins. High surface hydrophobicity of certain strains in our studies also suggests that various strains (maybe with different virulence properties) produce different lectins which react with glycoconjugates in gastric mucin, on gastric epithelial cells or intercellular junctions as well as in subepithelial mucosal tissues. Preliminary screening tests for interactions with fibronectin and other tissue matrix proteins have not yet given conclusive results for such nonhemagglutinin surface adhesins (Wadström and Baloda 1986). Further studies to define tissue invasion strategies by *H. pylori* are now under way. A number of both pathogens and indigenous microflora microbes suggest that lactosyl ceramide is a very common cell membrane attachment site for a great variety of organisms (Karlsson 1989), and that a multiple-step adhesion process is very common, involving more than one bacterial cell adhesin-receptor mechanism. In fact, electron microscope studies by Bode et al. (1988) demonstrate close adhesion to gastric epithelium with so-called pedestal formation and multiple-step binding as with some other enteric microbes (Wadström 1988).

Our recent findings indicate that *H. pylori* may produce at least two or three different hemagglutinins (Tables 1–3). It is too early to speculate how the microbe may use these putative cell adhesins in colonizing the stomach mucosa. However, it seems likely that one or two of these hemagglutinins allow the organism to make close contact with the stomach epithelium with pedestal formation similar to that reported by Knutton et al. (1989) for certain strains of enteropathogenic *E. coli* (EPEC). We have not been able to demonstrate fimbriae on prototype strains of the most common HA patterns (cells grown both on blood agar and in liquid media). To our knowledge fimbriae-like structures have not been demonstrated on *C. jejuni* or *Helicobacter*-like organisms except by Evans et al. from one strain of *H. pylori* expressing sialic-acid-specific hemagglutination. Thus, it is possible that *H. pylori* may produce both

Table 3. Inhibition of hemagglutination of *Helicobacter pylori* strains by glycoconjugates

	Helicobacter pylori strain and *erythrocyte species*				
	Strain 72		*Strain NCTC 11637*		
	Human	Sheep	Human	Sheep	Rabbit
Glycoconjugates					
Glycophorin type MN	I	I	I	I	I
Ganglioside type IV	(I)	(I)	–	–	(I)
Ganglioside type V	(I)	(I)	–	–	(I)
Disialoganglioside GD1a	(I)	(I)	(I)	–	(I)
Monosialoganglioside GM1	(I)	(I)	–	–	(I)
Trisialoganglioside GT1b	(I)	(I)	–	–	–
Monosialoganglioside GM2	(I)	I	–	–	(I)

[a] All gangliosides 2.5 mg/ml
I, total inhibition; (I), denotes partial inhibition

fimbrial and nonfimbrial surface hemagglutinins as uropathogenic strains of *E. coli.* It is even possible that such fimbrial and afimbrial agglutinins (AFAs) as on certain strains of *E. coli* may be genetically related (Labigne-Roussel and Falkow 1988). With these findings we have recently been screening *H. pylori* with different HA patterns for surface hydrophobicity by SAT. In brief, strains may be classified into two major groups (SAT values with high versus low surface hydrophobicity: SAT < 0.1 ammonium sulfate and > 1.0 *M* ammonium sulfate). No clear-cut correlation of high surface hydrophobicity to specific HA patterns has been found so far indicating the one or two specific fimbrial or afimbrial surface hemagglutinins expressing high surface hydrophobicity such as among enteropathogenic and uropathogenic *E. coli* (Wadström et al. 1984; Gonzalez et al. 1988). It is even possible that unrelated surface components such as outer membrane proteins (OMPs) like congo-red-binding proteins of various *Yersiniae* spp. and *Shigella* spp. determine surface hydrophobicity (Quadri et al. 1988). For this reason, we will now compare HA pattern, surface hydrophobicity, and plasmid profiles of selected strains of the various HA patterns since a number of fimbrial hemagglutinins as well as outer membrane proteins associated with virulence in *E. coli, Yersiniae,* and other enterics are mediated by plasmid genes. We also compared surface hydrophobicity by two other independent methods, i.e., hydrophobic interaction chromatography (HIC) on Octyl Sepharose and by two-phase partitioning in dextran polyethyleneglycol systems (Wadström et al. 1984). In brief, results of these studies showed that strains could be classified into various groups of cell surface hydrophobicity. It will now be interesting to investigate if the round dormant forms of *H. pylori* probably enriched in old laboratory cultures express higher surface hydrophobicity than ordinary vegetative cells in analogy to high surface hydrophobicity of dormant forms of various gram-negative marine microbes such as vibrios or spores of gram-positive bacteria. This area of research seems a fruitful area of exploration to obtain a better understanding of host-parasite interactions in acute and chronic gastritis with *H. pylori.* It seems most likely that penetration between epithelial gastric cells into the subepithelial tissues also involves lectin-like interactions maybe with cell adhesion molecules (CAMs) in the tight junctions and adhesion glycoconjugates in the basal membranes such as laminin and various proteoglycans.

Preliminary studies have shown that *H. pylori* of HA patterns I–III do not bind fibronectin, albumin, or fibrinogen. Studies are now in process to define other possible candidates for submucosal adhesion; processes may involve both carbohydrate protein (i.e., lectin like) and protein-protein interactions such as fibronectin and immunoglobulin binding to *staphylococci* and *E. coli* (Wadström and Baloda 1986; Höök et al. 1988). Sialoglycoconjugates are commonly also receptors for viral hemagglutinins colonizing the respiratory tract and other mucosal surfaces. Evans et al. (1989) recently reported that five American strains of *H. pylori* which adhered to mouse adrenal Y1 cells were inhibited by neuraminyl lactose and fetuin, while Lingwood et al. (1989) have detected a yet undefined glyceroglycolipid in lipid extracts of human red cells and human and pig gastric tissues which bind to Canadian isolates of *H. pylori.* From our present knowledge, it seems likely that two or more hemagglutinins of *H. pylori* use different glycolipids to colonize the gastric epithelium. We propose a model where the hemagglutinin/lectins interact with glycoconjugate, when the pathogen has rapidly moved down below the gastric mucin layer. Surface-active lipids cause (amphotheric-saturated phospholipids) a form of hydrophobic lining over the epithelium and make the normal gastric epithelium noncorrodible by luminal acids (Lichtenberger 1987). To allow rapid capturing and uptake by the gastric mucin layer, high surface hydrophobicity of *H. pylori* may be important. However, in order to rapidly penetrate the gastric mucin layer it seems likely that surface hydrophobic protein(s) may be turned on and off by specific genetic regulations, such as hydrophobic surface fimbrial hemagglutinins of various enteropathogenic *E. coli* (Wadström and Trust 1984). Studies on how growth conditions affect expression of hemagglutinins and surface hydrophobicity are now under way. Finally, we may speculate that strains with different hemagglutinins and hydrophobic properties expressed under various *in vitro* and *in vivo*-like growth conditions may be coregulated with other putative virulence factors such as *H. pylori* cytotoxins. Such coexpression of surface hemagglutinins and operon-regulated toxins are common among tissue-invasive strains of *E. coli,* and other calcium-regulated adhesins in *Yersinia enterocolita.* Since *H. pylori* seem to lack cell-invasive properties as virulent *Yersiniae* and *Shigellae* and enteroinvasive *E. coli,* it seems more likely that hemagglutinins may determine colonization of the gastric epithelium and penetration between the epithelial cells. However, these lectins may also interact with carbohydrate moieties in subepithelial tissue such as proteoglycans, fibronectin, laminin, and tissue collagens (Höök et al. 1988).

Acknowledgments. I would like to acknowledge T.J. Trust, University of Victoria, Victoria BC, Canada, R. Brossmer, University of Heidelberg, FRG, F. Megraud, University of Bordeaux, France, and colleagues in the department for collaboration in defining the virulence properties of *H. pylori:* P. Aleljung, F. Ascencio, J. Guruge, Å. Ljungh, P. O'Toole, and S. Whei.

References

Albertsson P-A (1978) Partition between polymer phases. J Chromatogr 159:111–122

Bode G, Malfertheiner P, Ditschuneit P (1988) Pathogenic implications of ultrastructural findings; *Campylobacter pylori* related to gastrointestinal disease. Scand J Gastroenterol 23: suppl 142, 25–39

Booth BA, Sciono CV, Finkelstein RA (1986) Adhesins of *Vibrio cholerae*. In: Mirelman D (ed) Microbial lectins and agglutinins. Wiley, New York, pp 169–182

Carlsson Å, Emödy L, Ljungh Å, Wadström T (1989) Carbohydrate receptor specificity of haemagglutinins of *Campylobacter pylori*. In: Megraud F, Lamonliatte H (eds) Gastroduodenal pathology and *Campylobacter pylori*. *Excerpta Medica Int Congress Series Nr 847*, Elsevier, Amsterdam, pp 375–378

Duguid J, Old DC (1980) Adhesive properties of Enterobacteriaceae. In: Beachey E (ed) Bacterial adherence. Receptors and recognition. Chapman and Hall, pp 186–217

Emödy L, Carlsson Å, Ljungh Å, Wadström T (1988) Mannose resistant haemagglutination of *Campylobacter pylori*. Scand J Infect Dis *20*:353–354

Evans DJ Jr, Moulds JJ, Graham DY (1988) *N*-Acetylneuraminyllactose-binding fibrillar haemagglutinin of *Campylobacter pylori:* a putative colonization factor antigen. Infect Immun *56*:2896–2906

Gonzalez EA, Blanco J, Baloda S, Wadström T (1988) Relative cell surface hydrophobicity of *Escherichia coli* strains with various recognized fimbrial antigens and without recognized fimbriae. Bact Hyg *269*:218–236

Hazell SL, Lee A, Brady L, Hennesey W (1986) *Campylobacter* and gastritis association with intracellular species and adaption to an environment of mucus as important facts in colonization of gastric epithelium. J Infect Dis *153*:658–663

Höök M, Switalski L, Wadström T, Lindberg M (1988) Interactions of pathogenic microorganisms with fibronectin. In: Mosher P (ed) *Fibronectin*. Academic, New York, pp 295–308

Karlsson KA (1989) Animal glycosphingolipids as membrane attachment sites to bacteria. Annu Rev Biochem *58*:309–350

Knutton S, Baldwin T, Williams PH, McNeish AS (1989) Actin accumulation at sites of bacterial adhesion to tissue culture cells: the basis of a new diagnostic test for enteropathogenic and enterohemmorhagic *Escherichia coli*. Infect Immun *57*:1290–1298

Labigne-Rousell A, Falkow S (1988) Distribution and degree of heterogenity of the afimbrial-adhesin-encoding operon (afa) among pathogenic *Escherichia coli*. Infect Immun *56*:640–648

Lichtenberger LM (1987) Membranes and barriers: With a focus on the gastric mucosal barrier. Clin Invest Med 10:181–188

Lindahl M, Brossmer R, Wadström T (1987) Carbohydrate receptors specific to K99 fimbriae of enterotoxigenic *Escherichia coli*. Glycoconjugate J *4*:51–58

Lindahl M, Faris A, Wadström T, Hjerten S (1981) A new test based on "salting out" to measure relative surface hydrophobicity of bacterial cells. Biochim Biophys Acad *677*:471–476

Lingwood CA, Law H, Pellizzari A, Sherman P, Drumm B (1989) Gastric glycerolipid as a receptor for Campylobacter pylori. Lancet II, 238–241

Nakazawa T, Kennishi H, Takemoto P, Shigeda M, Kochiyama T (1989) Haemagglutination properties of *Campylobacter pylori*. In Takemoto T, Kawai K, Shimoyama T (eds) *Campylobacter pylori* and gastrointestinal diseases. Tokyo International Symposium on *Campylobacter pylori*, Taisho Pharmaceutical Co, pp 87–91

Qadri F, Hossain SA, Cizar I, Haider K, Ljungh Å, Wadström T, Sack DA (1988) Congo red binding and salt agglutination as indicators of virulence in *Shigella* species. J Clin Microbiol *26*:1343–1348

Sjöberg PO, Lindahl M, Fröman G, Porath J, Wadström T (1988) Isolation and characterization of CS 2 sialic acid specific lectons of enterotoxigenic *Escherichia coli*. Biochem J *255*:105–111

Wadström T (1987) *Aeromonas* and *Plesiomonas*-enteric infections and fecal carriage. Experientia *43*:362–364

Wadström T (1988) Adherence traits and mechanisms of microbiological adhesion in the gut. *Bailleies Clin Trop Med Commun Dis 3*:417–433

Wadström T, Aleljung P (1989) Molecular mechanisms of bowel colonization. In: Midvedt T, Grubb R, and Nolin E (eds) "The regulative and protective role of the normal microflora". Macmillan, Houndsmills, London, pp 35–46

Wadström T, Baloda SB (1986) Molecular aspects on small bowel colonization by enterotoxigenic *Escherichia coli*. Microeco Ther *16*:243–255

Wadström T, Sjöberg P-O, Lindahl M (1984) Sialic acid specific lectins of enterotoxigenic *Escherichia coli*. In: Bog-Hansen TC, Breborowicz (eds) Lectins. vol 4, de Gruyter, Berlin, pp 417–423

Wadström T, Switalski LM, Speziale P, Rubin K, Ryden C, Fröman G, Faris A, Lindberg M, Hökk M (1985) Binding of microbial pathogens to connective tissue fibronectin: an early step in the localized and invasive infections. In: Jackson GG, Thomas H (eds) *Bayer-Symposium VIII*, Springer, Berlin Heidelberg New York, pp 193–207

Wadström T, Trust TJ (1984) Bacterial surface lectins. In: Jeljaszewicz J, Easman CSF (eds) Medical microbiology, vol 4. Academic, London, pp 287–334

Discussion

Graham: Both of the two previous speakers in their excellent presentations discuss some of the material from our laboratory. We absolutely agree that there are no fimbria structures – there are fibrillae, not fimbriae. Our work is continuing, but it is very clear that we have demonstrated fibrilla structures to bind through a specific sugar. Our most recent paper, which should have just now appeared, is with cell lines and extends our observations into cell lines. We have shown that the same findings hold; at least this story is quite consistent. All our material has not been published in proceedings of meetings such this one but in refereed journals. I think it will hold up. We will see whether the area is slightly more complicated, but at least this will be one of the important in vivo adhesins of *H. pylori.*

Lee: I would just like to make a general comment. It is always very important to remember that we are dealing here totally with in vitro systems. One talks as though really the adhesion pedestal is a major part, which clearly it is, but as one looks at the pictures, *H. pylori* is in a different number of states within the gastric mucosa, and certainly not all the organisms are adhering by a pedestal. What is really coming out now is that when one starts to look at determinants of pathogenicity of highly evolved pathogens – and this is clearly a highly evolved organism – the organisms adapt in a way that switches genes on off. It may well be that one of the problems in trying to correlate in vitro systems with what is happening in vivo is that in the particular unique environment of the stomach the organism may be switching on different adhesins or different factors that allow it to swim through mucus, and it is very difficult to mimic this. I think this is something that we always must remember when we are trying to interprete in vitro data, because it is not just *H. pylori* sticking by adhesion pedestals. There is much more going on in the stomach than this.

Wadström: I would like to return to Dr. Graham's comment. I have been in microbial pathogenesis for a number of years, and it is becoming more and more complex in all areas. So I do not want to be misunderstood here that our work necessarily disagrees with that of Evans, and I really think that it can be a very complex story. It may be very similar to *E. coli.* I would like to recommend Knuften's beautiful study on pedestal formation with enteropathogenic *E. coli.* I propose a model in which fibrilla-like proteins may be involved in initial colonization in the mucus layer. But I would like to stress again that fibrillae or fimbriae have never been shown in *E. coli* or any other enteropathogen to produce such close binding to epithelial cells as may be very important in *H. pylori* colonization. This is a two- or three-step model for *H. pylori* gastric colonization. This will give us much more work to do, and I would like to see more scientists recruited into this complex area.

Slomiany: I would like to make a comment on the role of mucins in the inhibition of agglutination of red cells by *H. pylori.* From our data it appears that because of the low content of sialic acid, mucin is not able to cause inhibition of erythrocyte agglutination by *H. pylori.* Another comment is that in our studies we have found that the common feature of *H. pylori* agglutinins is the recognition of lactosyl moiety bearing acidic substituent at C-3 of the terminal galactose residue. This substituent could be either sialic acid or a sulfate ester group.

Tytgat: Do bismuth salts interfere actively with hemagglutination or adhesion of these bacteria?

De Koster: I don't know.

Mégraud: Dr. Slomiany, can you answer this question?

Slomiany: I would like to answer the question. We have performed hemagglutination assays in the presence of bismuth subcitrate (De-Nol) and found that this agent has no effect on the hemagglutination of red blood cells by *H. pylori.*

Petersen: It is quite clear that the additional problem has two parts: one is the bacteria, and the other has something to do with surface cells. And I wonder whether there is any knowledge about the effect of varying maturity of these cells? How are the additional properties influenced by growth stimulation? Is there any information about the effect of hormones or, particularly, prostaglandins?

De Koster: All of these are quite interesting questions, but we do not have answers today.

Wadström: A group in Toronto has just reported in *Lancet* their having produced hemagglutinins in liquid medium, while we have produced hemagglutinins on solid surfaces. A number of microbes produce hemagglutinins only when grown on solid medium under special conditions. There is still much to learn about the regulation of surface hemagglutinins and other virulence factors of *H. pylori.*

Menge: I have learned from the literature that the expression of adhesins depends largely on the cultural conditions used in the microbiological laboratories. Is it possible that the different results obtained in Dr. Graham's and Dr. Wadström's laboratories are due to different microbiological techniques used for cultivating *H. pylori?* What do you think about this, Dr. Graham?

Graham: I agree.

Cytotoxic Activity of *Helicobacter pylori*

M. GREGOR[1], H. MENGE[2], M. WARRELMANN[3], G. BORNHÖFT[4], and E. O. RIECKEN[1]

Introduction

Helicobacter pylori is a direct cause of chronic active type B gastritis [1–3, 5, 6]. Furthermore, the presence of *H. pylori* is a necessary condition for gastritis-associated chronic recurrent duodenal ulcer disease [2]. The pathogenic mechanisms by which *H. pylori* generates these manifestaations are not well understood.Several factors have been proposed to explain the pathogenic properties of *H. pylori*. One of the putative virulence factors in *H. pylori* culture medium appears to be a protein that causes non-lethal intracellular vacuolization in a number of cell lines. Leunk et al. reported the existence of such a heat-labile protein with a molecular weight well above a hundred thousand which could be neutralized by specific antisera [7]. This cytopathic factor was found to be present in 66.6% of *H. pylori* strains isolated from patients with peptic ulcer disease [4]. The purpose of our study was to quantify the frequency of infection with cytotoxic *H. pylori* in a group of consecutive patients and to correlate the production of this cytotoxin with the clinical syndrome, the endoscopic findings, and the histological appearance of the antral mucosa in those patients.

Patients and Methods

Fifty-seven consecutive patients attending for diagnostic gastrointestinal endoscopy were included in the study. All were referred for the evaluation of upper abdominal complaints. Four antral biopsies were obtained from each patient. In each case, two specimens were fixed in 10% buffered formol saline and processed routinely. Sections were evaluated histologically following a conventional stain with hematoxylin and eosin. The two further biopsies from each patient were put on Columbia chocolate agar with Skirrow supplement (vancomycin, trimethoprim, polymyxin B) plus amphotericin B, and were incubated under microaerophilic conditions at 37°C for 5–7 days (Gas-Pac-System, Anaerocult C). The appearance of small translucent

[1] Abteilung für Innere Medizin mit Schwerpunkt Gastroenterologie, Universitätsklinikum Steglitz, Freie Universität Berlin, Hindenburgdamm 30, 1000 Berlin 45, FRG
[2] Medizinische Klinik II, Krankenanstalten der Stadt Remscheid, Akademisches Lehrkrankenhaus der Universität Bonn, Hans Potyka-Str. 28, 5630 Remscheid, FRG
[3] Institut für Medizinische Mikrobiologie, Freie Universität Berlin, Hindenburgdamm 27, 1000 Berlin 45, FRG
[4] Institut für Pathologie, Universitätsklinikum Steglitz, Freie Universität Berlin, Hindenburgdamm 30, 1000 Berlin 45, FRG

H. Menge et al. (Eds.)
Helicobacter pylori 1990

colonies consisting of typically gram-negative spiral rods with positive urease, catalase, and oxidase reactions was considered to be a positive result. Thereafter, all *H. pylori* isolates were grown in brain-heart infusion (BHI) broth supplemented with fetal calf serum 10% v/v, hemin 5 μg/l, and the Skirrow mixture of antibiotics plus amphotericin B. Incubation was for 3 days at 37°C in a microaerophilic atmosphere.

For cytotoxin assay, broth-culture filtrates (0.22-μm pore filter, Millipore) of strains were added to HeLa cells (1.5×10^4/well preincubated for 24 h in 24-well culture plates) in vitro at dilutions of 1:1, 1:2, 1:4 and 1:10 using Earle's modified eagles medium supplemented with 25 m*M* HEPES, 10% fetal calf serum, and 2 m*M* glutamine as cell culture medium. Uninoculated, supplemented BHI-broth was used as a negative control, and a culture filtrate of *H. pylori* (NCTC 11637) served as a positive control. 24 and 48 h after the addition of broth-culture filtrate, HeLa cells were examined by phase-contrast microscopy for the presence of intracellular vacuolization. Cytotoxin assays scored positive if more than 50% of the cells exhibited intracytoplasmic vacuolization.

Results and Discussion

The normal appearance of HeLa cells before the addition of the broth-culture supernatant is shown in Fig. 1A. 12 h after the addition of the cytopathic broth-culture

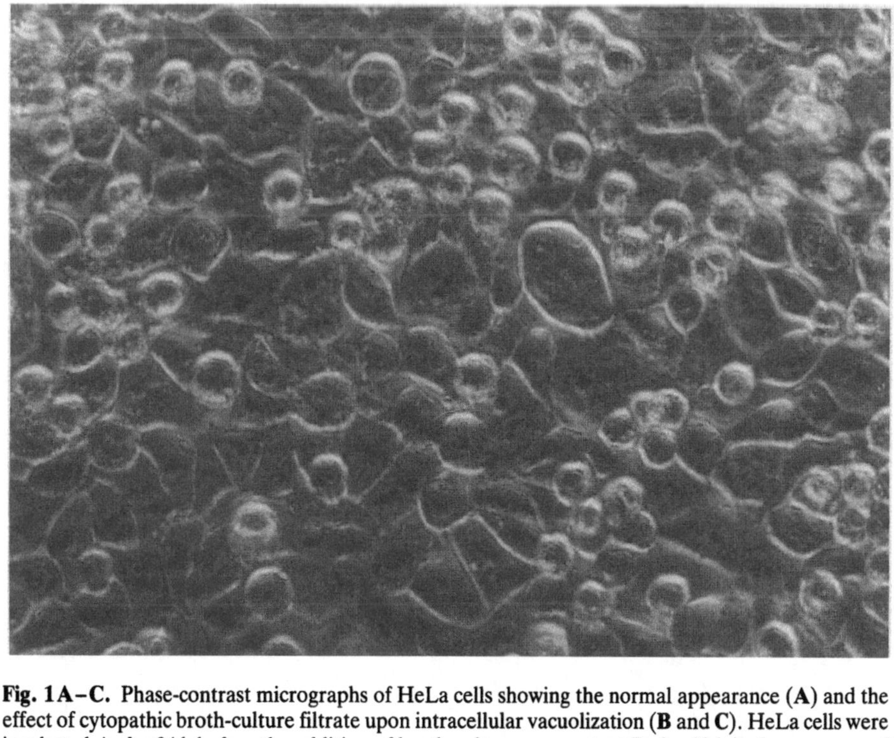

Fig. 1A–C. Phase-contrast micrographs of HeLa cells showing the normal appearance (**A**) and the effect of cytopathic broth-culture filtrate upon intracellular vacuolization (**B** and **C**). HeLa cells were incubated **A:** for 24 h before the addition of broth-culture supernatant **B:** for 12 h in the presence of BHI broth-culture filtrate of *H. pylori* and **C:** for 24 h in the presence of BHI broth-culture filtrate of *H. pylori*

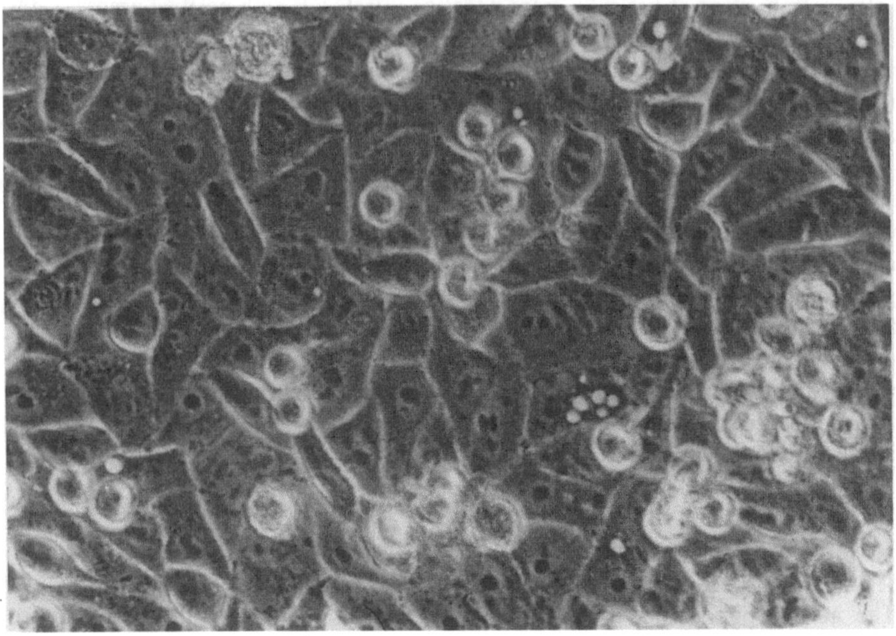

Fig. 1B

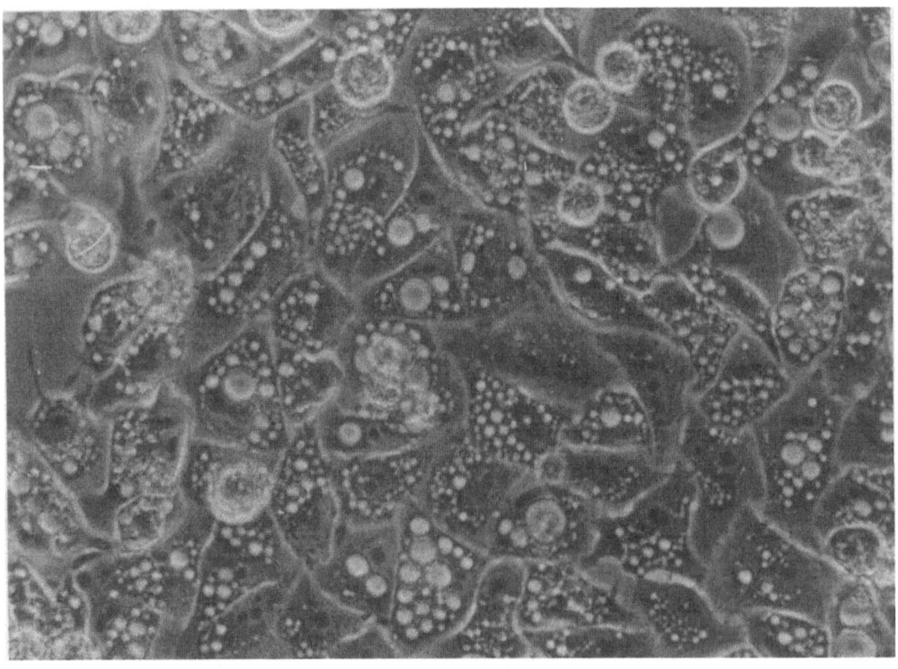

Fig. 1C

Table 1. Evaluation of *H. pylori* colonization by microbiology in antral biopsies of 57 patients and cytotoxic activity of *H. pylori* isolates

	no. of patients	
Total no. of patients tested (n = 57)		
female/male[a]	37/20	
H. pylori (+) (n = 24)		
culture (+)	24	
CLO-test (+)	23	
Cytotoxin (+)	14	(60.9%)
Cytotoxin (−)	9	(39.1%)

[a] age range, 20–85 years; mean age 54.2 years

filtrate *H. pylori* has initiated the intracellular vacuolization process in some of those cells, which has reached maximal levels by 24 h in some cases (Fig. 1B, C).

Cytotoxic activity was stable when broth-culture filtrates were heated at 56°C for 30 min. However, heating of broth-culture filtrates at 70°C for 30 min resulted in complete loss of cytopathic activity, which could also be blocked by acidification indicating this factor to be protein in nature. In a preliminary experiment, we started to purify this protein using gel filtration of concentrated *H. pylori* (NCTC) broth-culture filtrate on a Sepharose CL 6 B column followed by SDS-polyacrylamide gel electrophoresis. These data suggest that the cytopathic protein has a molecular weight of above 800000, which may indicate either a multiunit molecule or a molecule which is linked to a carrier protein.

Overall, *H. pylori* strains were cultured from antral mucosa of 24 patients under microaerophilic conditions. In 23 of these cases the CLO test was also positive. We tested 23 *H. pylori* strains for the presence of cytotoxic activity. Intracellular vacuolization of HeLa cells was observed in 60.9% of the isolates tested following incubation with broth-culture supernatant for 24 h (Table 1). In no case did the concentration of broth-culture filtrate reveal cytotoxic activity that was not detectable before concentration. However, when we passaged five cytotoxin-negative *H. pylori* strains 25 times, two of those five became cytotoxin-positive following the 15th and 18th subcultivation, respectively, which may reflect either the existence of a switch-on mechanism or the possible effect of mutation during such a subcultivation strategy.

The sex and age distribution of the patients as well as their clinical symptoms were no different in either of the two groups of cytotoxin-producing and cytotoxin-negative strains (Table 2). Of the 23 strains tested for intracellular vacuolization, six were from

Table 2. Cytotoxigenicity of *H. pylori* strains isolated from 23 patients

	Cytotoxin (+)	Cytotoxin (−)	Total (n = 57)
female	8	7	37
male	6	2	20
age (years) 20–39	1	2	12
40–59	7	2	22
60–79	4	4	16
> 80	2	1	7

Table 3. Cytotoxigenicity of *H. pylori* strains isolated from 23 patients with various endoscopic diagnoses

Endoscopic appearance	Cytotoxin (+)	Cytotoxin (−)
normal gastric mucosa	3	3
"antral gastritis"	9	4
ulcer duodenal	1	1
gastric	1	1

Table 4. Cytotoxigenicity of *H. pylori* strains isolated from 23 patients with chronic antral gastritis

Antral gastritis	Cytotoxin (+)	Cytotoxin (−)
mild	2	1
moderate	8	6
severe	4	2
active	10	6
nonactive	4	3

patients with gastroduodenal mucosa which appeared to be normal, and 13 were from patients with subjective mucosal appearances such as erythema, friability, and swelling of the antral mucosa without any signs of erosions or hemorrhages (Table 3). With regard to peptic ulcer disease, however, we can not draw any conclusion about a possible association between cytotoxic activity and peptic ulcer disease because of the low number of ulcer patients included.

Of the 24 *H. pylori*-positive patients, 23 had histological signs of antral gastritis of varying degrees, with active gastritis in 16 of the patients. Again, there were no statistically significant differences between the degree of the activity of gastritis and the identification of cytotoxin-secreting *H. pylori*-strains as revealed by intracellular vacuolization of HeLa cells (Table 4).

In conclusion, the pathogenic significance, if any, of this nonlethal vacuolization factor is not clear and remains to be established. The question whether such a factor may contribute to the development of inflammation should be evaluated following the isolation and detailed characterization of this protein. The understanding of the existence of cytotoxic variability between different infecting strains of *H. pylori* may help to answer many important questions about the role of *H. pylori* in gastritis and in peptic ulcer disease.

References

1. Bartlett JG (1988) Campylobacter pylori: factor or fancy. Gastroenterology 94:229–238
2. Börsch GMA (1989) Clinical significance of Campylobacter pylori. Eur J Gastroenterol Hepatol 1:27–33
3. Dooley CP, Cohen H (1988) The clinical significance of Campylobacter pylori. Ann Intern Med 108:70–79
4. Figura N, Guglielmetti P, Rossolini A et al. (1989) Cytotoxin production by Campylobacter pylori strains isolated from patients with peptic ulcers and from patients with chronic gastritis only. J Clin Microbiol 27:225–226
5. Graham DY (1989) Campylobacter pylori and peptic ulcer disease. Gastroenterology 96:615–625
6. Graham DY, Klein PD (1987) Campylobacter pyloridis gastritis: the past, the present, and speculations about the future. Am J Gastroenterol 82:283–286
7. Leunk RD, Johnson PT, David BC, Kraft WG, Morgan DR (1988) Cytotoxic activity in broth-culture filtrates of Campylobacter pylori. J Med Microbiol 26:93–99

Discussion

Graham: Let me give you a different model for another type of experiment that would address the same question, something we tried to do with the people at Procter and Gamble and I know that Marty Blaser is trying it also. I don't know what the answers are because it's all coded at the present time. Patients who have these toxin-producing strains make antibodies that block this reaction. So, therefore, one could more easily evaluate patients with gastric ulcer, duodenal ulcer, or non-ulcer dyspepsia and asymptomatics with infection and see the how many the toxin is actually active in by looking for antibodies. One can do a bigger, probably better, experiment more rapidly to see if this toxin relates to a specific disease entity. We've been trying that for about a year but haven't got any answers back.

Gregor: You are perfectly right: to measure the circulating antibodies against such a particular cytotoxic protein would be very appropriate to evaluate the prevalence of infection with *H. pylori* secreting a nonlethal vacuolization factor in various upper gastrointestinal disease states. However, so far, the only antisera which have been reported by Leunk et al. to neutralize the cytotoxic activity of *H. pylori* have been raised in rabbits against different preparations of *H. pylori* as well as broth-culture filtrate [7].

Slomiany: Is it possible that your toxin effect is due to some enzymatic activities elaborated by *H. pylori,* let's say a lipase activity, and what you are observing is the enzyme acting on these cells and not the toxin? How would you distinguish between these two?

Gregor: At the moment, we can not rule out this possibility for sure in particular because, as I mentioned already, the cytopathic factor is heat-sensitive as well as acid-sensitive.

Slomiany: That could indicate again that the observed effect might be due to enzymatic activity, rather than to cytotoxic activity.

Gregor: I agree, that we do not have a lot of information about the biochemical nature of this cytotoxic factor. For this reason, we have to await further information which comes from the isolation and purification of this cytopathic protein.

Blessing: Have you measured the pH of the supernatant and what is the purification procedure of the protein factor.

Gregor: The pH of the supernatant was 7.3. The purification method we have used so far includes a concentration step by ultrafiltration as well as various chromatographic procedures which means gel-permeation chromatography and ion exchange chromatography. We tried to use HPLC techniques but unfortunately we ran into problems with our bioassay system.

Wyatt: You've explained to us that there was no difference in the degree of inflammatory infiltration in the biopsies from the patients with cytotoxin positive and negative strains of *H. pylori.* Did your histopathologist also try to assess whether there was any difference in cellular degeneration of the surface epithelial cells, since that might be more expected from the effects on cells in vitro?

Gregor: No, we have not yet tried to assess any difference in cellular degeneration of the surface epithelial cells. But this should be done in particular by electronmicroscopy to evaluate also whether there are any signs of intracellular vacuolization.

Malfertheiner: Dr. Gregor, you first said that the cytopathic effects you observed might be related to a switch-on/switch-off effect. Wouldn't it then be an easy way to prove this by doing serial examinations from different phases of your cultures. Then, your answer would probably be that all bacteria produce this cytopathic effect. At a certain point of their growth they might have it, and at another time not.

Gregor: Yes, so far, we have done such passaging with five cytotoxin-negative *H. pylori* strains and two of those strains showed a switch-on of cytotoxic activity. Doing the same with five cytotoxin-positive strains, we never found a switch-off of cytotoxic activity.

Megraud: Maybe all strains produce cytotoxin, but sometimes at low levels, and you can only find it if you study broth after concentration.

Gregor: I agree. However, none of the broth-culture filtrates in our series which were cytotoxin-negative became cytotoxin-positive following a concentration procedure.

Malfertheiner: If all strains have the capacity to be cytopathic at a certain point, it would make it understandable that you don't find clinical, endoscopical, and histological differences. Of course, what we see in the patient is a long-term condition difficult to correlate with an in vitro experiment.

Gregor: I think, we are not in the position today to draw the conclusion from our experiment that all strains really have the capacity to be cytopathic.

Graham: I think it's dangerous to use the switch-on/switch-off analogy in this context. Surface proteins come and go, and you can turn them on or you can turn them off. What you're talking about here is possibly emergence of a new strain or a substrain that was in very low concentration in your initial inoculum. It is much more complicated when you're talking about multiple generations of bacteria that all develop or lose a new property.

Helicobacter pylori and Gastric Mucus Integrity*

B. L. Slomiany, V. L. N. Murty, J. Piotrowski, S.-L. Wang, and A. Slomiany

Introduction

A unique property of gastric mucosa is its ability to withstand the insults imposed by the luminal contents and to resist the challenge by invading bacteria. Although there is no general agreement as to the mechanism of mucosal protection, the consensus is that this phenomenon is multicomponential in nature, and includes at least three major defense perimeters, which are the mucus-bicarbonate zone, the cell membranes of gastric epithelium, and the mucosal blood flow [1–4]. Hence, the brunt of luminal insults, at least in the initial stage, falls on the mucus layer, which constitutes the only identifiable physical barrier between the gastric lumen and the surface epithelial cells of the mucosa. The integrity of this defense perimeter depends upon a delicate dynamic equilibrium, controlled by factors affecting the synthesis, secretion, and breakdown of its constituents [3, 5, 6]. While this equilibrium is maintained successfully under normal physiological conditions, injury to the mucosa ensues when aggressive forces overcome factors that control mucosal defense.

Although disintegration of the mucus coat has been known to occur with gastric disease, the process was attributed exclusively to the enhanced activity of intragastric pepsin [7]. More recent data, however, provided a strong argument that a bacterial factor, namely infection by *Helicobacter pylori,* may be responsible for the weakening of gastric mucus gel integrity. As *H. pylori* resides in the proximity of the surface of the gastric epithelium, protected from the corrosive luminal contents by a thick coat of mucus, and yet exhibits free mobility in this viscous environment, our studies concentrated for some time on the enzymatic activities of this microorganism toward mucus gel constituents. The results of these investigations suggest that *H. pylori* elaborates extracellular protease and lipases capable of mucus gel lipids and glycoprotein degradation.

Mucus Gel Organization

Understanding the role of mucus layer in gastric mucosal defense, and how its integrity is compromised by the aggressive forces, requires a thorough knowledge of mucus gel organization. Although the matrix of the gel arises through noncovalent

* This work was supported by USPHS grant #DK21 684-13 from the National Institute of Diabetes and Digestive and Kidney Diseases and Grant #AA05 858-08 from the National Institute on Alcohol Abuse and Alcoholism, National Institutes of Health.

H. Menge et al. (Eds.)
Helicobacter pylori 1990

Table 1. Chemical composition of gastric mucus

Component (mg/100 mg)	Species			
	Man	Pig	Dog	Rat
Protein	63.7	64.2	65.7	58.4
Glycoprotein	14.8	15.1	12.6	18.6
Lipids	18.2	17.6	18.9	21.3
Covalently bound fatty acids	0.2	0.3	0.2	0.3

interaction between mucus glycoprotein molecules, the mucus coat is not a single entity, but a heterogeneous mixture of the proteins, glycoproteins, and lipids which arrive to the mucosal surface through the process of glandular secretion, serum element transudation, and cell exfoliation (Table 1). In gastric lumen environment these constituents, and lipids in particular, enter into heterotypic interaction with mucus glycoprotein and thus affect the physical, chemical, and functional properties of mucus coat. Two types of interactions between lipids and mucus glycoprotein are distinguished: one in which lipids remain associated with the glycoprotein through hydrophobic forces, and the other involving fatty acids which exist in a covalent linkage with the glycoproteins [5, 6, 8–10]. The data on the topography of lipids associated with mucus glycoprotein polymer indicate that phospholipids interact with the glycoprotein through the nonglycosylated regions, while the interaction with glycolipids and neutral lipids, such as triglycerides, cholesterol, and cholesteryl esters, appears to involve the peripheral regions of mucus glycoprotein polymer molecule [3, 8].

The extent to which the associated lipids enter into the heterotypic interaction with mucus glycoprotein is apparently determined by the content and distribution of covalently bound fatty acids. The topography data indicate that at least four covalently bound fatty acids are present on the nonglycosylated regions of the glycoprotein polymer and one in the proximity of the amino terminal of each glycoprotein subunit [3, 11]. Increasing evidence suggests that both types of lipids play an important role in the maintenance of gastric mucus gel integrity [3, 9, 11–13]. A clear concept is, thus, emerging according to which mucus glycoprotein polymer through its various hydrophobic and hydrophilic regions forms a dynamic continuum with other components of other mucus (Fig. 1). The concept of dynamic organization of gastric mucus implies that the integrity and strength of mucus gel could be disrupted not only through mucin degradation, but also through changes in mucus gel lipid composition. This is an important distinction, since until now the prevailing view was that mucus constituents other than mucin constitute the impurities which contribute little to mucus gel function, and the data on the role of lipids and proteins in mucus function were even considered controversial [14]. With the concept of dynamic organization of gastric mucus in mind, we studied the nature of changes brought by *H. pylori* infection in mucus gel mucin as well as its lipids.

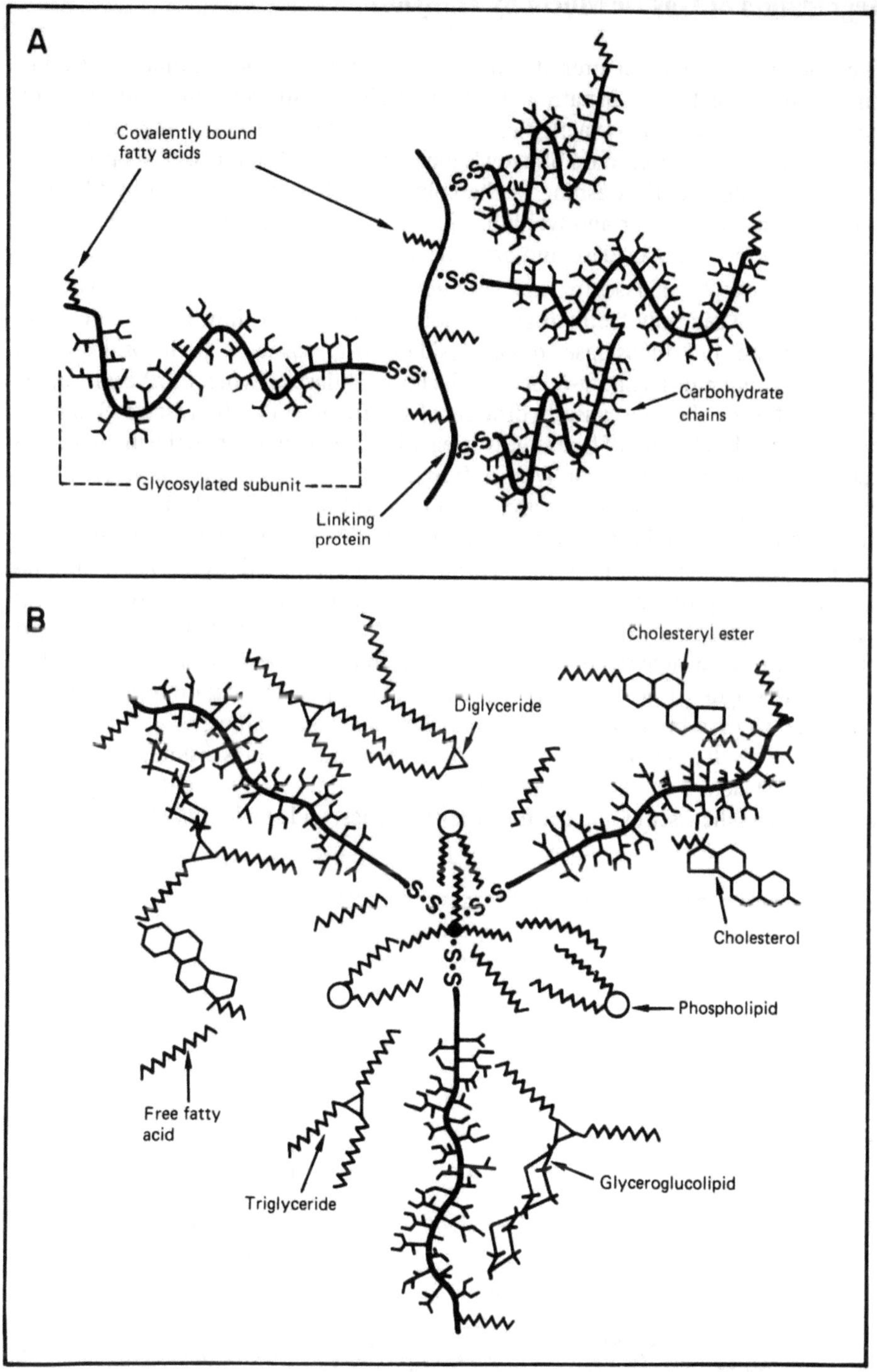

Fig. 1A, B. Diagrammatic representation of the dynamic model of gastric mucus glycoprotein organization. **A** side view; **B** top view

Degradation of Gastric Mucin by *H. pylori*

Since the loss of mucus gel integrity due to excessive degradation of mucus glycoprotein is a prominent feature in pathology of gastric disease, studies were conducted into the protease and glycosidase activities of *H. pylori*. The extracellular material elaborated by *H. pylori*, cultured on Skirrow's medium from antral mucosal biopsies, was obtained through gentle washing of the colonies with saline followed by filtration through sterilization filter and lyophilization. Such obtained powder was examined immediately for its glycosidase and protease activities.

Assays of exoglycosidase enzyme activities conducted with a battery of synthetic substrates revealed only feeble β-galactosidase activity, and showed the absence of neuraminidase, α-*L*-fucosidase, α-galactosidase, α-glucosidase, β-glucosidase, β-*N*-acetylglucosaminidase, and α-*N*-acetylgalactosaminidase enzyme. Furthermore, the *H. pylori* filtrate did not cause hydrolysis of gastric mucin carbohydrate chains, as evidenced by the absence of free sugars release [15]. However, when the incubate was examined on gel chromatography, a shift in mucin elution profile characteristic for proteolytic degradation of mucus glycoprotein was observed (Fig. 2). Parallel experiments with albumin indicated that the *H. pylori* filtrate caused extensive degradation of the protein. This apparent protease exhibited maximum activity at pH 7.0 and was capable of rapid proteolysis of albumin, as well as gastric mucin. The enzyme was pH sensitive and its activity dropped by 60% at pH 3.0, 50% at pH 5.0, and 45% at pH 8.0. The protease activity of the filtrate was found to be associated with a low molecular weight (< 50 K) protein fraction and, upon examination with various inhibitors, showed behavior typical of metalloproteinase (Table 2).

Since the result of *H. pylori* protease action on gastric mucin is disintegration of the polymeric structure of the glycoprotein and formation of glycopeptides which no longer possess the viscous and gel-forming properties, and exhibit only limited hydro-

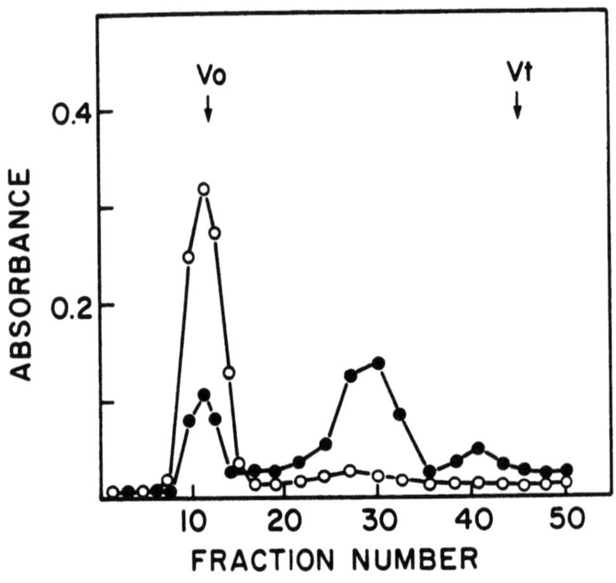

Fig. 2. Bio-Gel A-50 column chromatography in 6*M* urea-0.05*M* sodium phosphate buffer, pH 7.0, of gastric mucus glycoprotein before (○) and after (●) incubation with *H. pylori* filtrate. Fractions were monitored for carbohydrate by the phenol-H_2SO_4 method

Table 2. *H. pylori* protease characterization

Agent	Activity (%)
Control	100
α-2-Macroglobulin (3 μg)	9.5
Zincov (0.4 m*M*)	30.5
Phenylmethylsulfonyl fluoride (1 m*M*)	100
Ethylenediaminetetraacetic acid (1 m*M*)	26.2

gen ion retardation capacity [16], the erosion of mucus glycoprotein polymer, which constitutes the gel matrix, may, indeed, be of dire consequence to the mucosal integrity. The *H. pylori,* thus, by affecting degradation of deeper levels of the mucus gel drastically reduces the dimension and physicochemical qualities of acid-bicarbonate mixing zone required for luminal acid dissipation. As a consequence, the integrity of the mucus coat, due to challenge on the luminal side by acid and pepsin, and on the mucosal side by *H. pylori* protease, becomes severely undermined and renders the stomach epithelium vulnerable to damage by luminal contents.

Lipolytic Activity of *H. pylori*

As many pathogenic microorganisms, in addition to proteases, are known to produce extracellular lipases which are involved in microbial pathogenicity [17, 18], and since the integrity and strength of gastric mucosal defense depend also upon its lipid constituent [3, 6, 16], the extracellular material elaborated by *H. pylori* was examined for its capability of mucosal lipid degradation. This led to the identification of two lipolytic enzymes, namely, triglyceride lipase and phospholipase A_2. By following the release of fatty acid, it was found that the lipase attains its maximum activity at 37°C and the pH of 7.2. In the case of phospholipase A_2, maximum conversion of phosphatidylcholine substrate to free fatty acid and lysophosphatidylcholine was attained at the pH range of 7.0–7.4 and 37°H. Both enzymes were sensitive to low pH and temperature variation [19, 20].

The results obtained with neutral lipids of gastric mucus revealed that incubation with *H. pylori* filtrate led to substantial changes in the proportion of individual components (Table 3). These were reflected in a 15% increase in free fatty acids, a

Table 3. Effect of *H. pylori* filtrate on the neutral lipid composition of rat gastric mucus

Neutral lipid	% of total neutral lipids: Control	% of total neutral lipids: *H. pylori* filtrate incubate
Free fatty acids	48.8	56.2
Mono- and diglycerides	6.3	17.6
Triglycerides	23.6	4.9
Cholesterol	11.1	11.3
Cholesteryl esters	10.2	10.0

Table 4. Effect of *H. pylori* filtrate on the phospholipid composition of rat gastric mucus

	% of total lipid phosphate	
Phospholipid	Control	*H. pylori* filtrate incubate
Phosphatidylcholine	29.1	8.7
Phosphatidylethanolamine	14.3	3.5
Phosphatidylserine	3.8	3.2
Phosphatidylinositol	4.3	3.6
Sphingomyelin	12.5	12.6
Lysophosphatidylcholine	15.9	37.2
Lysophosphatidylethanolamine	0.3	11.5
Phosphatidylglycerol	8.7	8.9
Phosphatidic acid	3.6	3.5
Diphosphatidylglycerol	3.5	3.7
Unidentified	4.0	4.2

2.8-fold increase in mono- and diglycerides, and a 4.8-fold decrease in triglycerides. Examination of gastric mucus phospholipids following incubation with *H. pylori* filtrate showed the conversion of phosphatidylcholine and phosphatidylethanolamine to the corresponding lysophospholipids (Table 4). Compared with the controls, the *H. pylori* filtrate-incubated phospholipids showed a 3.3-fold decrease in the content of phosphatidylcholine and a 4.1-fold decrease in phosphatidylethanolamine; at the same time, the content of lysophatidylcholine increased 2.3-fold and that of lysophosphatidylethanolamine 38-fold [19].

Thus, with respect to its lipolytic activities, *H. pylori* shares characteristics common to the majority of pathogenic microorganisms, which are known to produce large amounts of extracellular lipase and phospholipase enzymes [17, 18]. These enzymes apparently play an important role, not only in pathogen proliferation, bbut alsoappear to be active components of toxins and, hence, influence the pathogenic potential of the microorganism [17, 18, 21, 22]. As mucus lipids and phospholipids, in particular, contribute to the integrity and resilience of gastric mucosal defense [3, 12], and are involved in the maintenance of hydrophobic lining of the stomach [11, 23], the alterations in lipids caused by *H. pylori* lipases may be of serious consequence to the mucosal defense. Furthermore, an increase in lysolecithin level due to *H. pylori* phospholipase A_2 offsets the ratio of this lipid to other phospholipids, leading to a drastic change in the lytic activity of the lysophospholipid toward gastric epithelium and the mucus coat [24, 25]. The lipolytic activity of *H. pylori* could, thus, be detrimental at the same time to two major elements of mucosal defense: namely, the mucus layer and the cell membranes of gastric epithelium.

Effect of Antiulcer Agents on *H. pylori* Mucus-Degrading Enzymes

Since a number of mucosal strengthening agents used in ulcer therapy are known to exert their beneficial action through strengthening the mucosal integrity and enhancement of the physicochemical properties of mucus defense perimeter [3, 12, 26–28], an evaluation of these drugs' effect on the *H. pylori* protease and lipase enzymes could

Table 5. Effect of mucosal strengthening agents on the degradation of gastric mucus by *H. pylori* protease

Agent	Maximal concentration (g/liter)	Proteolytic activity inhibition (%)
Sucralfate	10	0
Sofalcone	1.0	3–5
Geranylgeranylacetone	1.0	10–12
Colloidal bismuth subcitrate (De-Nol)	1.0	37

aid in a more rational approach to ulcer therapy. The results of *H. pylori* protease assays in the presence of several mucosal strengthening agents are summarized in Table 5. The data showed that the only appreciable (Fig. 3) inhibitory activity occurred with colloidal bismuth subcitrate (De-Nol). Marginal inhibitory effects were observed with geranylgeranylacetone and sofalcone, while sucralfate did not show measurable effects on the protease activity. From the results of preincubation, it appears that the mechanism of inhibition of gastric mucus proteolysis by De-Nol results from the drugs' interaction with mucus, rather than with the protease [29]. The antiproteolytic activity of De-Nol was dose dependent and attained its maximal inhibitory effect at a concentration of 1×10^{-1} g/liter, at which point a 37% decrease in mucus proteolysis occurred. It is noteworthy that this concentration of De-Nol is readily achieved with the normal dose (4 × 300 mg De-Nol tablets/day) during ulcer therapy.

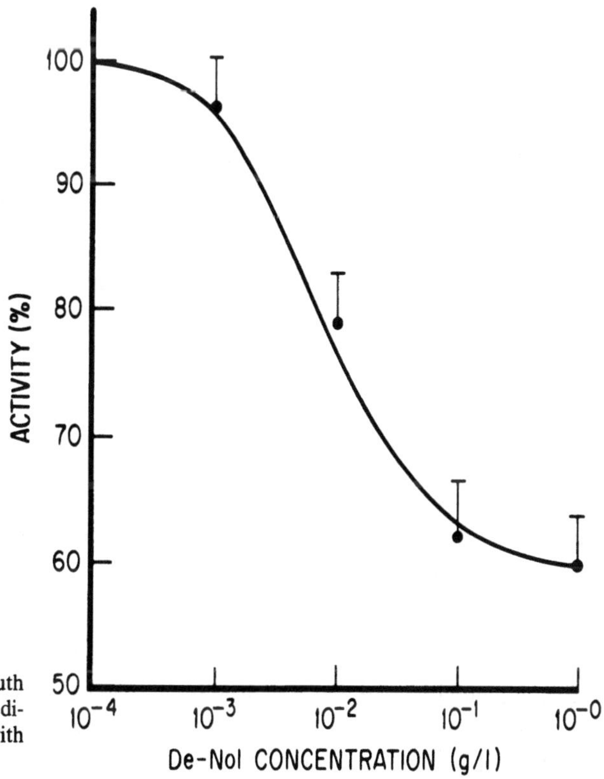

Fig. 3. Effect of colloidal bismuth subcitrate concentration on the digestion of gastric mucus with *H. pylori* protease

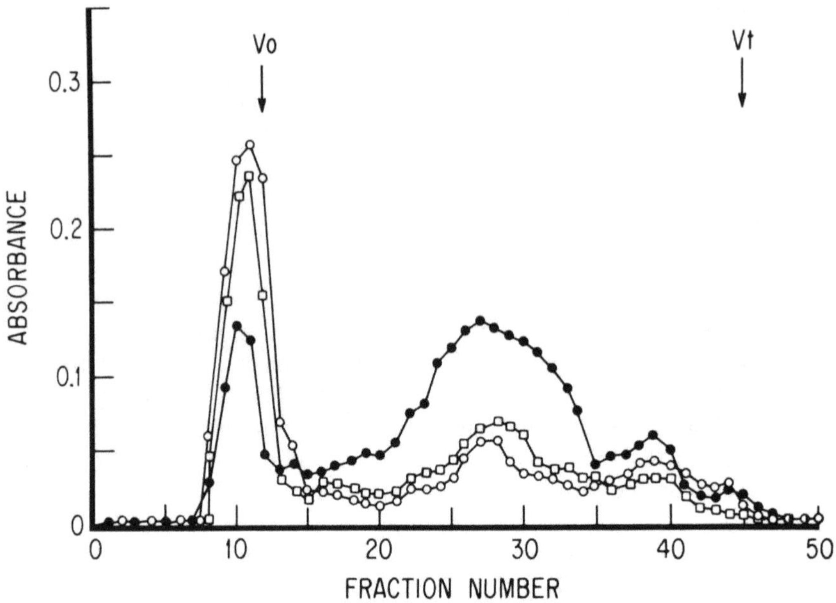

Fig. 4. Bio-Gel A-50 column chromatography in 6*M* urea-0.05*M* sodium phosphate buffer, pH 7.0, of intact gastric mucus (○), and the mucus following incubation with *H. pylori* protease in the absence (●) and in the presence (□) of colloidal bismuth subcitrate. Fractions were monitored for carbohydrate by the phenol-H_2SO_4 method

The effectiveness of De-Nol on the *H. pylori* protease action toward gastric mucin is illustrated in Fig. 4. The high-molecular-weight undegraded mucus glycoprotein polymer was found to be predominant in the mucus prior to *H. pylori* protease incubation, while following incubation with *H. pylori* the low molecular weight degraded form of mucin dominated. However, inclusion of De-Nol in the incubation mixture prevented the degradation of mucin by *H. pylori* protease. This finding extends our knowledge as to the mode of beneficial action of colloidal bismuth subcitrate in promoting the healing of gastric and duodenal ulcers, and sheds light on the underlying mechanism. Apparently, this drug, due to its antiproteolytic activity, counteracts the excessive degradation of mucus coat by pepsin from the luminal side [30], and by *H. pylori* protease from the epithelial side. It may well be that, even without total *H. pylori* eradication, De-Nol is able to keep in check the rampant damage of the mucosal integrity by neutralizing the protease elaborated by this bacteria, as well as that of intraluminal pepsin. This could account for the lower recurrence rate of duodenal ulcer following De-Nol therapy.

The data on the effect of antiulcer mucosal strengthening agents on the lipolytic activity of *H. pylori* are limited to De-Nol and sofalcone [19, 20]. The results obtained with sofalcone indicate that this drug is capable of inhibition of gastric mucus triglyceride degradation (43%), but has little, if any, inhibitory effect on the activity of *H. pylori* phospholipase A_2 [31]. Since neutral lipids of gastric mucus contribute little to

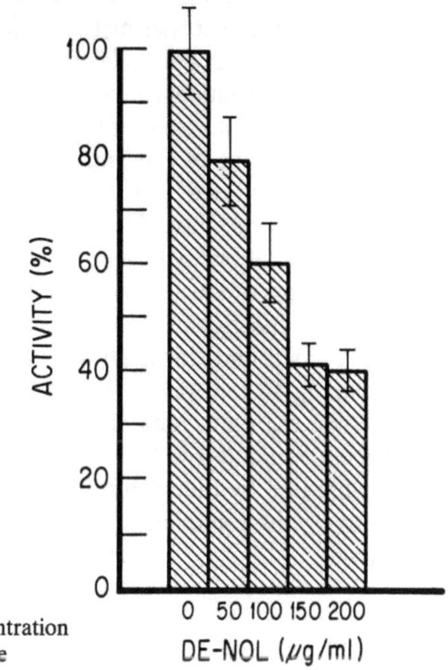

Fig. 5. Effect of colloidal bismuth subcitrate concentration on the phospholipase A_2 activity of *H. pylori* filtrate

the physicochemical properties of mucus gel, it may be concluded that the beneficial action of sofalcone, in promoting the healing of gastric and duodenal ulcers, could be due only in part to the drug's ability to keep in check the activities of the enzymes elaborated by *H. pylori* which otherwise are highly detrimental to the mucosal integrity.

In contrast to sofalcone, De-Nol exerts its inhibitory action on both *H. pylori* lipases. The rate of inhibition of triglyceride lipase activity appears to reach maximum effect (21%) at a De-Nol concentration of 150 µg/ml [32]. In the case of phospholipase A_2 activity, the inhibition of phospholipid degradation in the presence of De-Nol attains the level of 60% (Fig. 5). Therefore, the beneficial action of colloidal bismuth subcitrate in ulcer healing could be the result of the drug's ability to counteract the activities of protease and lipase enzymes associated with bacterial proliferation, thus causing *H. pylori* eradication. It should be borne in mind, however, that virulence of many microorganisms does not depend on their enzymatic activities alone, as the heat-inactivated lipases are also highly detrimental to the host defense [17, 18, 21]. Whether De-Nol is capable of affecting the latter phenomenon remains to be established.

Conclusions

Although the clinical data provide increasingly convincing indications that *H. pylori* is a causitive factor in gastritis and peptic ulcer, the advances toward the clear understanding of this bacterium pathogenic action are slow in forthcoming. Conceivably, *H. pylori*, having a niche bordering two major perimeters of gastric mucosal defense, could detrimentally affect mucus layer as well as surface cells of gastric epithelium. Indeed, the mucosa of patients infected with *H. pylori* shows massive infiltration with polymorphonuclear leukocytes and lymphocytes, and the bacteria appear to penetrate the tight junctions of the epithelial cells [33]. Furthermore, recent findings provide leads that sulfated and sialic acid containing glycolipids of epithelial cell membranes serve as receptors for *H. pylori* colonization of gastric mucosa [33–35]. Alterations brought about by *H. pylori* in mucus gel are also obvious and include such consequences as loss of mucus coat continuity, its patchy appearance, and reduction in thickness. Identification of the enzymes elaborated by *H. pylori* which are clearly detrimental to lipids and mucus glycoproteins of the gastric mucus coat provides an important clue as to the way by which this pathogen undermines gastric mucosal integrity. While the pathogenic consequences of *H. pylori* colonization of gastric mucosa almost certainly result from many facets, the findings that the mucolytic enzymes elaborated by the bacterium are subject to inhibition by certain mucosal strengthening agents could aid in a more rational approach to *H. pylori*-associated gastric disease.

References

1. Silen W (1987) Gastric mucosal defense and repair. In: Johnson LR (ed) Physiology of the gastrointestinal tract, 2nd edn. Raven, New York, pp 1055–1069
2. Flemstrom G (1987) Gastric and duodenal mucosal bicarbonate secretion. In: Johnson LR (ed) Physiology of the gastrointestinal tract, 2nd edn. Raven, New York, pp 1011–1029
3. Slomiany BL, Sarosiek J, Slomiany A (1987) Gastric mucus and the mucosal barrier. Dig Dis 5:125–145
4. Szabo S, Pihan G, Triers S (1986) Alteration in blood vessels during gastric injury and protection. Scand J Gastroenterol 21[Suppl 125]:92–96
5. Slomiany A, Takagi A, Slomiany BL (1985) The synthesis and secretion of gastric mucus glycoprotein by mucosal cells cultured in the presence of ethanol. Arch Biochem Biophys 236:654–666
6. Slomiany BL, Piasek A, Sarosiek J, Slomiany A (1986) The role of surface and preformed intracellular mucus in gastric mucosal protection against hydrogen ion. Scand J Gastroenterol 20:1191–1196
7. Glass GBJ, Slomiany BL (1977) Derangement of biosynthesis, production and secretion of mucus gastrointestinal injury and disease. In: Elstein M, Parke DV (eds) Mucus in health and disease. Plenum, New York, pp 311–347
8. Witas H, Slomiany BL, Zdebska E, Kojima K, Liau YH, Slomiany A (1983) Lipids associated with dog gastric mucus glycoprotein. J Appl Biochem 5:16–24
9. Slomiany A, Jozwiak Z, Takagi A, Slomiany BL (1984) The role of covalently bound fatty acids in the degradation of human gastric mucus glycoprotein. Arch Biochem Biophys 229:560–567
10. Slomiany A, Witas H, Aono M, Slomiany BL (1983) Covalently linked fatty acids in gastric mucus glycoprotein of cystic fibrosis patients. J Biol Chem 258:8535–8538
11. Gwozdzinski K, Slomiany A, Nishikawa H, Okazaki K, Slomiany BL (1988) Gastric mucin hydrophobicity: effects of associated and covalently bound lipids, proteolysis and reduction. Biochem Int 17:907–917
12. Bilski J, Sarosiek J, Murty VLN, Aono M, Moriga M, Slomiany A, Slomiany BL (1987) Enhancement of the lipid content and physical properties of gastric mucus by geranylgeranylacetone. Biochem Pharmacol 36:4059–4065

13. Slomiany BL, Murty VLN, Carter SR, Slomiany A (1986) Effect of covalently bound fatty acids and associated lipids on the viscosity of mucus glycoprotein in cystic fibrosis. Digestion 34:275–280
14. Allen A (1981) Structure and function of gastrointestinal mucus. In: Johnson LR (ed) Physiology of the gastrointestinal tract. Raven, New York, pp 617–639
15. Slomiany BL, Bilski J, Sarosiek J, Murty VLN, Dworkin B, VanHorn K, Zielenski J, Slomiany A (1987) *Campylobacter pyloridis* degrades mucin and undermines gastric mucosal integrity. Biochem Biophys Res Commun 144:307–314
16. Sarosiek J, Slomiany A, Slomiany BL (1988) Evidence for weakening of gastric mucus integrity by *Campylobacter pylori.* Scand J Gastroenterol 23:585–590
17. Barrett-Bee K, Hayes Y, Wilson RG, Ryler JF (1985) A comparison of phospholipase activity, cellular adherence and pathogenicity of yeasts. J Gen Microbiol 131:1217–1221
18. Rollof J, Braconier JH, Soderstorm C, Nillson-Ehle P (1988) Interference of *Staphylococcus aureus* lipase with human granulocyte function. Eur J Clin Microbiol Infect Dis 7:505–510
19. Slomiany BL, Nishikawa K, Piotrowski J, Okazaki K, Slomiany A (1989) Lipolytic activity of *Campylobacter pylori:* effect of sofalcone. Gastroenterology 94:399
20. Slomiany BL, Murty VLN, Piotrowski J, Okazaki K, Slomiany A (1988) Effect of colloidal bismuth subcitrate (De-Nol) on the lipolytic activity of *Campylobacter pylori.* Am J Gastroenterol 83:1029
21. Rollof J, Hedstrom SA, Nilsson-Ehle P (1987) Lipolytic activity of *Staphylococcus aureus* strains from disseminated and localized infections. Acta Pathol Microbiol Immunol Scand A, B 95:109–113
22. Brockerhoff H, Jensen RG (1974) Lipolytic enzymes. Academic, New York
23. Lichtenberger LM, Graziani LA, Dial EJ, Butler BD, Hills BA (1983) Role of surface-active phospholipids in gastric cytoprotection. Science 219:1327–1329
24. Slomiany BL, Sarosiek J, Liau YH, Laszewicz W, Slomiany A (1986) Lysolecithin affects the viscosity, permeability and peptic susceptibility of gastric mucin. Scand J Gastroenterol 21:1073–1079
25. Slomiany BL, Glass GBJ, Kojima K, Banas-Gruszka Z, Slomiany A (1982) Effect of lysolecithin on the constituents of gastric mucus. In: Chandler EN, Elder JB, Elstein M (eds) Mucus in health and disease, vol 2. Plenum, New York, pp 163–174
26. Slomiany BL, Laszewicz W, Slomiany A (1986) Effect of sucralfate on the viscosity of gastric mucus and the permeability to hydrogen. Digestion 33:146–151
27. Slomiany BL, Liau YH, Mizuta K, Slomiany A (1987) Fatty acylation of mucin by gastric mucosa: effect of sofalcone and sucralfate. Biochem Pharmacol 36:3273–3276
28. Tytgat GNJ (1987) Colloidal bismuth subcitrate in peptic ulcer: a review. Digestion 37:31–41
29. Sarosiek J, Bilski J, Murty VLN, Slomiany A, Slomiany BL (1989) Colloidal bismuth subcitrate (De-Nol) inhibits degradadation of gastric mucus by *Campylobacter pylori* protease. Am J Gastroenterol 84:506–510
30. Bilski J, Sarosiek J, Nishikawa H, Slomiany A, Slomiany BL (1988) Colloidal bismuth subcitrate (De-Nol) inhibits peptic degradation of gastric mucus. Am J Gastroenterol 83:1029
31. Slomiany BL, Nishikawa H, Piotrowski J, Okazaki K, Slomiany A (1989) Lipolytic activity of *Campylobacter pylori:* effect of sofalcone. Digestion 43:33–40
32. Slomiany BL, Kasinathan C, Slomiany A (1989) Lipolytic activity of *Campylobacter pylori:* effect of colloidal bismuth subcitrate (De-Nol). Am J Gastroenterol 84:1273–1277
33. Graham DY (1989) *Campylobacter pylori* and peptic ulcer disease. Gastroenterology 96:615–625
34. Slomiany BL, Piotrowski J, Samanta A, VanHorn K, Slomiany A (1989) Gastric mucosal sulfatides and sucralfate inhibit agglutination of erythrocytes by *C. pylori.* Am J Gastroenterol 84:1169
35. Slomiany BL, Piotrowski J, Samanta A, VanHorn K, Murty VLN, Slomiany A (1989) *Campylobacter pylori* colonization factor shows specificity for lactosylceramide sulfate and GM_3 ganglioside. Biochem Intern 19:929–936

Discussion

Hazell: I am sure that you have had these questions before, and that you have the answers. I would like you to address the issue of the time course of your studies. You indicate periods of 24–48 h before obtaining significant changes in terms of breakdown of the mucus, considering that the stomach is in a dynamic state where mucus is being continually produced. Also, with particular regard to phospholipase activity, phospholipase is notorious for being affected by steric factors and the enzyme configuration. I would like some comment on phospholipase activity as it relates to the mucus in its native state.

Slomiany: With respect to *H. pylori* protease, the data which you are referring to are on viscosity and hydrogen ion retardation. I agree that one begins to observe changes only following longer periods of exposure to *H. pylori* filtrate. However, if proteolytic activity of *H. pylori* is measured by more sensitive methods, such as trinitrophenylation, the proteolytic degradation of mucin is observable within 30 min of incubation. Concerning the mucus being continuously produced and renewed, I would like to point out that we are just approximating the possible in vivo conditions, and that it is quite possible that in situ the enzyme may be considerably more active that in our test tube assay. As to the phospholipase issue, it is clear that lysolecithin was generated. This compound is well known to have a detrimental effect on gastric mucosal integrity, and a number of people consider this lipid to be a contributing factor in the etiology of gastric disease. About a year ago, when we reported on phospholipase A_2 of *H. pylori* at the AGA meeting, Raedsch from this country communicated that patients with *H. pylori* have a higher concentration of lysolecithin in their gastric juice. This past May during the AGA meeting, his group showed that *H. pylori* contains phospholipase A_2 activity. How do these enzymes affect the mucus gel? It is well known that the generation of lysolecithin is mucolytic to mucus gel, as evidenced by the loss of gel viscosity and by its ability to retard hydrogen ion diffusion. Furthermore, what I think is even more important, is that lysolecithin is a very potent lytic agent capable of cell lysis. So the lysolecithin produced by the action of *H. pylori* enzyme could easily compromise gastric mucosal integrity.

Graham: This morning we heard phenomenology related to the concept that if I can measure it in the laboratory, it must have something to do with the disease. When I look in a stomach and see a white coating on the mucosa upon gastric secretory studies, and I immediately spin the fluid, I get this nice, thick gelatinous stuff at the bottom; this is the mucus gel, and what one works with is the soluble stuff in the top. Is this correct?

Slomiany: No Sir!

Graham: Is that right?

Slomiany: Yes, but I think we have little misunderstanding to clarify. When you open the stomach, what you see is adherent mucus gel existing in equilibrium with that in solution. The soluble mucus is simply discarded since it represents the degraded mucus components. Now, you have mucus gel which adheres to the mucosal surface, and this is what we use in our studies.

Graham: How do you get that from people?

Slomiany: We are working mainly with animals. It is a little more difficult to obtain undegraded mucus from humans, but there are some adventurous gastroenterologists in Europe who apparently are able to collect the gastric mucus under buffering conditions. Obviously the best source would be through access to human surgical discards.

Graham: So you are working with that gelatinous insoluble stuff?

Slomiany: Yes, that gel can be recovered either by gentle scraping or with sodium chloride buffered to pH 7.0. The gel consistency is observed at concentrations above 30 mg/ml; below this concentration one is dealing with solution.

Graham: Are your experiments done with that in natural state or in the diluted state?

Slomiany: With the exception of studies on viscosity and hydrogen ion permeability, measurements are made using mucus at 10 mg/ml.

Graham: One-third of the concentration that would spontaneously form what we are talking about – is this correct?

Slomiany: Yes.

Graham: I am not saying that what you do is not important, but that the pictures which you show do not relate to what I mean by gels.

Veldhuyzen van Zanten: Did you also test the effect of *H. pylori* on bismuth subsalicylate (Peptobismol)?

Slomiany: No, we did not. However we did study preparations of bismuth subcitrate (De-Nol) and bismuth subnitrate. The inhibitory activity of the latter appears to be about 30% lower than that of the former.

Wadström: Your discovery of phospholipase A_2 in *H. pylori* was very interesting, for this is a very rare enzyme among microbes; most microbes produce phospholipase, which is often a very potent cytolytic and hemolytic toxin. So, my question is, could this phospholipase A_2 that you are working with be hemolytic and have cytolytic effects also on other cells?

Slomiany: That was actually what I was alluding to in my comments to the previous speaker. It is possible, and has actually been shown be Rollof and others in Sweden, that the virulence of many pathogenic organisms is preserved even when the enzymatic activity is destroyed. This means that even if you inactivate the enzyme activity, the detrimental effect on that particular protein will persist.

Lee: As you know, we have argued that *H. pylori* is one of a group of organisms specifically adapted to mucus, particularly as regards moving in a viscous environment. Organisms do things only if there is something in it for them. What I would like to know is, what do you consider all of this enzyme activity to be for. How is it useful to the organism? Because they will only do it if it is useful to them. And secondly, why is it that not everyone with antral gastritis has a gastric ulcer?

Slomiany: As regards to your second question, I am not a clinician and must leave you to worry about that. Concerning your first question, it is obvious that the functions performed by living organisms are directed towards survival. Therefore it is possible that some of the enzymes elaborated in *H. pylori* facilitate its movement within the gel environment, whereas others, such as protease activity might reflect the need of bacteria for nutrients.

Sipponen: Do you have any data about structure and function of mucus in gastritis with or without *H. pylori* infection? Such experiments would be very important because gastritis itself influences the structure and function of mucus on the gastric surface.

Slomiany: You are quite right, it would be interesting to compare the mucus gel from healthy individuals with that from patients with *H. pylori,* with respect to mucin molecular forms of distribution.

Sipponen: If your theory about the role of *H. pylori* is correct, differences should be found in the mucus before and after the eradication of the bacterium.

Slomiany: I am looking forward to collaborating with you in obtaining samples from those two groups. Possibly we could also establish this kind of collaboration with some people within the United States.

Nwokolo: You have just presented data to suggest that De-Nol may in some way protect the integrity of gastric mucus by inhibiting the enzymes derived from *H. pylori.* What I want to ask is, first, what concentrations of De-Nol did you use, and, secondly, do you think that this effect is due to the bismuth metal contained in De-Nol or to the secondary structure of this compound?

Slomiany: The question of what is the active component of various bismuth preparations comes up over and over again. At this point it is clear that the preparations which are colloidal appear to be more active, and that is where the CBS belongs. I can not answer whether the bismuth itself would cause a similar effect, but bismuth preparations have been known for ages to be potent bacteriocidal agents. Browsing through the book from the last symposium, I understand that the effect of bismuth preparations is due to bismuth itself, since under the acidic pH of the stomach the colloidal bismuth subcitrate and other preparations dissociate. Regarding concentrations, those used in our studies ranged from 150 to 200 μg/ml. This concentration can easily be achieved with the normal dose of De-Nol, which is 300 mg four times daily under ulcer therapy. Actually, our data indicate that one does not need this much to achieve the discussed effects in the in vitro assays. The in vivo situation obviously may be different.

Helicobacter pylori and Other Gastric Spirilla: Similarities and Differences*

A. Lee and J. Fox

The Stomach as a Specialized Ecological Habitat

Microbiologists interested in the microbial flora of the gastrointestinal tract have traditionally ignored the stomach. Due to the harsh environment resulting from acid secretion, conditions were considered to be hostile to permanent colonization by bacteria although it was accepted bacteria could survive passage into the lower bowel. An exception was the work of Savage (1980), who showed the gastric mucosa of rodents to be permanently colonized with acid-tolerant lactobacilli and yeasts. However, the isolation of *Helicobacter pylori* and its association with gastroduodenal disease has focussed interest on bacteria in the stomach and it is now clear that many animal species have similar bacteria colonizing their gastric surfaces, i.e. humans, dogs, cheetahs, cats, monkeys, ferrets, rats (Lee 1989a). One characteristic of the microbial ecology of harsh environments is so called low species diversity; that is, very low numbers of species are present at any one time (Alexander 1971). This is a consequence of the need for specialized adaptations being required to live in that site. This is certainly so in the stomach where usually one and at the most three bacterial species are found together. Thus most animals with bacteria inhabiting the gastric mucus have only one species present. In humans the species normally present is *H. pylori.* As more bacteria are isolated from other animal species it is important to compare their properties with *H. pylori* in order to be better able to identify those factors that are essential for gastric colonization and those which might be involved in the initiation of gastroduodenal disease. The aim of this short article is to review the current knowledge on the gastric spirilla other than *H. pylori* and highlight any differences and similarities.

Gastric Spirilla

Helicobacter pylori

This bacterium is shown in Fig. 1. Our hypothesis is that this is the human gastric spirillum although there have been reports that the organism has been found in the stomachs of primates in captivity (Newell et al. 1988) and pigs housed in contact with their Mexican family owners (Rivera et al. 1989). The question remains whether these

* This work is supported by a grant from the National and Medical Research Council of Australia

H. Menge et al. (Eds.)
Helicobacter pylori 1990

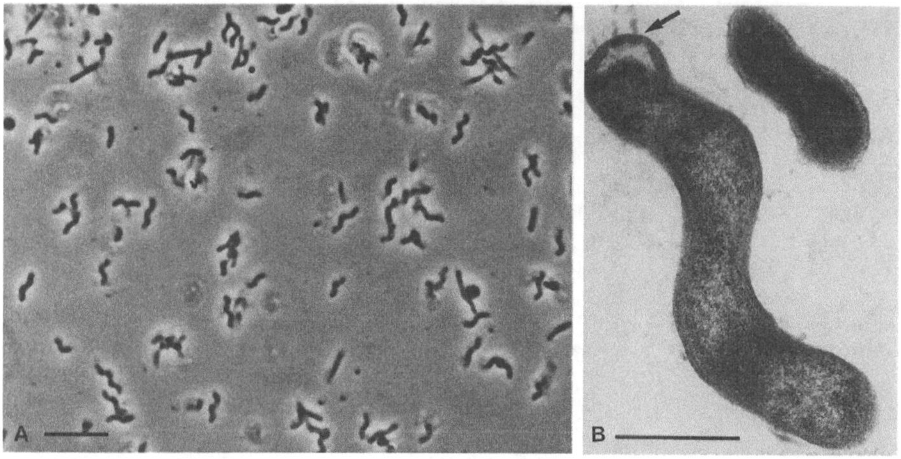

Fig. 1A, B. Pure culture of *Helicobacter pylori* showing spiral morphology. **A** Phase contrast microscopy, *bar,* 5 µm; **B** Transmission electron microscopy; *bar,* 0.5 µm. Note the insertion sites of the multiple polar flagella *(arrow)*

animals had acquired the organism from their human handlers, i.e. no non-human reservoir has yet been found.

Helicobacter mustelae

This organism isolated from the ferret stomach by one of us is to some extent atypical in that it is not a spiral. Occasionally curved forms are seen but on culture and in vivo it is a small rod-shaped-like organism (Fox 1986) (Fig. 2).

CS1-Like Bacteria

CS1 is the temporary name given to a spiral organism isolated by us from the cat stomach (Lee et al. 1988) (Fig. 3). The characteristic periplasmic fibrils occurring singly or in pairs make the organism easily identifiable in vivo. A similar organism has been reported in the dog stomach (Henry et al. 1987).

"Gastrospirillum"

This is another highly spiralled helical organism that is also seen in the gastric mucosa of cats and dogs. A very similar form has been found in the stomach of most primates so far examined (Fig. 4). This is distinct from CS1 in that the periplasmic fibrils are not present. This bacterium is the only one of the gastric bacteria described, other than *H.*

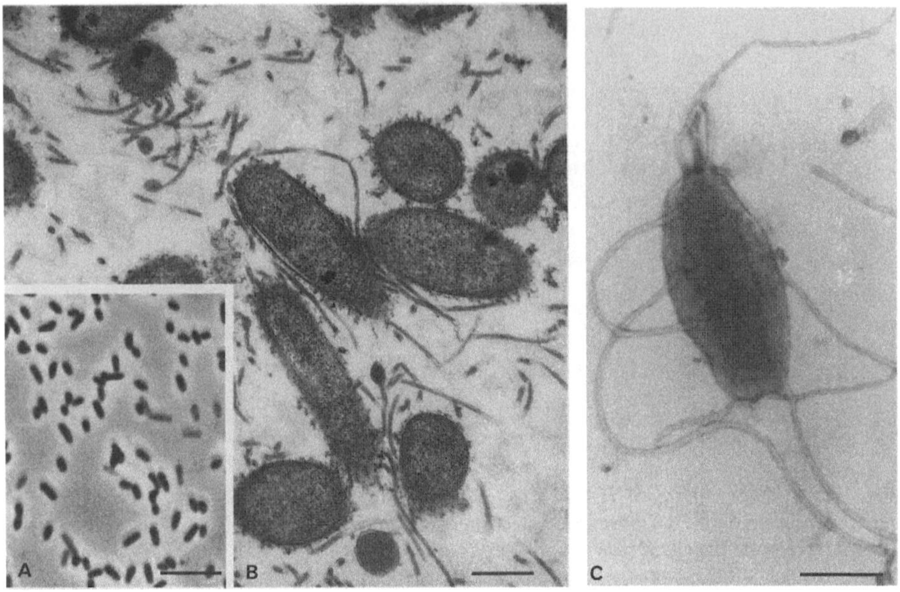

Fig. 2A–C. Pure culture of *Helicobacter mustelae* showing rod-shaped morphology and long polar and lateral flagella. **A** Phase contrast microscopy; *bar,* 1 μm; **B, C** transmission electron microscopy; *bar,* 0.2 μm

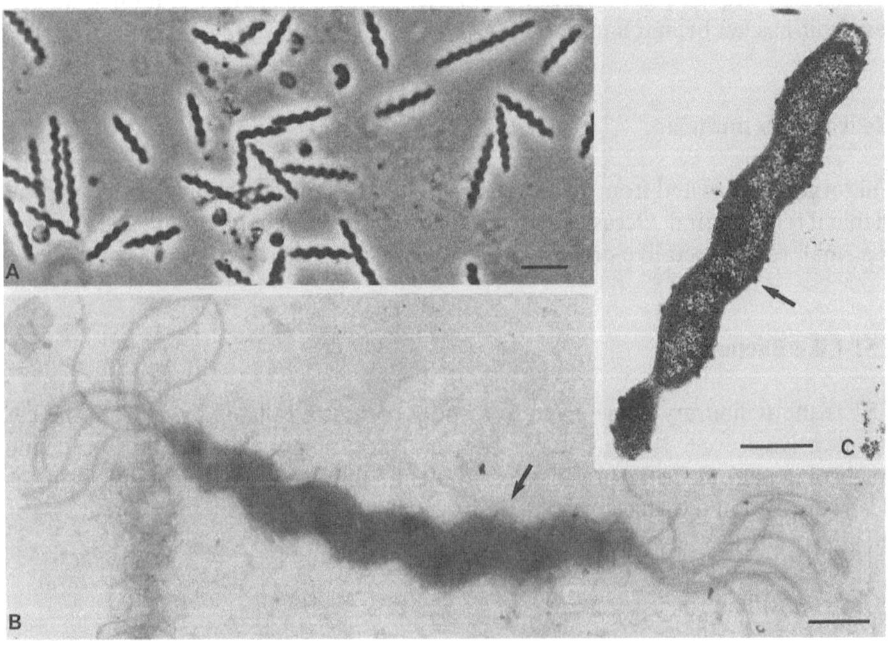

Fig. 3A–C. Pure culture of CS1, a helical bacterium isolated from the stomach of a cat showing spiral morphology, bipolar tufts of flagella and periplasmic fibrils. **A** Phase contrast microscopy; *bar,* 2 μm; **B, C** transmission electron microscopy; *bar,* 0.5 μm. The periplasmic fibrils occurring in pairs are shown by the *arrow*

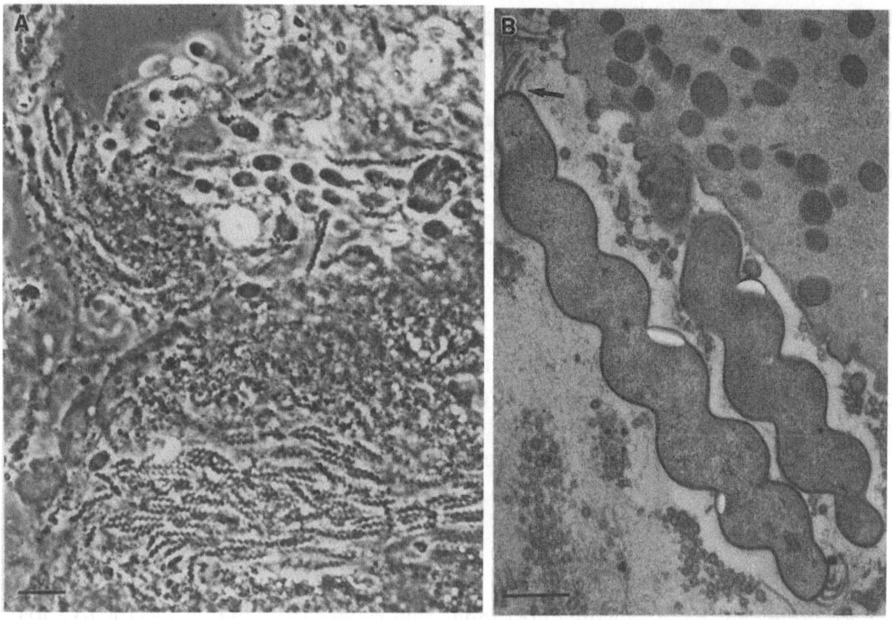

Fig. 4 A, B. In vivo culture of *Gastrospirillum hominis* in stomach of a mouse. **A** Phase contrast microscopy of scrapings of the gastric mucosa of a colonized mouse showing the spiral shape of the organism and the very large number of bacteria that pack the gastric pits; *bar*, 5 μm. **B** Transmission microscopy of a thin section of the gastric mucosa of a colonized mouse showing two bacteria. On the top organism the bipolar tufts of flagella can be clearly seen *(arrow)*

pylori, that has been seen in the human stomach and thus is worthy of special interest (Dent et al. 1987; Lee et al. 1989b). The organism has not been cultured using conventional techniques but we have managed to keep isolates from mandril and macaque monkeys, humans, cats and dogs alive in the rodent stomach (Dick et al. 1989). The name *"Gastrospirillum hominis"* was suggested for the human organism by McNulty (McNulty et al. 1989).

Similarities and Differences in the Gastric Spirilla

Morphology

As can be seen from the figures already presented, there are considerable differences in the morphology of these organisms. *H. pylori,* CS1 and *Gastrospirillum* have a spiral shape which has been postulated to give the organisms an ability to penetrate gastric mucus (Lee and Hazell 1988); however, the latter two organisms have a much more helical morphology. In contrast, *H. mustelae* has no obvious spiral shape. The flagella arrangements are also different. *H. pylori* has a single tuft of up to seven polar

Table 1. Similarities and differences between the gastric spirilla

Morphology	Shape	Turns	Flagella number	Location
Helicobacter pylori	Spiral	1–3	4– 7	Unipolar
CS1-like	Helical	5–7	10–17	Bipolar
Gastrospirillum	Helical	4–5	10–12	Bipolar
Helicobacter mustelae	Rod	0–1	4– 8	Polar and lateral

flagellae while CS1 and gastrospirillum have fascicles of up to 12 flagellae at both ends. *H. mustelae* has an unusual arrangement with several lateral flagellae being obvious. The other striking difference between these bacteria is the periplasmic fibrils of the CS1-like bacteria. These differences are summarized in Table 1.

Host Specificity

These organisms have a distinct host range that ranges from highly specific to apparently non-specific. Current knowledge is summarized in Table 2. There are many experiments to be done but clearly *H. pylori* and *H. mustelae* have a much more restricted host range than CS1 and *Gastrospirillum.*

Table 2. Similarities and differences between the gastric spirilla

Host specificity	Human	Pig	Non-human primate	Cat	Dog	Ferret	Rodent
Natural infection							
Helicobacter pylori	+++	?+	?+	–	–	–	–
CS1-like	–	–	–	+	+	–	–
Gastrospirillum	++	?	+++	+++	+++	–	–
Helicobacter mustelae	–	–	–	–	–	++++	–
Experimental infection							
Helicobacter pylori	+++	++	++	?	++	–	–
CS1-like	?	?	?	?	++++	?	+++
Gastrospirillum	?	?	?	?	?	?	++++
Helicobacter mustelae	?	?	?	?	?	++++	–

+++, heavy colonization; ++, moderate colonization; +, seen in small numbers; ?, not known

Physiological

The three organisms that have been cultured to date share many physiological features as summarized in Table 3. All are microaerophilic and are strongly urease positive, they do not ferment carbohydrates, are catalase and oxidase positive and

Table 3. Similarities and differences between the gastric spirilla

Physiology	
Shared properties	
	Microaerophilism
	Urease
	Oxidase
	Catalase
	Alkaline phosphatase
	Non-fermentation of carbohydrates
	Hippurate not hydrolysed
	H_2S not produced
Differences	
	Leucine aminopeptidase *(H. mustelae* negative)
	Nitrate reductase (*H. pylori* negative)
	Glutamate dehydrogenase (CS1 negative)

share many other enzymes. However, there are some differences, thus *H. mustelae* lacks nitrate reductase unlike the others whilst CS1 lacks the glutamate dehydrogenase shown by both *H. mustelae* and *H. pylori.* All we know about *Gastrospirillum* at present is that it is strongly urease positive.

Specificity for the Stomach

Helicobacter clearly does not thrive in the environment of the lower bowel and is not easily cultured from faeces. In the gnotobiotic pig model of *H. pylori* infection, colonization was only found in the stomach (Krakowka et al. 1987). Recent experiments by us to be reported in greater detail later would suggest that specificity for the stomach is characteristic of all the gastric spirilla both in natural and laboratory infection. This is shown in Table 4. This apparent specificity for the environment of

Table 4. Similarities and differences between the gastric spirilla

Tissue specificity	Stomach	Duodenum	Jejunum	Ileum	Cecum	Colon	Rectum
Helicobacter pylori							
Natural human	+++	±	–	–	–	–	–
Experimental pig	++	–	–	–	–	–	–
CS1							
Experimental dog	+++	–	–	–	–	–	–
Experimental mice	+++	–	–	–	–	–	–
Experimental rat	+++	–	–	–	–	–	–
Gastrospirillum							
Experimental mice	++++	–	–	–	–	–	–
Helicobacter mustelae							
Natural infection	+++	–	–	–	–	–	–

+++, heavy colonization; ++, moderate colonization; +, seen in small numbers; –, no colonization

gastric mucosae is consistent with the idea of the gastric spirilla being a highly evolved group of specialized bacteria. These four groups of bacteria appear very fragile and ball up into spherical forms as cultures age and thus are unlikely to be excreted in the faeces in significant numbers as they would not survive the trip down the small and lower bowel.

Ability To Cause Gastritis

Given the irrefutable proof of *H. pylori* as the major aetiological agent in histological gastritis a fundamental question to be answered is whether or not the other gastric bacteria have similar pathogenic potential. Experiments undertaken by us in Boston and to be reported in detail elsewhere show that these other organisms do have the potential to induce both an acute and chronic inflammatory cellular response. Results on the histopathology of both natural and experimental infections are summarized in Table 5.

The gastric mucosa of the majority of adult dogs and cats examined have heavy infiltrations of mononuclear cells often aggregated into lymphoid-like germinal centres and this is classified as lymphocytic gastritis. It has been previously suggested this chronic gastritis was due to gastric spirilla known to colonize these stomachs in high numbers (Henry et al. 1987). Experiments with pure cultures of CS1 in germ-free dogs carried out in the laboratory of Dr. Steve Krakowka proved conclusively the organisms had this inflammatory potential. Figure 5 shows the lymphoid response of the dog gastric mucosa to 1 month's colonization with CS1. This was similar but more marked than that obtained by Krakowka and Lambert in gnotobiotic pigs (Krakowka et al. 1987; Lambert et al. 1987).

Of probably more importance is the response of the germ-free mouse stomach to colonization with CS1. A striking acute inflammatory response was observed resulting in crypt abscesses not unlike those seen in early *H. pylori* infection. Over a period of weeks this response modified to an active/chronic infection as observed with *H. pylori* in humans. Examples of the acute response are seen in Fig. 6. In the ferret

Table 5. Similarities and differences between the gastric spirilla

Ability to induce gastritis	Active gastritis (polymorphs present)	Chronic only gastritis (mononuclear response)	Active/chronic
Helicobacter pylori			
Natural (human)	+	?	+
Experimental (pig)	+	+	–
CS1			
Natural	?	+	±
Experimental dog	?	+	±
Experimental GF mice	+	–	+
Helicobacter mustelae			
Natural (ferret)	?	+	–
Gastrospirillum			
Natural (human)	?	+	+

+, present; ?, not known; –, absent

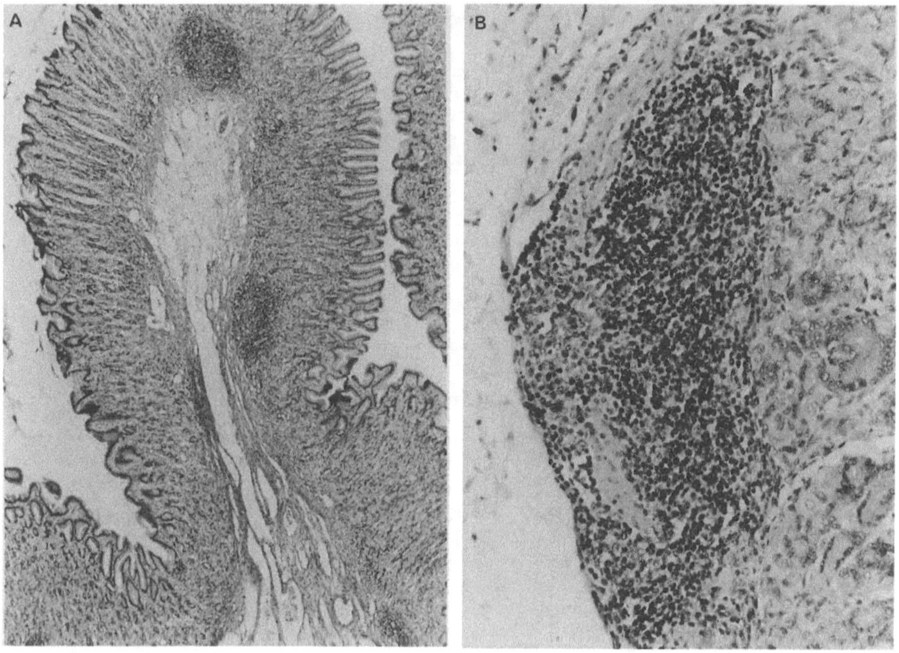

Fig. 5 A, B. Sections of the stomach of a 5-week-old germ-free beagle dog 4 weeks after oral inoculation of a pure culture of the gastric spirillum CS1 showing extensive mononuclear cell infiltration. **A** An area of fundus that showed large numbers of lymphoid nodules in the subglandular portion of the mucosa. Four nodules are seen in this field. In addition to the lymphoid nodules there is a mild to moderate diffuse mononuclear cell infiltrate in the subglandular portion of the mucosa, H & E, × 200. **B** High-power view of a lymphoid nodule showing focal extension through the muscularis mucosa into the underlying submucosa. A few plasma cells are intermixed with the lymphocytes in the subglandular infiltrates and lymphoid nodules, H & E, × 2000

stomach a distinct histopathology is seen in response to *H. mustelae*. The responses of the human gastric mucosa to *Gastrospirillum* will be discussed in more detail by Heilmann in the following chapter.

Evolutionary Relatedness

The analysis of the 16S ribosomal RNA sequence of these organisms has revealed perhaps the most important similarity (Paster, Lee, Dewhirst, Fox, and Ferrero, submitted for publication). Ribosomal RNA is a highly conserved molecule as its function has remained constant over the evolution of prokaryotic organisms. This close similarity reflects a common evolution. When compared with all the *Helicobacter*-like organisms grown from the gastrointestinal tract, the bacteria most closely related to *H. pylori* are firstly CS1 and secondly *H. mustelae*. This is unlikely to be coincidence and presumably is a reflection of the evolution of a distinct cluster of gastric bacteria early on in mammalian evolution.

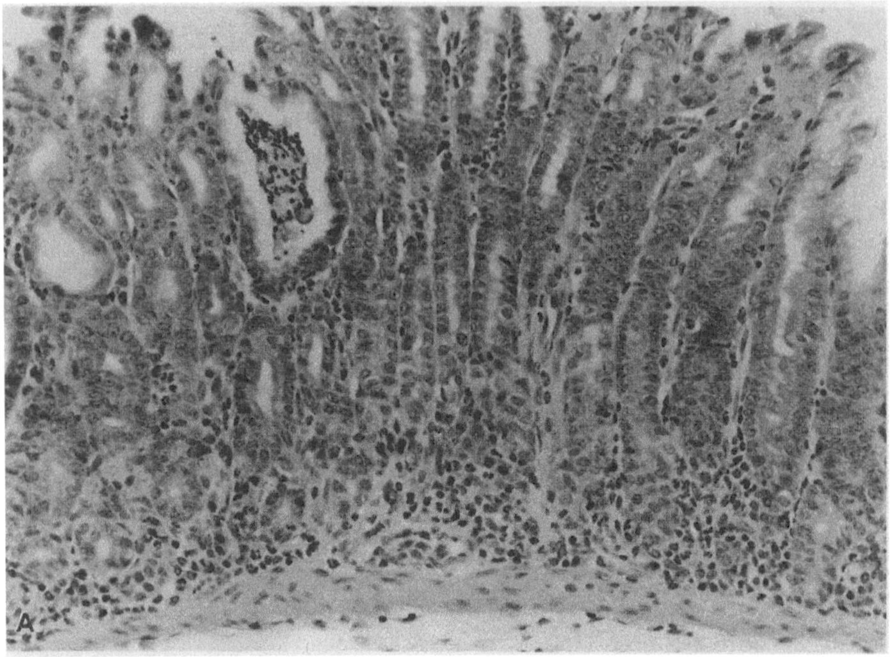

Fig. 6

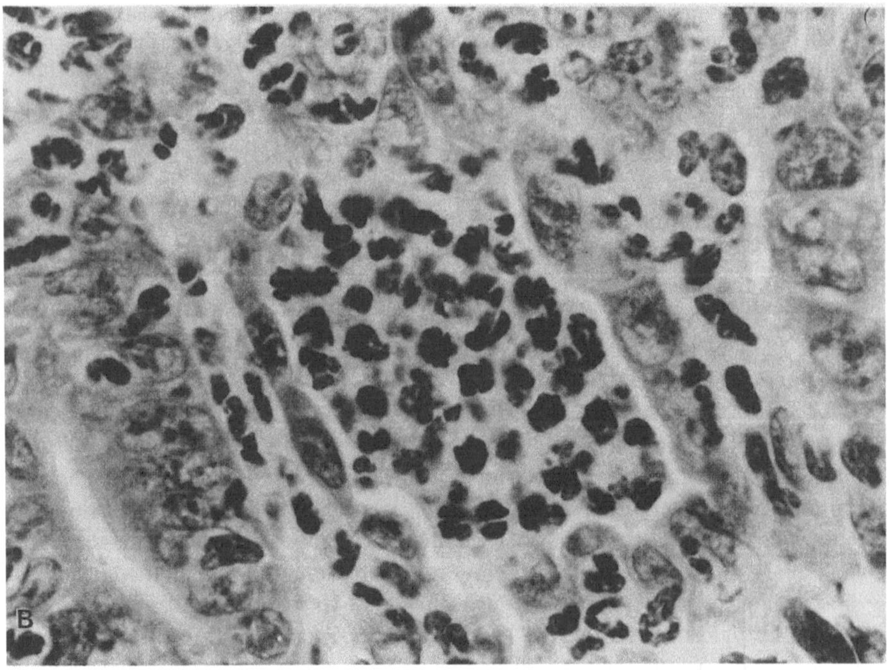

Fig. 6

Gastric Spirilla as a Single Genus

Despite some of the phenotypic differences described above, *H. pylori* and *H. mustelae* are officially recognized as belonging to the same genus. The close similarity of 16S ribosomal RNA sequences is consistent with this. Previously others have suggested *Campylobacter* was not the true home for these bacteria and suggested a new genus be created (Romaniuk et al. 1987). Goodwin and colleagues have officially transferred both these organisms to the new genus *Helicobacter* (Goodwin et al. 1989). As mentioned above, CS1 and these two bacteria form a tight cluster with an average level of homology of 94.5%, therefore we are suggesting that CS1 belongs to the newly formed genus *Helicobacter* and we will propose the name *"Helicobacter felis"* (Paster, Lee, Dewhirst, Fox, and Ferrero submitted for publication). Thus the stomach has been the site for the evolution, possibly from primitive mucus colonizers, of a group of highly specialized bacteria still closely related enough to fall in the one genus. When we finally grow *Gastrospirillum* I predict that it too will probably fall within this same genus.

Conclusion

On balance, there are more similarities between *Helicobacter pylori* and the non-*Helicobacter pylori* gastric spirilla than differences. The limited host range of *Helicobacter pylori* makes extensive animal experimentation difficult; however, with the other organisms particularly *Helicobacter mustelae* and CS1 this is more feasible. Demonstration that they all belong to the same genus, now officially named *Helicobacter*, makes the study of these animal models, especially in defining the nature of gastritis, all the more relevant to human gastroduodenal disease.

Acknowledgements. We would like to thank Jani O'Rourke for the production of the photomicrographs of bacteria and Dr. Jim Murphy for the histopathological studies. Hazel Mitchell, Richard Ferrero, Nada Heinene, Elizabeth Dick, Stephen Danon and Nerissa Lee all contibuted in some way to this work. Also, the help of Dr. Mel Dickson of the exellent Biomedical Electron Microscopy unit at the University of New South Wales is acknowledged.

Fig. 6A,B. Sections of the glandular mucosa of the stomachs of germ-free mice following oral inoculation of a pure culture of the gastric spirillum CS1. **A** Tissue from an animal 2 weeks postinfection showing diffuse infiltration of polymorphonuclear leucocytes in the subglandular area composed of a mixture of eosinophils and neutrophils with focal extension of these cells into the lamina propria. Mononuclear lymphocytes are also seen, H & E, × 2000. **B** Tissue from an animal 4 weeks postinoculation. A moderate mixed leukocytic infiltrate was present in the glandular mucosa but was most marked in the subglandular area. The mononuclear cell component was composed of a mixture of lymphocytes and macrophages; the polymorphonuclear cell infiltrate was composed of eosinophils and neutrophils. This field shows one of the small microabscesses often seen within the lumen of the glands

References

Alexander M (1971) Microbial ecology. Wiley, New York

Curry A, Jones DM, Skelton-Stoud P (1989) Novel ultrastructural findings in a helical bacterium found in the baboon *(Papio anubis)* stomach. J Gen Microbiol 135:2223–2231

Dent JC, McNulty CAM, Uff JS, Wilkinson SP, Gear MWL (1987) Spiral organisms in the gastric antrum. Lancet II:96

Dick E, Lee A, Watson G, O'Rourke J (1989) Use of the mouse for the isolation and investigation of stomach-associated, spiral-helical shaped bacteria from man and other animals. J Med Microbiol 29:55–62

Fox JG, Edrise BM, Cabot EB, Beaucoge C, Murphy JC, Prostak KS (1986) *Campylobacter*-like organisms isolated from gastric mucosa of ferrets. Am J Vet Res 47:236–239

Goodwin CS, Armstrong JA, Chilverts T, Peters M, Collins MD, Sly L, McConnell W, Harper WES (1989) Transfer of *Campylobacter pylori* and *Campylobacter mustelae* to *Campylobacter* gen. nov. as *Campylobacter pylori* comb. nov. and *Campylobacter mustelae* comb. nov. respectively. Int J Syst Bacteriol 39(4):397–405

Henry GA, Long PH, Burns JL, Charbonneau DL (1987) Gastric spirillosis in beagles. Am J Vet Res 48:831–836

Krakowka S, Morgan DM, Kraft WG, Leunk RD (1987) Establishment of gastric *Campylobacter pylori* infection in the neonatal gnotobiotic piglet. Infect Immun 55:2789–2796

Lambert JR, Borromeo KJ, Pinkard H, Turner CB, Smith ML (1987) Colonisation of gnotobiotic piglets with *Campylobacter pyloridis* – an animal model? J Infect Dis 155:1344

Lee A (1989a) *C. pylori* and CLO in animals. Overview of mucus colonizing organisms. In: Rathbone B, Heatley V (eds) *Campylobacter pylori* and gastroduodenal disease. Blackwell, Oxford, pp 246–260

Lee A (1989b) Human gastric spirilla other than *C. pylori*. In: Blaser M (ed) *Campylobacter pylori* in gastritis and peptic ulcer disease. Igaku-Shoin, New York 225–240

Lee A, Hazell SL (1988) *Campylobacter pylori* in health and disease: an ecological perspective. Microbiol Ecol Health Dis 1:1–16

Lee A, Hazell SL, O'Rourke J, Kouprach S (1988) Isolation of a spiral-shaped bacterium from the cat stomach. Infect Immun 56:2843–2850

Lee A, Eckstein RP, Fevre DI, Dick E, Kellow JE (1989) Non *Campylobacter pylori* spiral organisms in the gastric antrum. Aust NZ J Med 19:156–158

McNulty CAM, Dent JC, Curry A, Uff JS, Ford GA, Gera MWL, Wilkinson SP (1989) New spiral bacterium in gastric mucosa. J Clin Pathol 42:585–591

Newell DG, Hudson MJ, Baskerville (1988) Isolation of a gastric campylobacter-like organism from the stomach of four rhesus monkeys, and identification as *Campylobacter pylori*. J Med Microbiol 27:41–44

Rivera E, Luqueno V, Clava JJ, Ruiz-Palacios GM (1989) Exposure to swine, a risk factor for human *Campylobacter pylori* infection (abstract P1–45). Vth International Workshop on Campylobacter infections, Puerto Vallarta, Mexico 25th February–1 March 1989

Romaniuk PJ, Zo Howaska B, Trust TK, Lane DJ, Olsen GJ, Pace NR, Stahl DA (1987) *Campylobacter pylori*, a spiral bacterium associated with human gastritis, is not a true *Campylobacter*. s pp J Bacteriol 169:2137–2141

Savage DC (1980) Adherence of normal flora to mucosal surfaces. In: Beachey EH (ed) Bacterial adherence. Chapman and Hall, London, pp 33–49

Further Observations on Human Spirobacteria

K. L. Heilmann and F. Borchard

The intensive search for *Helicobacter pylori* in gastric biopsies has led to the discovery of spiral organisms, different from *H. pylori*, in the human gastric mucosa [1–5]. Spiral-shaped microorganisms were described in the gastric mucosa of various mammalian species as early as 1893, but not in humans [6–8, 10]. They seem to be widely distributed in nature and may be found to colonize nearly 100% of the gastric mucosa of adult cats, dogs, and monkeys [9]. Infection of the human species, however, seems to be an exceptionally rare event. Dent and McNulty [1], the first to describe the infection in humans, found three cases of infection in 1300 biopsies, i. e., in about 0.23%. This corresponds almost exactly to the percentage of cases of infection found in our own study, 27 cases in 11909 gastric biopsies, which were designed to examine and screen patients for *H. pylori* over a period of 18 months. The higher incidence of 0.6% and 0.7% discovered in smaller series seems to be unrealistic, though the organism is very easy to miss.

This organism for which McNulty et al. [10] proposed the name *Gastrospirillum hominis* and which no one has yet been able to culture, can be recognized in routinely processed hematoxylin and eosin (HE)-stained sections as weakly-staining spirals, differing in form and size clearly from *H. pylori*. It stains very well with different silver stains such as Steiner's or Whartin-Starry's stains. *G. hominis* is gram-negative and occurs either as a single organism or in small groups, localized underneath the mucus layer, above the surface cells, and frequently deep within the foveolae (Fig. 1). It never occurs in such great numbers as *H. pylori* and appears mostly in the antral and rarely in the corpus mucosa, where it can be identified light microscopically within parietal cells, as demonstrated by Bizzozero [6]. In one case, *G. hominis* and *H. pylori* occurred together, as reported by the French group [5].

In scanning electron microscopy (SEM), the organisms are aggregated in small clusters of 3–10, some of them lying parallel close to each other on the mucosal surface. Most of the organisms are straight, some of them are bent (Fig. 2). In transmission electron microscopy (TEM), some of the organisms have pointed, some blunted ends (Fig. 3). At the blunted ends, an insertion complex is visible with up to 12 flagellae (Fig. 4). The flagellae have swollen ends, and their variable form with partial parallel course and partial cord-like twisting suggests the mobility of these organelles. There are no axial filaments and no periplasmic fibers. *G. hominis* may be seen on the surface of antral and corpus mucosa below the mucus layer, sometimes adhering to the membranes of the surface cells without a preference for the tight junctions. At the point of adherence, there is kinking and partial destruction of the microvilli. As in light microscopy, the organisms are seen intracellularly, where they probably cause

H. Menge et al. (Eds.)
Helicobacter pylori 1990

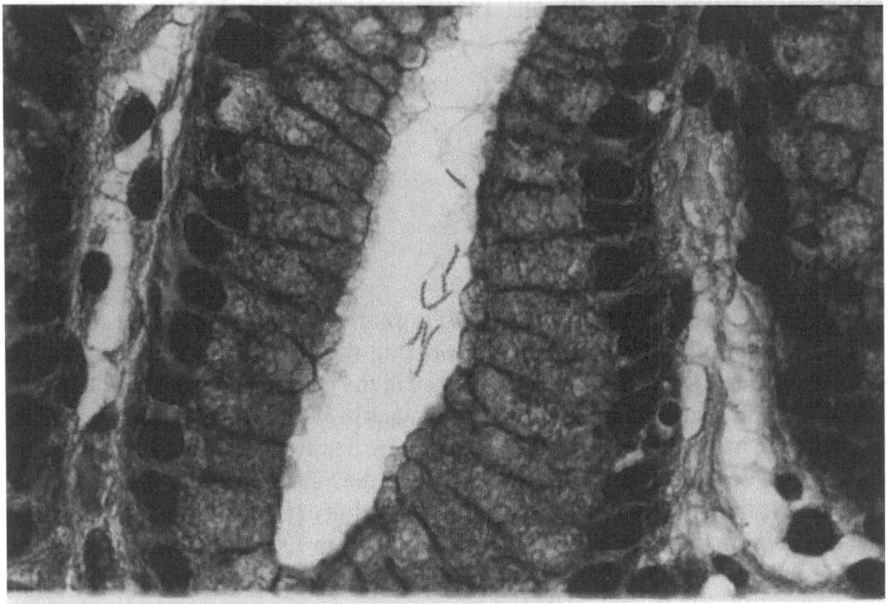

Fig. 1. *G. hominis* in a gastric pit in the antral mucosa. H & E, × 800

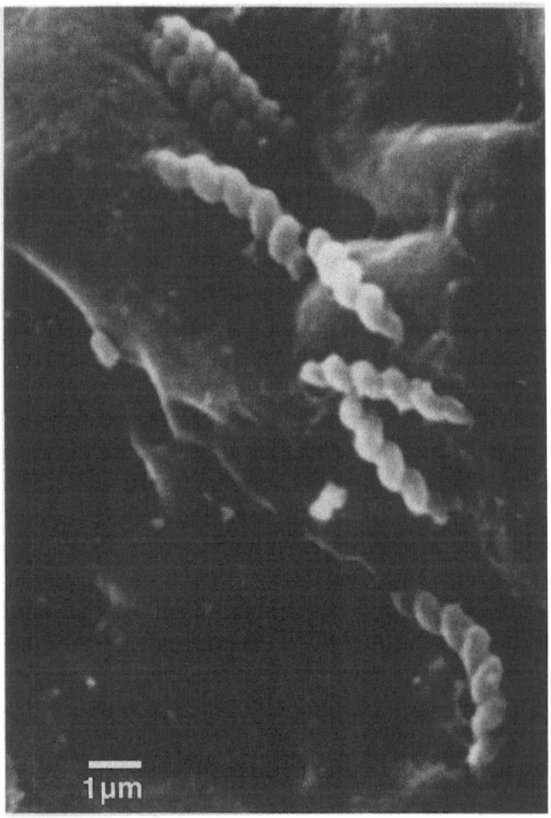

Fig. 2. *G. hominis* on the mucosal surface of the gastric body; most are straight, a few bent, and some lie parallel close to each other. SEM

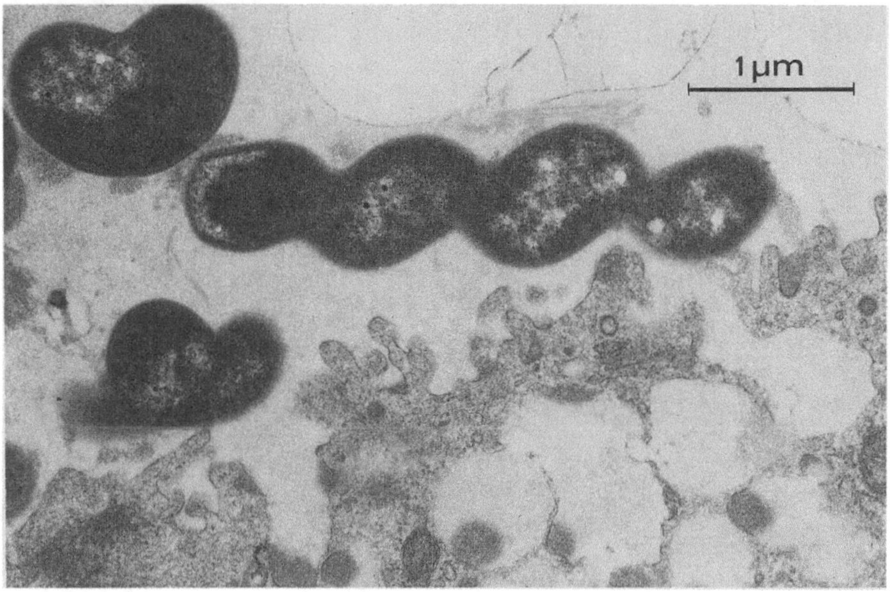

Fig. 3. A few *G. hominis* lying on the surface of a mucopeptic cell. Degeneration of microvilli. Note varying bacterial diameter. TEM × 32000

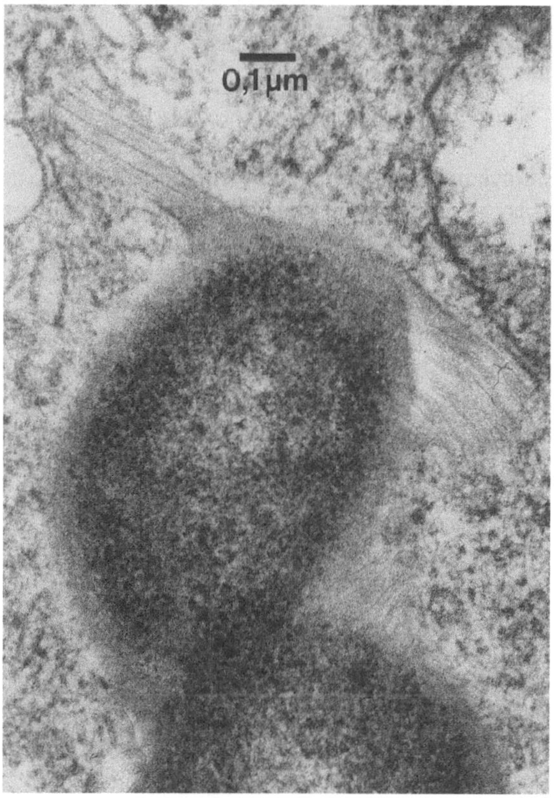

Fig. 4. Ends of intracellular *G. hominis* with flagellar apparatus next to mitochondria. Filaments with cord-like twisting or parallel course. TEM × 110000

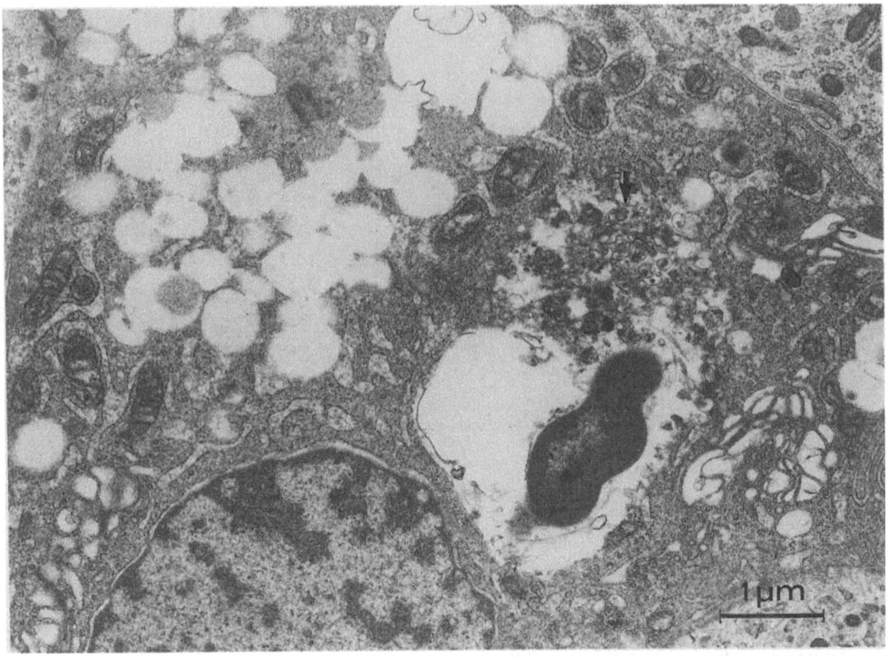

Fig. 5. Degenerative changes of an antral mucopeptic cell next to *G. hominis* invasion: formation of a large vacuole with microvesicular desintegration of organelles *(arrow)*, dilatation of the SER and mild mitochondrial swelling. TEM × 20500

mitochondrial swelling and formation of cytoplasmic vacuoles around the bacteria (Fig. 5). They can be identified in parietal, mucopeptic, and even endocrine cells.

In contrast to the hitherto known behavior of spirilla in animals, the presence of *G. hominis* in humans seems to be associated with an inflammatory reaction. In 27 of our 30 cases, active gastritis grade 1 or 2 with intraepithelial and interstitial granulocytes and a lymphoplasmocellular infiltrate was observed. Only three patients just had chronic gastritis with no granulocytic component. In most cases, the inflammatory response was less severe than in *H. pylori* infection. Twenty-three patients, i.e., 86% of them showed clinical symptoms of non ulcer dyspepsia, which in seven cases lasted less than 1 month and in five cases up to 1 year. In five cases, a biopsy urease test was positive.

Eight patients were treated with bismuth salts. In all patients, relief of the symptoms was seen. In biopsies taken between 30 days and 138 days after administration of the bismuth salts, the organisms were no longer detected. The granulocytes disappeared completely, whereas the lymphoplasmocellular infiltrate decreased in most cases during this relatively short observation period. The same developments were observed in the cases of both *H. pylori* and *G. hominis* infection. However, *H. pylori* was still present after therapy (Table 1).

G. hominis can probably survive for a long period of time in the stomach, as two of our cases may demonstrate. The organisms were detected in one case in a biopsy from

Table 1. Bismuth-induced changes in gastritis associated with *G. hominis*. (Data from the Institute of Pathology, Landshut, 1989)

Patients Age (years)	Sex	Therapy	GSH B	GSH A	GRAN B	GRAN A	LY/PLA B	LY/PLA A	Interval (days)
28	F	Bi-ss/28	+	−	++	−	+	+	55
41	F	Bi-ss/28	+	−	++	−	++	+	45
50	F	Bi-ss/28	+	−	+	−	+	+	138
21	M	Bi-ss/28	+	−	+	−	+	+	30
26	M	Bi-ss/28	+	−	++	−	++	+	30
50	M	Bi-ss/28	+	−	++	−	++	+	50
52	M	Bi-ss/28	+	−	++	−	++	−	79
60	M[a]	Bi-ss/28	+	−	++	−	++	+	35

GSH, *G. hominis;* GRAN, granulocytes; LY/PLA, lymphoplasmocellular infiltrate; B, before therapy; A, after therapy

[a] Double infection with *G. hominis* and *H. pylori*. *H. pylori* persisted after the treatment

1979, which was restained and reexamined, and in the other case, in a biopsy from 1985. In both cases there was chronic active gastritis, which did not change significantly.

Comparing the behavior and morphology of the spiral-shaped microorganisms found in humans with those seen in animals, many similarities become apparent.

We examined gastric biopsies and postmortem specimens of six dogs and 25 cats. All dogs harbored spiral-shaped bacteria, the presence of which was associated with a mild form of gastritis (Fig. 6). Of 25 cats, only 20 showed spiral bacteria; four of these

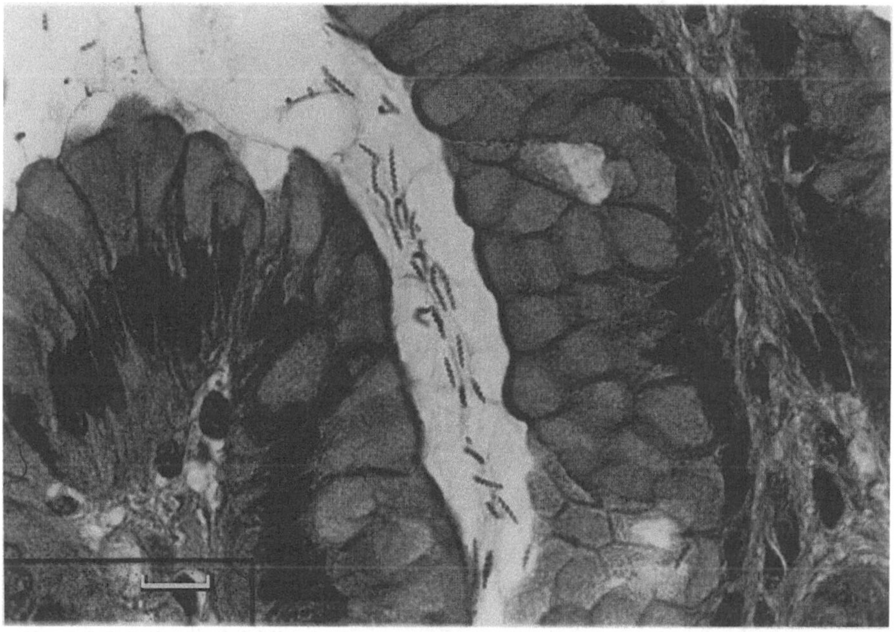

Fig. 6. Spirillae in the foveolae of a dog stomach. H & E × 800

Table 2. Ultrastructural features of spiral organisms derived from human and cat. (Data from the Institute of Pathology, Landshut, 1989)

	Human	Cat
Length	5.16 μm	5.92 μm
Diameter	0.79 μm	0.76 μm
Wave length	1.01 μm	1.16 μm
Amplitude	0.97 μm	1.19 μm
Windings	6.6 /O	6.6 /O[a]

[a] O = Organism

cases showed chronic and 12 of them chronic active gastritis. Of the five cases without the organisms, three showed gastritis and two normal mucosa. Ultrastructurally, the spiral bacteria in animals are almost identical with their human counterparts (Table 2). They colonize the surface and also appear intracellularly, where they cause mitochondrial swelling (Fig. 7, 8).

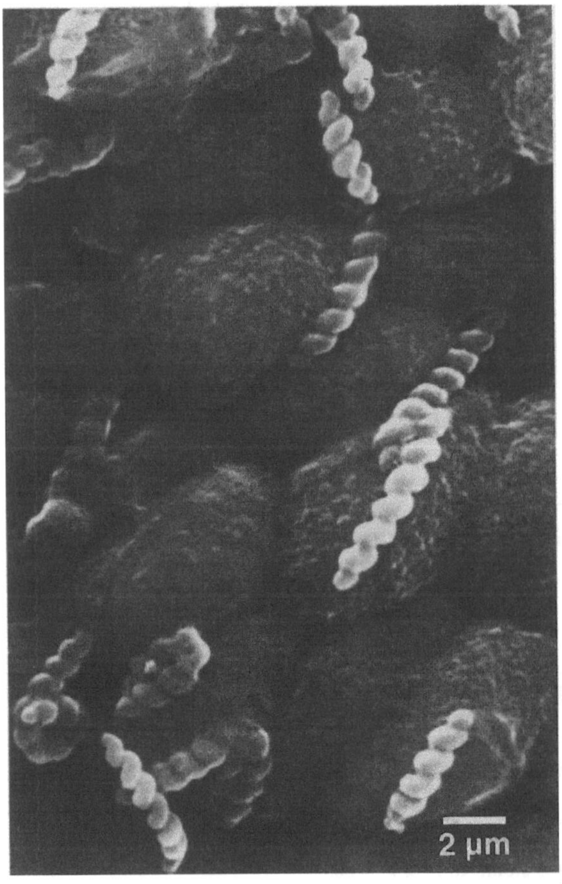

Fig. 7. Spirillae on the mucosal surface of a cat stomach. Note the similarity to the human organisms as shown in Fig. 2. SEM

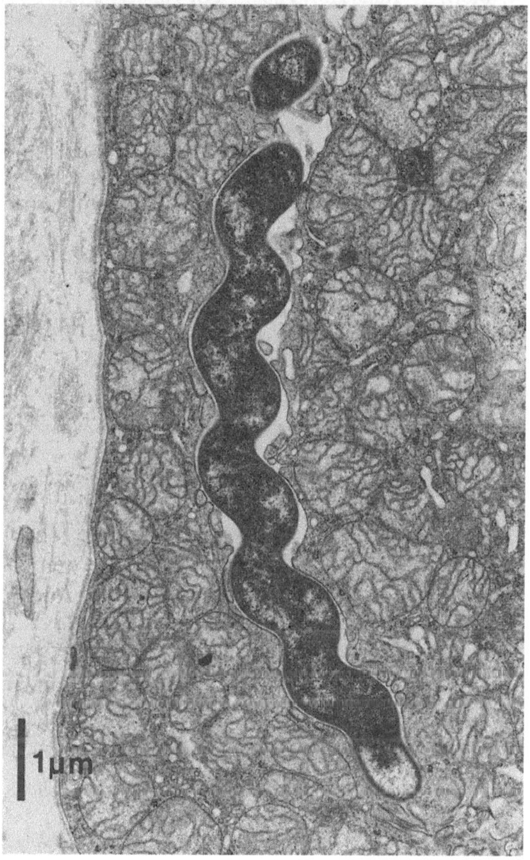

Fig. 8. Spirillum in the canaliculus of a parietal cell in a cat stomach. TEM × 20500

Infection of the human gastric mucosa with spiral-shaped organisms seems to be associated with an inflammatory response similar but less severe than that seen in *H. pylori* infection. Gastritis associated with *G. hominis* is a rare event, accounting for only 0.23% of all gastric biopsies. It seems possible to eliminate the organisms with bismuth salts. Despite many morphological similarities between the organisms found in humans and domestic animals, it is not clear whether domestic animals transmit the bacteria to humans.

References

1. Dent JC, McNulty CAM, Uff JC, Wilkinson SP, Gear MWL (1987) Spiral organisms in the gastric antrum. Lancet II:96
2. Heilmann KL (1988) Spirochätenähnliche Organismen in der menschlichen Magenschleimhaut. Dtsch Med Wochensch 113:1298–1299
3. Dye KR, Marshall BJ, Frierson HF, Guerrant RL, McCallum RW (1988) Gastritis in a human due to infection with an organism resembling the cat gastric spirillum. Gastroenterology 94:A108

4. Morris A, Rafiq AM, Thomsen L, Vanderwel M, Hollis B (1988) Tightly spiral shaped bacteria in the human gastric antrum – are they urease positive? 1st meeting of the European campylobacter pylori study group. Bordeaux
5. Morvan J, Vialette G, Lamouliatte H, Teyssou R, Seurat PL, Carteron B, Megraud F (1988) Spiral bacterial different from campylobacter pylori observed in human stomach tissue. 1st meeting of the European campylobacter pylori study group. Bordeaux
6. Bizzozero G (1893) Über die schlauchförmigen Drüsen des Magen-Darm-Kanals und die Beziehungen ihres Epithels zu dem Oberflächenepithel der Schleimhaut. Arch Mikr Anat 42:82
7. Weber AF, Hase O, Sautter JH (1958) Some observations concerning the presence of spirilla in the fundic glands of dogs and cats. Am J Vet Res 18:677–680
8. Kasai K, Kobayashi R (1919) Stomach spirochetes occuring in mammals. J Parasitol 6:1
9. Lee A, Hazell S (1988) Campylobacter pylori in health and disease: an ecological perspective. Microbiol Scol Health Dis 1:1–16
10. McNulty CM, Dent J, Curry A, Uff JS, Ford GA, Gear MWL, Wilkinson SP (1989) New spiral bacterium in gastric mucosa. J Clin Path 42:585

Discussion

Vaira: Dr. Heilmann, did you have any chance to do an ELISA test on your patients?

Heilmann: No, not yet.

Vaira: I ask because we saw something similar in children with duodenal ulcers with negative *H. pylori.* Our microbiologist, Dr. Holton in London, found that the IgG level to *H. pylori* was very, very low. It may be interesting to see whether in your patients you also find low titer against *H. pylori.*

Menge: Dr. Lee and Dr. Heilmann, you investigated higher developed animals such as dogs and cats, but there are some smaller animals such as some kinds of ants and bugs which harbour spirobacteria in their intestine. Do you by chance know whether they are similar to those that you have found?

Lee: What I was talking about was the idea of this evolution of the organisms. I had a long talk with an expert in mammalian evolution, and he said, "What you have got to do is go back to the roots of it all and find a frog and a reptile." And so we are about to do this, adding the kangaroo, because this is very interesting in terms of evolution. I know that kangaroos are loaded in their rectal mucosa with spiral organisms, but I have never looked at the stomach. So, this is about to take place.

Börsch: I think the observation that bismuth compounds eradicate the spirals *(Gastrospirillum hominis)* is very important since we know that bismuth compounds do not eradicate *H. pylori.* We have often wondered whether this might be due to pharmacokinetic properties of bismuth, but your observations suggest that this resistance might be an intrinsic property of the bacteria themselves: that *H. pylori* is rather resistant to bismuth, and that the other ones *(G. hominis)* do respond. I think this observation is very important.

McNulty: We treated a patient with bismuth subcitrate (De-Nol) and then with metronidazole, and the organism was not eradicated. Either the organism is more difficult to eradicate than *H. pylori,* or apparent clearance is followed by multiplication and relapse.

Heilmann: I did not say eradicate – I said eliminate. I do not know yet whether there is really an eradication after bismuth treatment. We stained all the biopsies with silver stain and tried to find the organisms. In no case could *Gastrospirillum* be found.

Lee: I have just a quick comment in terms of the animals there. Looking at the clearance of these organisms in the animals, it parallels that with the use of antimicrobials against *H. pylori.*

Ober: I have a question related not to the organisms but to the changes of the mucosa. Do the mice, dogs, and rats always get gastritis, or do some of them also get ulcers? As was mentioned earlier, it is unclear why some humans get ulcers and others merely widespread inflammations.

Heilmann: Cats and dogs get ulcers, but very rarely. The veterinarian with whom I work can confirm this. He operated on bleeding ulcers in dogs and cats. But at present we have not studied the specimens for these organisms, and in our current series we have no case with an ulcer.

Lee: To comment on this, I think it may partially be a matter of numbers. Certainly with any of the animals – and clearly the germ-free dogs have no ulcers – we are dealing at this stage with relatively low numbers, and so one would not expect to see it. But the thing we do not know about and certainly need to look more at is the issue of gastric metaplasia because we are talking about things going on in the duodenum. We know that occasionally these organisms can colonize a duodenum, but not all. Krakowka's work has also shown that some of the pigs had *H. pylori* in the duodenum. But the possible association with metaplasia has not been looked at. I think this is a critical question, and we need to do a lot more work before we can answer it.

Sipponen: When you see the colonization of the *Gastrospirillum hominis,* is it mixed with that of *H. pylori?*

Heilmann: In one case I identified both organisms. Dr. Stolte told me that he has had two cases, and Dr. Mégraud has also had cases. So, this phenomenon exists, but I think it is rather rare. Usually the two appear alone.

Newell: I would like to clarify one point. In the nonhuman primates that we have investigated, approximately 50% have this helical gastric organism, and certainly not all of them have gastritis. *Helicobacter* infection does not appear to cause significant gastritis in rhesus monkeys or baboons.

Börsch: I have a question for Dr. Lee. What happens to gastric spiral bacteria in humans or in experimental animals when the natural gastric environment changes, for instance by acid reduction, or other gut bacteria invasion. Do they disappear?

Lee: I cannot answer the question. It is obviously something that we will consider, but at this stage we are only trying to determine where they colonize in the germ-free animals and to understand the histopathology. Now that we see what happens, there is obviously much more to be done.

Varkonyi: Dr. Lee mentioned that *Helicobacter* infection occurs only in the stomach and not in the duodenum. I would like to argue with this statement because we are doing routinely lower part duodenal biopsies to determine disaccharidase activities in the duodenum in the case of contaminated small bowel syndrome. In about 5% of the cases we could find *Helicobacter* in the lower part duodenal biopsy materials.

Lee: Is it certain that we are talking about *H. pylori* here? It is well known that these organisms can colonize gastric metaplasia in the bulb, and with large numbers it is not surprising if some organisms come through the duodenum. I have never seen this, and I certainly would be interested if one actually sees tissue association, considering what is seen with the gastric metaplasia. In the duodenum it is literally a one-cell difference between the organism on the gastric cell and the adjacent duodenal cell. So, I would be very surprised if those organisms are genuinally colonizing the lower duodenal mucosa.

Wyatt: It has been my impression when looking at the spiral organisms that they tend to be free within the gastric pits rather than being surface associated therefore giving quite a different sight than *H. pylori.* Yet in the scanning electron micrographs that you showed they seem to be attached to the cell surface. First, which way of looking at this gives a more genuine representation of the situation in vivo? And secondly, could you make some comments as to how often you see adherence pedestals or cell attachments being formed by the various organisms that you have described?

Lee: I am convinced that the two are totally different. I do not believe that either CS1 or *Gastrospirillum* adhere to tissue. In our recent paper on one of the human cases (in fact in the human case we got the organism from a mouse) we commented on the clear distinction to the organism lying in the lumen. Certainly, I think this is the trouble with the electron micrographs; you obviously get the odd organism that looks as though it adheres, and there are wonderful photographs of *C. jejuni* showing that it adheres like mad, but it probably does not. So I believe that in the slides you showed, the *Gastrospirillum* and *H. pylori* demonstrated the very point. They showed all the *Gastrospirillum* in the lumen, and they certainly showed some of the *H. pylori* in the lumen mucus but a lot a more attached to the cells.

Heilmann: I have to confirm this. I think the light-microscopic picture is really more correct than the electron-microscopical picture.

Animal Models of *Helicobacter pylori* Gastritis*

S. Krakowka, D. R. Morgan, K. A. Eaton, and M. J. Radin

Introduction

Ideally, an animal model of gastritis associated with infection by *Helicobacter pylori* should: possess the essential features of the human disease including susceptibility to human isolates of *H. pylori,* be widely available to investigators, be easily manipulated (e.g., endoscopy, therapy) and should not be in a species that is endangered, expensive, or perceived as special by animal welfare activists. To date, none of the available models fulfills all of these criteria. Nonetheless, substantial progress in delineating the course of infection by *H. pylori* in nonhuman species has occurred in the past several years. It is the intent of this short review to evaluate the data available critically and to make projections for specific future directions with the available model species.

Common Laboratory Animals

Shortly after general acceptance of *H. pylori* as a human gastric pathogen, a series of oral inoculation studies into mice, rats, guinea pigs, rabbits, and dogs were performed. In spite of use of recent clinical isolates and high doses of inocula, gastric colonization was not achieved nor was chronic active gastritis produced (Goodwin et al. 1986; Morgan et al. 1988). Parenteral inoculation of rodents produced transient bacteremia and 72-h colonization in spleen and liver; no subsequent invasion of gastric tissue was detected (Ehlers et al. 1988). In contrast, intraperitoneal inoculation of H. pylori or sterile cell-free bacterial lysates was lethal in mice (Hupertz and Czinn 1988). For the former, live organisms were not recovered from tissues of the moribund mice. The toxic factor was not bacterial lipopolysaccharide but rather a trypsin and heat-sensitive cytotoxic protein. In spite of these negative data, one investigator has reported successful colonization of gnotobiotic rats for 9 days even though others have failed to establish a germ-free rodent model of infection (Adrian Lee 1989, personal communication). Thus, these data, in aggregate, indicate that the likelihood of rodents supporting *H. pylori* infection is remote.

* This research was supported by a grant from the Procter and Gamble Company and fellowship 1F32 A107938-01 (Eaton), NIH-PHS

H. Menge et al. (Eds.)
Helicobacter pylori 1990

Ferrets

Ferrets are excellent laboratory research animals. In addition to large litter sizes, ferrets are generally tractable and are easily subjected to gastric endoscopy and biopsy. Further, they are susceptible to a variety of pathogens of human and veterinary medical importance. In 1986, Fox and colleagues reported the isolation of a *Helicobacter sp.* from a ferret with gastric ulceration (Fox et al. 1986). Subsequent study of this *Helicobacter*-like organism has revealed a high incidence of gastric colonization, gastric ulcers, and attendant diffuse or multifocal lymphoplasmacytic cellular infiltrates most prominent in the pylorus (Tompkins et al. 1988; Fox et al. 1988). The organism responsible for these lesions, while closely resembling *H. pylori*, is sufficiently different in guanine and cytosine content, protein profiles, and DNA homology to be considered a separate species, recently named *H. mustelae* (Fox and Lee 1989).

Concurrent gastritis or colonization by *H. mustelae* renders conventionally raised ferrets unsuitable as experimental host species for infection by *H. pylori*. Recently, marginal success in raising germ-free ferrets was reported (Bell and Manning 1989). Hand-raising kits in laminar flow hoods is currently being evaluated; recent experiences are promising (Fox, J 1989, personal communication). It will be important to determine if *H. mustelae*-free ferrets are susceptible to colonization with *H. pylori*.

Primates

In many respects, primates are the ideal animal substitute for the study of human infectious disease. Not only is there great anatomical and physiological similarities but many human investigative reagents are extensively cross-reactive with their primate counterparts, obviating the need to develop them for in-depth study. Disadvantages of primates include expense and the need for specialized housing and facilities, inaccessibility to many investigators, and the sensitivity of these species in the public arena.

Both naturally occurring and experimentally induced bacterial gastritis were described in rhesus monkeys *(Macaca mulatta)* (Bronsdon and Schoenknecht 1988; Newell et al. 1988; Baskerville and Newell 1988). Chronic gastritis is characterized by mucus depletion and nodular to diffuse lymphoplasmacytic cellular infiltrates restricted largely to the superficial mucosa. Organisms recovered from naturally infected monkeys appear indistinguishable from human strains of *H. pylori*. Similarly, pigtailed macaques *(Macaca nemestrina)* harbor *H. pylori* and infected individuals exhibit achlorhydria and lesions typical of human type B gastritis. In a small survey series, cynomolgus monkeys appear to harbor the agent though apparently less frequently than the rhesus monkey (Euler et al. 1989). Baboons do not appear to be colonized by *H. pylori*. Unlike the human disease, the gastric inflammatory lesions ascribed to *H. pylori* in primates appear to be chiefly composed of mononuclear cells, not neutrophils.

Thus while the evidence for susceptibility of primates, particularly rhesus monkeys, is undisputed, many of these studies may be compromised by the coprophagic habits of primates and concurrent infection with *C. jejuni*, *C. coli*, *C. fetus*, and several other species of gastric spiral bacilli.

Gnotobiotic Piglets

In 1987, we (Krakowka et al. 1987) and Lambert et al. (1987) independently reported that gnotobiotic piglets were susceptible to gastric colonization with human strains of *H. pylori.* These studies were prompted in part because of the apparent insusceptibility of conventional animals and in part because the pig is a functional monogastric species with dietary habits and gastric, anatomical, and physiological characteristics similar to man (Kurihara-Bergstrom et al. 1986). As an experimental animal, piglets have several desirable features including large litter size (n = 8–15), dietary self-sufficiency within hours after birth, and a well-studied mucosal immune system.

Many features of human gastric disease are reproduced in piglets challenged with *H. pylori.* Colonization is chiefly restricted to the stomach, although organisms have been recovered occasionally from the esophagus and duodenum. The bacteria can be recovered from gastric mucus and gastric juice as well as from mucosal swabs or tissue fragments collected from the cardia, fundus, antrum, and pylorus. The bulk of the organisms are found between the mucus layer and superficial mucus-secreting gastric epithelia closely apposed to epithelial surfaces. Occasional foci of organisms can be demonstrated in dilated gastric pits. The organism has never been found in intraepithelial sites or below the lamina propria.

Gross and microscopic lesions are prominent in piglets examined 21 days after infection and beyond. Most infected piglets demonstrate excessive accumulations of gastric mucus with entrapped milk curd. Close examination of gastric mucosa reveals small (1–2 mm) raised clusters of lymphoid follicles. These follicles, most prominent in the cardia at the junction of the nonglandular and glandular stomach, tend to follow the lesser curvature of the stomach along prominent rugal folds. Ulcers or erosions in the glandular stomach are not present although occasional "stress" erosions may be present in the squamous portion of the nonglandular stomach. These latter lesions are nonspecific in etiology and frequently encountered as asymptomatic lesions in pigs of all ages. In our studies, the lesion is seen in uninfected controls though at a lower frequency than in infected littermates.

Diffuse or multifocal lymphoplasmacytic cellular infiltrates involving the lamina propria and occasionally obliterating gastric pits are the histopathological hallmarks of infection. Transient, mild, and inconsistent neutrophilic infiltration may precede this lesion. Transmigrating mononuclear cells are frequently seen underlying colonies of organisms. Gastric mucus contains degenerate cells of gastric epithelial and leukocyte origin.

Gastric epithelia also display a series of alterations from the normal which, when combined with other data, appear typical for this disease. Tissue sections stained for polysaccharides by the PAS method show moderate to marked mucus depletion. Epithelia overlying inflammatory foci exhibit cytoplasmic vacuolation and subtle but distinct single-cell necrosis. The former may be observed in uninfected controls but is quantitatively much less prominent (Eaton et al. 1989). The only extragastric lesion detected thus far in piglets is hypertrophy and hyperplasia of lymphoid tissues including Peyer's patches and tonsils. This lesion no doubt reflects activation of the mucosa-associated immune system by *H. pylori* infection.

Infected piglets (but not controls) respond immunologically to *H. pylori* by mounting both a local and systemic humoral immune response to antigens of *H. pylori*

(Krakowka et al. 1989; Eaton et al. 1990). In sera, the IgM-based responses which predominate early are gradually replaced by vigorous IgG antibodies. Serum IgA responses are modest but detectable from 14 days after infection onward. Gastric secretions and bile collected from infected piglets but not littermate controls contain *H. pylori*-specific IgA and trace amounts of IgG. Western blot analyses revealed that the response is complex with as many as 20 distinct bands present (Krakowka, S 1989, unpublished work). Preliminary data collected in a long-term study indicate that peripheral blood lymphocytes are responsive to crude *H. pylori* antigens (Krakowka et al. 1989).

Space limitations and dietary constraints preclude maintaining infected piglets much beyond 45–50 days of age. In a recently completed pilot study (Eaton et al. 1990), piglets infected as gnotobiotes were transferred to a specific pathogen-free environment 3 weeks after infection and then examined for organisms 6, 8, and 12 weeks after infection. In spite of subsequent colonization with *Lactobacillus sp., H. pylori* was recovered in eight of ten piglets (three of three at 87 days). Restriction endonuclease digests of DNA recovered from the challenge inocula and the isolates recovered from infected piglets were identical, indicating that the reisolates were not environmental contaminants or other unrelated *Helicobacter sp*. These findings greatly expand the utility of the model to include future studies of recrudescence following antimicrobial therapy, sequential endoscopic biopsy findings, and cofactor studies on gastric ulceration.

The utility of this model is best demonstrated, however, by its use in defining bacterial virulence factors and its value for testing, in vivo, various experimental (and proprietary) therapeutic agents. Four potential virulence factors have been suggested for *H. pylori.* These include motility, adhesins, cytotoxin, and urease activity (Morgan and Leunk 1989). In a recently completed study, the relative virulence of three different strains varying in toxin production and motility was determined (Eaton et al. 1989). A nontoxigenic nonmotile strain (T×30a) was avirulent; a weakly motile toxigenic strain (60190) was moderately virulent whereas a highly motile toxigenic strain (26695) was highly virulent. Further in combination infection experiments (simultaneous infection with 60190 and 26695), only 26695 was recovered; the isolates exhibited enhanced motility when compared with parental inocula. Thus motility appears to be a prime bacterial virulence factor whereas production of exotoxin appears to be a secondary virulence factor. The role of adhesins and urease remains to be tested.

Piglets tolerate daily treatment with a variety of antimicrobial agents and bismuth salts quite well. It must be noted that they rapidly learn to object to orally administered tablets and capsules. In short-term treatment studies (10 days), patterns of drug efficacy and failure mimic those obtained in human clinical studies. What remains to be determined, however, is if successfully treated piglets experience a high incidence of recrudescence following cessation of treatment as occurs in humans.

Finally, it should be noted that Engstrand et al. (1989) recently reported successful colonization of five of seven weanling barrier-raised piglets. Gastric lesions produced in these animals were similar to those described above. These investigators utilized endoscopy and biopsy to monitor the course of infection, thereby demonstrating the feasibility of these techniques for sequential monitoring of the disease process.

Gnotobiotic Dogs

A recently completed study demonstrated that *H. pylori* will colonize neonatal gnotobiotic dogs for at least 30 days (Radin et al. 1990). Five of seven pups were orally challenged with *H. pylori* at 7 days of age. The two remaining pups were contact exposed to the infected littermates from PID 23 onward. Organisms were recovered from the stomachs of all seven pups as well as the oropharynx and rectum in one instance each, and the esophagus and duodenum in two instances each at necropsy on PID 30. Microscopic lesions (focal to diffuse lymphoplasmacytic infiltrates) were typical of *H. pylori* gastritis except that neutrophilic and eosinophilic infiltrates were more prominent than that observed in piglets. Much remains to be defined with this model given the potential usefulness of dogs in long-term studies either as gnotobiotes or as conventionalized animals.

Discussion and Conclusions

This brief review has summarized the information currently available on nonhuman animal models of gastritis induced by *H. pylori.* None of the species evaluated completely replicates the spectrum of human disease associated with *H. pylori.* It is noteworthy that the hallmark microscopic lesion identified in human gastric tissue is superficial chronic active gastritis. Most studies report that neutrophils are the most obvious inflammatory cell component in humans although lymphofollicular gastritis is now recognized as typical of infection by *H. pylori* (Dixon et al. 1988). In none of the animal species evaluated, except perhaps the rhesus monkey, are neutrophilic infiltrates a prominent part of the histopathological spectrum. There are several potential explanations for this discrepancy. It could be that the isolates used to challenge animals, even though of human origin, have lost their ability to attract neutrophils to the site(s) of colonization. Alternatively, humans may be unique regarding chemotactive responsiveness to *H. pylori.* Thirdly, it may be that neutrophilic gastritis occurs only in immune individuals subject to repeated localized infection of gastric mucosa derived from occult or hidden sites such as gastric mucus. In any event, neutrophilic gastritis as it occurs in humans is an unusual manifestation of a persistent bacterial infectious disease.

A second feature of human disease not shared thus far in the developed animal model systems is the close association between bacterial colonization and gastroduodenal ulceration. In this regard, ferrets infected with *H. mustelae* come closest to the human counterpart. Ulcerogenesis associated with *H. pylori* gastritis likely requires interaction with secondary factors such as stress, alcohol and tobacco abuse, use of nonsteroidal anti-inflammatory drugs, and poor dietary habits. Resistance of the gastric mucosa to ulceration depends upon the anatomical arrangement of the mucosa as well as the interaction of multiple physiological processes. Healthy goblet cells secrete mucus and bicarbonate ions, forming a "bicarbonate battery" that neutralizes protons diffusing toward the mucosa. In addition, the mucus barrier decreases mucosal contact with pepsin, microorganisms, and potentially harmful ingested substances. Endogenous prostaglandin production, especially of the E series, appears to mediate cytoprotection by enhancing mucus and bicarbonate ion secretion and/or by increasing gastric capillary blood flow which, in turn, supplies bicarbonate ions and essential nutrients. Disruption of any of the components of the mucosal barrier will result in decreased protection against acid and pepsin, predisposing to ulceration. These data suggest several mechanisms whereby ulcerogenic agents may interact to facilitate a breach in the mucosal barrier. Further, one can predict that several of these unknown factors, each innocuous alone, act in concert to initiate or perhaps perpetuate the disease process. If *H. pylori* is intimately associated with ulcerogenesis, then manipulation of available animal models with the variables of ulcerogenesis in mind should permit delineation of the pathogenesis of this important human disease.

References

Baskerville A, Newell DG (1988) Naturally occuring chronic gastritis and *C. pylori* infection in the rhesus monkey: a potential model for gastritis in man. Gut 29:465–472

Bell J, Manning D (1989) Derivation of gnotobiotic ferrets and oral inoculation with *Campylobacter jejuni.* Abstract 8 of the American Association of Gnotobiotics Meeting, Columbus, Ohio

Blaser MJ (1987) Gastric *Campylobacter*-like organisms, gastritis and peptic ulcer disease. Gastroenterology 93:371–383

Bronsdon MA, Schoenknecht FD (1988) *Campylobacter pylori* isolated from the stomach of the monkey *Macaca nemestroma.* J Clin Microbiol 26:1725–1728

Dixon MF, Wyatt JI, Burke DA, Rathbone BJ (1988) Lymphocytic gastritis – relationship to *Campylobacter pylori* infection. J Pathol 154:125–132

Eaton KA, Morgan DR, Krakowka S (1989) Virulence factors for *Campylobacter pylori.* Infect Immun 57:1119–1125

Eaton KA, Morgan DR, Krakowka S (1990) Persistence of *Campylobacter pylori* in conventionalized piglets. J Infect Dis 161:1299–1301

Ehlers S, Warrelmann M, Hahn H (1988) In search of an animal model for experimental *Campylobacter pylori* infection: administration of *Campylobacter pylori* to rodents. Zentralbl Bakteriol Mikrobiol Hyg [A] 268:341–346

Engstrand L, Jorgenson A, Schwan A, Gustavsson S (1989) A pig model for *Campylobacter pylori* gastritis-systemic antibody response. Abstract in gastroduodenal disease and *Campylobacter pylori,* University of Virginia, 10–12 May 1989

Euler GR, Zarenko GE, Moe JB, Ulrich RG, Schaadt S (1989) Naturally-occurring *Campylobacter pylori* (CP) infection in the cynomologus *(Macaca fascicularis)* and rhesus *(Macaca mulatta)* monkey. Abstract in gastroduodenal disease and *Campylobacter pylori,* University of Virginia, 10–12 May

Fox JG, Edrise BM, Cabot EB, Beaucage C, Murphy JC, Prostak KS (1986a) *Campylobacter*-like organisms isolated from gastric mucosa of ferrets. Am J Vet Res 47:236–239

Fox JG, Goad MEP, Hotaling LI (1986b) Gastric ulcers in ferrets. Lab Anim Sci 36:562

Fox JG, Cabot EB, Taylor NS, Larasway R (1988) Gastric colonization by *Campylobacter pylori* subsp. *mustelae* in ferrets. Infect Immun 56:2994–2996

Fox JG, Lee A (1989) Gastric *Campylobacter*-like organisms: their role in gastric disease in laboratory animals. Lab Anim Sci 39:543–553

Goodwin CS, Armstrong JA, Marshall BJ (1986) *Campylobacter pyloridis,* gastritis, and peptic ulceration. J Clin Pathol 39:353–365

Graham DY (1989) *Campylobacter pylori* and peptic ulcer disease. Gastroenterology 96:615–625

Hupertz V, Czinn S (1988) Demonstration of a cytotoxin from *Campylobacter pylori.* Eur J Clin Microbiol Infect Dis 7:576–578

Krakowka S, Morgan DR, Kraft WG, Leunk RD (1987) Establishment of gastric *Campylobacter pylori* infection in the neonatal gnotobiotic piglet. Infect Immun 55:2789–2796

Krakowka S, Eaton K, Morgan DR (1989) *Campylobacter pylori* gastritis in gnotobiotic piglets: persistence of gastric infection after conventionalization. In: G.M. Ruiz-Palacios (ed) Fifth Intl Workshop on *Campylobacter* infections, Feb 25–Mar 1, 1989, Puerto Vallerta, Mexico

Kurihara-Bergstrom L, Woodworth M, Feisrellin S, Beall P (1986) Characterization of the Yucatan miniature pig skin and small intestine for pharmaceutical applications. Lab Anim Sci 36:398–399
Lambert JR, Borromeo M, Pinkard KJ, Turner H, Chapman CB, Smith ML (1987) Colonization of gnotobiotic piglets with *Campylobacter pyloridis* – an animal model? J Infect Dis 155:1344
Morgan D, Leunk R, Krakowka S (1988) Animal models of gastritis induced by *Campylobacter pylori:* microbiology, histology, and serology. Annual meeting Am Soc Microbiol
Morgan DR, Leunk R (1989) Pathogenesis of infection by *Campylobacter pylori.* In: Blazer MJ (ed) *Campylobacter pylori* in gastritis and peptic ulcer disease. Igaku-Shoin, New York, pp 115–133
Newell DG, Hudson MJ, Baskerville A (1988) Isolation of a gastric *Campylobacter*-like organism from the stomach of four rhesus monkeys and identification as *Campylobacter pylori.* J Med Microbiol 27:41–44
Radin MJ, Eaton KA, Krakowka S, Morgan DR, Lee A, Otto G, Fox JG (1990) *Campylobacter pylori* gastric infection in gnotobiotic beagle dogs. Infect Immun in press
Reed KD, Berridge BR (1988) *Campylobacter*-like organisms in the gastric mucosa of rhesus monkeys. Lab Anim Sci 38:329–331
Tompkins DS, Wyatt JI, Rathbone BJ, West AP (1988) The characterization and pathological significance of gastric *Campylobacter*-like organisms in the ferret: a model for chronic gastritis? Epidem Inf 101:269–278

Discussion

Wyatt: One of the things that is quite striking in the human stomach with *H. pylori* is that inflammation in the antrum is often denser and more active than it is in the body. In duodenal ulcer patients, for example, we very often see *H. pylori* colonizing morphologically normal body mucosa. Do you notice the same distinction with anatomical sites in the stomachs of the animals that you've looked at?

Krakowka: We have just started to look at that in a quantitative manner. What I can tell you is that in the piglet, the inflammation is most prominent in the rugal folds along the lesser curvature of the stomach. The infection is most prominent in the same areas. Dr. Eaton is in the process of doing a bacterial count from half stomachs and from various sites. The number of organisms per unit area tend to follow the inflammation, in other words, it tends – again I'm speaking only of the piglet – to follow the lesser curvature rather than to occur down in the fundic region. Does that answer your question?

Wyatt: Yes, that's inflammation as assessed by the nodularity of the mucosa.

Krakowka: Yes, and by histopathologic examination as well.

Wyatt: My second question, if I may carry on is related to that. The photographs that you've shown us have shown quite substantial lymphoid aggregates in the mucosa, do you also see follicles with germinal centers.

Krakowka: One could argue that those lymphoid follicles are in fact germinal centers.

Wyatt: Do they have germinal centers?

Krakowka: My answer would be no. In addition to the very prominent lymphofollicular aggregates, there is a diffuse inflammation of the lamina propria which I did not show but which is very similar to the CS1 lesion that Professor Lee showed. I can tell you we are just starting into the histochemistry. The gastric mucosa contains many IgA-secreting plasma cells and very few IgM- and IgG-secreting plasma cells. That's where we are.

Wyatt: Thank you very much.

Westblom: Did you see lymphoid follicles in the dogs, and if so, were they similar to those you saw in the piglets?

Krakowka: Yes, we did. In fact, there were more neutrophils and eosinophils found in the gastric tissues of the dog than of the piglet. The most prominent feature of the inflammation was again these lymphoplasmacytic aggregates. These were not nearly as intense or severe as in the CS1 studies, which were done in parallel, but they were clearly there.

Sipponen: Possibly the follow-up of your animals is too short, but have you ever seen any atrophy or metaplasia following this inflammation in your animal models?

Krakowka: We have not seen that. That's a very important question, because one of the things that has always bothered me, is why do we not see gastric ulceration or other features of chronic active gastritis. It's my hope as we increase the number of animals that we follow up for a long period of time, that some of these very subtle lesions will appear. I need to learn how to endoscope 200-pound pigs among other things before we start investigating this in great detail.

Isotype and Specificity of Local and Systemic Anti-*Helicobacter pylori* Antibodies

D. G. Newell and A. R. Stacey

Introduction

The majority of patients known to be colonized with *Helicobacter pylori* elicit a significant circulating immune response (Newell and Rathbone 1989). Evidence suggests that a similar specific immune response exists at the gastric mucosal surface (Wyatt et al. 1986). Despite this response the organism persists in colonizing an immunologically hostile environment and will even recur after temporary clearance (Langenberg et al. 1986). Several reasons for the ineffectiveness of the immune response can be postulated:

1. Host factors:
   a) Immunoincompetence at the gastric mucosal surface
   b) Colonization of an immunologically privileged site
2. Bacterial factors:
   a) Antigenic drift
   b) Loss of antigen-antibody complexes from bacteria
   c) Non-specific immunoglobulin binding
   d) Mimicry of human antigens
3. Bacterial manipulation of host response:
   Stimulation of non-antigen-specific responses

Most of these reasons would be due to the capacity of the bacteria to avoid host antibodies but it is also possible that the host is incapable of mounting a response which is effective at the site of colonization. Little is known of the immunocompetence of the gastric mucosa during bacterial colonization. Therefore, we have investigated the types of antibodies produced by the host at various mucosal and systemic sites. Additionally we have begun to investigate the specificity of those antibodies using antigenic material, chromatographically fractionated from *H. pylori* sonicate and by western blotting. Because obtaining sufficient human material from some sites, like the mucosal surface, is impractical, we have also attempted to produce antibodies in larger quantities from immortalized local B cells.

Materials and Methods

Antibodies

Serum (50 patients), lymph nodes (2 patients), and gastric antral biospies (2 patients) were obtained from patients of known *H. pylori* status. Cells were dissociated from

H. Menge et al. (Eds.)
Helicobacter pylori 1990

lymph nodes and a mononuclear cell population prepared by centrifugation over Ficoll-Paque (Pharmacia Ltd). The isolated cells were then cultured overnight in RPMI 1640 with 10% fetal calf serum (FCS). The supernatant was retained for analysis. The cells (10^7) were incubated with Epstein-Barr virus (EBV) obtained from the cell line B95–8 for 2 h at 37 °H. The transformed cells were then cultured at 10^6 cells/ml in RPMI 1640 in 10% FCS. The growing cells were regularly passaged, dilution cloned, and screened for antibody production by ELISA against *H. pylori* whole cell sonicate.

Gastric antral biopsies were cultured by submersion in 1 ml RPMI 1640 medium containing 10% FCS for 3 days at 37 °H. The medium was replaced daily and the harvested medium stored at 4 °C with protease inhibitor [0.1 m*M* phenyl methyl sulfonyl fluoride (PMSF)] and 0.01% acide.

Antibody Isotype Analysis

The isotype of human anti-*H. pylori* antibodies in serum and culture supernatants was identified as previously described (Steer et al. 1987) using an indirect (ELISA) technique with mouse monoclonal anti-human IgG subclass antibodies or sheep anti-human class antibodies.

Antibody Specificities

Sonicates of *H. pylori* were fractionated by fast liquid protein chromatography (FPLC) as previously described (Stacey et al. 1989). The antibody specificity of serum or supernatants was determined by ELISA as previously described (Newell et al. 1987) using the FPLC fractions at 5 µg/ml on the solid phase. SDS-PAGE gels of *H. pylori* acid-extractable material, whole cell sonicate or FPLC fractions were electroblotted onto nitrocellulose and immunolabelled as previously described (Newell et al 1987), except for the supernatants, where greater sensitivity was obtained using a gold-silver enhancement detection system (Janssen Ltd).

Results

In the serum of patients colonized with *H. pylori* the major class of immune response was IgG. Many, but not all of the patients induced a specific IgA response but few showed any detectable specific IgM. The major IgG subclass of the systemic antibody response was IgG1 though the majority of patients also had specific IgG2 (Fig. 1). There was a small, but significant ($P = 0.01$) rise in the IgG4-specific antibodies but no IgG3. In contrast, the major class of specific antibodies in supernatant from the lymph node cells cultured overnight was of the IgA isotype with, again, no detectable IgM. A similar isotype pattern was observed in the supernatants from the cultured gastric biopsies. The IgG1 antibodies were raised in the lymph node material but no detectable IgG2, IgG3, or IgG4 antibodies were observed.

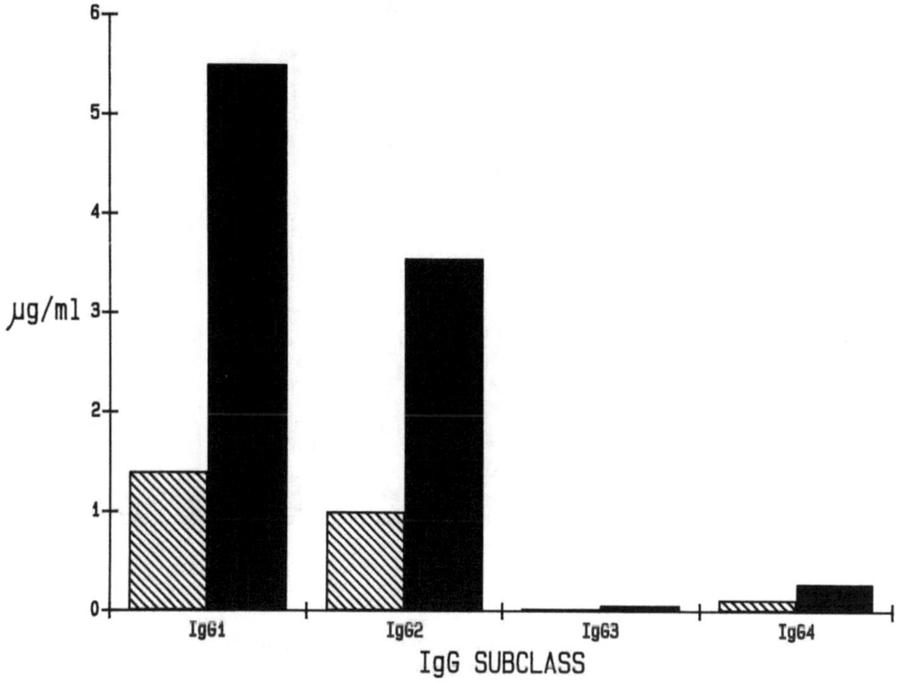

Fig. 1. Serum anti-*H. pylori* IgG subclass antibodies. ▨, *H. pylori*-negative patients; ■, *H. pylori*-positive patients

After culture with EBV the lymph node lymphoid cells grew as small clumps of cells. These clumps of cells produced anti-*H. pylori* antibody of the IgM isotype, for a period of up to 5 months in culture.

The specificities of antibodies in the serum and supernatants from lymph node cells, transformed lymph node cells and gastric biopsies, as demonstrated by ELISA against the FPLC fractions of *H. pylori* are shown in Fig. 2. The results indicate that the antibodies of the serum, lymph node, and gastric mucosa had essentially the same antigenic profiles, reacting strongly with fractions 14–15 and 17–18. These fractions contain the urease and flagella proteins respectively. Serum antibodies reacted predominantly on western blots of these fractions, with the 61K, 56K and 28K polypeptides of urease and the 54K polypeptide of flagellin. Notably the immortalized cells from the lymph node only produced antibodies reacting with the flagella fraction. This antibody-containing material immunolabelled only a 54K polypeptide band in protein profiles of *H. pylori* whole cells and fractions 17–18.

Conclusions

As expected the major class of antibody response in the serum was IgG but in the local mucosal tissues of the gastric mucosa and the draining lymph nodes specific IgA

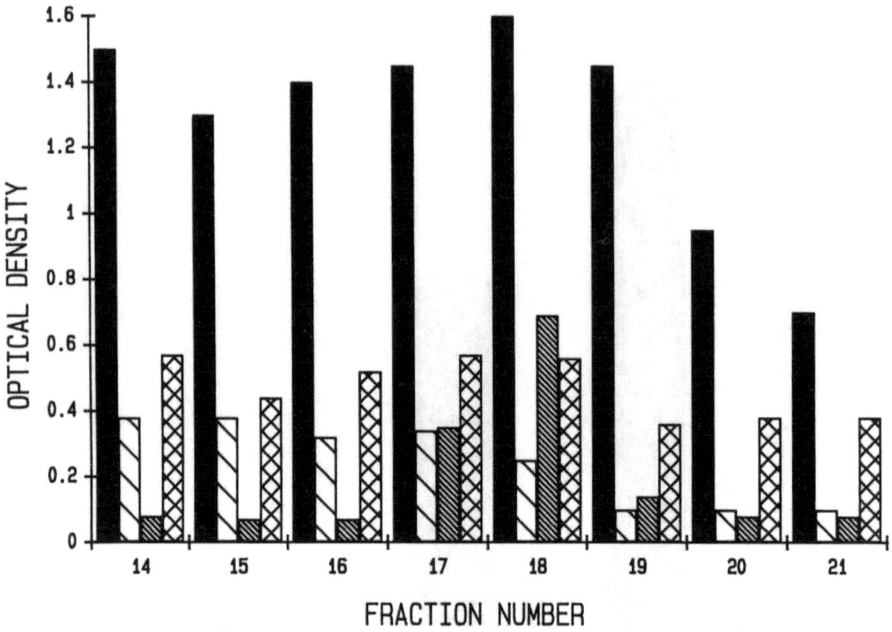

Fig. 2. Specificity of serum and local antibodies against FPLC fractions (14–21) of *H. pylori*. Note fractions 14 and 15 contain the urease while fractions 17 and 18 contain the flagella. ■, serum; ◻, lymph node supernatant; ▨, lymph-node-transformed cells supernatant; ⊠ gastric biopsy supernatant

predominated. Mucosally produced IgA is actively transported through the epithelial cells after binding to a polymeric Ig receptor expressed on the serous membrane. Once at the luminal surface proteolytic enzymes cleave the complex, leaving the IgA protected from further enzyme activity by secretory piece. It is reasonable to assume therefore that the specific IgA observed at the gastric surface is active at the luminal surface. Secretory IgA is effective at mucosal surfaces mainly by binding to the bacterial surface, thereby inhibiting the adherence to epithelial tissue. Although it would not be expected that there was a mechanism for IgG transport across the gastric mucosa, specific IgG is obviously produced locally and a transsudate apparently enters the lumen, where its half-life would be relatively short. Most of this locally produced IgG is of the IgG1 subclass. An important effector mechanism of IgG1 is the fixation of complement and the activation of the complement cascade once bound to antigen. Such a mechanism could mediate some of the inflammatory reactions observed during *H. pylori*-associated gastritis. The specific IgA, IgG2, and IgG4 would contribute little to such a mechanism. Recently, Valnes and Brandtaeg (1989) have used immunohistological techniques to identify the subclass of IgG-producing immunocytes within the gastric mucosa of patients with gastritis. Interestingly they found that IgG1 immunocytes predominated in antral specimens and that IgG3 as well as IgG2 immunocytes were also present. Because of its structure IgG3 is extremely susceptible to proteolysis, which could account for the absence of IgG3 antibody activity in our studies.

It is obvious from these results that the gastric mucosa is immunocompetent, reacting to the antigenic stimulus at the mucosal surface by presenting antigen and initiating an immunocyte response of the isotypes suitable for preventing and eliminating colonization by the bacterium. However, that response is obviously ineffective. It is, therefore, important to identify the antigenic specificity of the antibodies produced locally. The major advantage of using chromatographically fractionated bacterial material is that the antigens are present in their native form while western blotting can only detect antibodies directed against continuous epitopes. Using this material we have identified the urease- and flagella-containing fractions as the major antigens involved in the induction of the immune response at the mucosal surface and draining lymph nodes. Moreover, this antigen profile reflects the specificity observed with serum antibodies. We can now further investigate the specificity of that response using western blotting and/or radioimmunoprecipitation. Furthermore, we have demonstrated that local antibody-producing cells can be immortalized to produce larger quantities of antibody for more detailed study of their efficacy, such as in the inhibition of bacterial adherence or mobility.

Our results so far suggest that the host mounts an adequate immunoglobulin response to the infection. It would appear, therefore, that persistent colonization of the gastric mucosa with *H. pylori* is dependent on efficient bacterial defense factors rather than host immunoincompetence. However, these local B-cell responses require help and regulation, which involves the proliferation of antigen specific T cells. Such T cells must contribute significantly to the cellular components of gastritis. Immunopathological events may, therefore, be a consequence of *H. pylori* colonization of the gastric epithelium.

References

Langenberg W, Rauws EAJ, Widjokusumo A, Tytgat GNJ, Zanen HC (1986) Identification of *Campylobacter pylori* isolates by restriction endonuclease DNA analysis. J Clin Microbiol 24:414–417

Newell DG (1987) Human antibody responses to the surface protein antigens of *Campylobacter pyloridis*. Serodiagn Immunother 1:209–217

Newell DG, Rathbone BJ (1989) The serodiagnosis of *Campylobacter pylori* infection – a review. Serodiagn Immunother 3:1–6

Stacey AR, Newell DG (1989) The development of antigens for improved serodiagnostic tests of *Campylobacter pylori* associated gastritis. In: Megraud F, Lamouliatte H (eds) Gastroduodenal Pathology and *Campylobacter pylori*. Excerpta Medica, Amsterdam pp 193–195

Steer HW, Hawtin PR, Newell DG (1987) An ELISA technique for the serodiagnosis of *Campylobacter pyloridis* infection in patients with gastritis and benign duodenal ulceration. Serodiagn Immunother 1: 253–259

Valnes K, Brandtaeg P (1989) Subclass distribution of mucosal IgG-producing cells in gastritis. Gut 30:322–326

Wyatt JI, Rathbone BJ, Heatley RV (1986) Local immune response to gastric *Campylobacter* in non-ulcer dyspepsia. J Clin Pathol 39:863–870

Discussion

Westblom: Have you looked at interleukin response in the gastric mucosa?

Newell: No, we haven't. We have not yet looked at interleukins or any antigen-specific T cell responses. The investigation of the cellular immune responses will depend on the development of techniques to isolate and expand antigen-specific immunocompetent cells from the gastric mucosa.

Tytgat: Are there other infectious conditions where despite a seemingly adequate immune response the pathogens survive?

Newell: There are other chronic infections of the gastrointestinal tract. The intestinal parasites are good examples of pathogens surviving host immune responses and residing in the gastrointestinal tract for long periods. In *H. pylori* infections we are observing a chronic life-long exposure of the host to an antigen load which can be enormous. We know very little about the ability of the gastric mucosa to respond to such antigens. I would like people to see this infection as a unique model of immune responsiveness at a mucosal surface. We are only just beginning to appreciate the complexity of this immune response, to recognize organisms' ability to avoid that response. There is considerably more work to be done.

Section 2

Epidemiology of *Helicobacter pylori*

Survival of *Helicobacter pylori* in the Aquatic Environment

U.E.H. Mai, M. Shahamat, and R.R. Colwell

A large body of information has by now accumulated concerning the worldwide distribution of *Helicobacter pylori* and its association with chronic gastritis and peptic ulcer disease [1]. However, only a relatively small amount of clinically relevant information is available concerning the transmission and potential reservoirs of *H. pylori.* Of the many questions still to be answered concerning the basic microbiology of this organism and its transmission, are questions as fundamental as whether *H. pylori* survives in the aquatic environment, and if so, whether it remains infective under environmental conditions. If *H. pylori* is maintained in the viable state under such environmental conditions, it may undergo physiological changes that enhance or ensure survival. Parameters that may play a role in the survival of *H. pylori* in the natural environment include temperature, pH, nutrient concentration, oxygen saturation, and salinity.

Previous work in our laboratory suggests that bacteria, when adapting to a new environment, may undergo morphological and physiological changes, and that some species undergo dormancy. Dormancy is defined as a rest period or reversible interruption of the phenotypic development of an organism [2, 3]. A dormant stage may involve the formation of spores, as in the case of gram-positive bacteria, or the ability of nonsporulating gram-negative bacteria, such as *Pseudomonas* spp., *Salmonella* spp., and *Escherichia coli,* to remain viable under adverse environmental conditions [2, 4, 5]. During the dormant stage these bacteria undergo morphological changes that result in transformation from a rod shape to small coccoid cells. Several investigators have demonstrated this phenomenon in both laboratory and field conditions [6, 7]. Dormant cells do not grow on standard bacteriological media; consequently, alternative methods for detecting and enumerating these bacteria are required, including radiolabeled substrate uptake [8, 9], detection of respiratory activity [10, 11], and differential staining [12–14].

To address the issue of whether dormancy occurs in *H. pylori,* we first sought to determine whether it enters a viable but dormant state under adverse environmental conditions. The following experimental design was employed. Vegetative cells of spiral-shaped *H. pylori* – grown on blood agar plates (blood agar base number 2 Oxoid plus 7% horse blood), suspended in sterile water, and incubated at 4°C for variable periods of time – were enumerated by both plate and direct microscopic counting.

Figure 1 shows results of a representative experiment. The total cell count, employing acridine orange staining (AODC) remained constant over the observed period. However, the viable count was zero after 10–20 days. Thus by standard bacteriological methods the organism was clearly nonculturable. Morphologically, the original population of vegetative spiral-shaped *H. pylori* at the beginning of the experiment

H. Menge et al. (Eds.)
Helicobacter pylori 1990

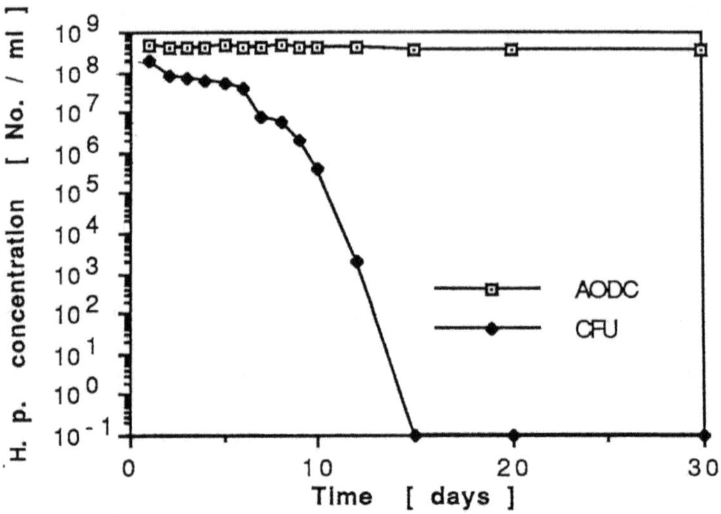

Fig. 1. H. pylori suspended in sterile water for 30 days. ⊡: total cell counts (aeridine orange staining, AODS), ◆: culturable organisms (colony forming units, (FU)

were curved rods, and these changed to closely coiled, horseshoe-shaped, and finally coccoid forms at the end of the 20-day incubation period. The latter persisted during the long-term extension of the experiment. Evidence for the viability of these cells, which were in a nonculturable state, was provided using thymidine incorporation. The metabolic activity of *H. pylori* was monitored under substrate depriviation, i.e., oligotrophic conditions with initial maximum thymidine uptake coinciding with the large number of viable, culturable cells. The persisting measurable uptake of thymidine indicates the presence of cells that remain viable and metabolically active, but not culturable (Fig. 2). Similar results were obtained employing *E. coli* cultures under similar experimental conditions. During the nonculturable stage, thymidine uptake provided evidence of metabolic activity. Also, the transformation of vegetative *H. pylori* from rod-shaped cells to coccoid cells under conditions of substrate limitation and reduced temperature of incubation was demonstrated by altering osmolarity and other parameters.

To determine whether transformation of *H. pylori* was possible from the dormant stage to the "vegetative," infective spiral-shaped stage (i.e., actively growing cells) *H. pylori,* aged in sterile river water for 1 year and incubated at 4°C, was used in the following experiments. The substrate concentration of the cell suspension was increased according to the protocol shown in Fig. 3. Using a liquid medium visible growth was observed by day 14, and on day 30 the urease reaction was positive. Finally, by day 37 spiral-shaped bacteria were recoverable on the solid phase of the biphasic (liquid/solid) medium used in the experiment.

From results obtained to date, we draw the following conclusions. Under conditions unfavorable for growth of *H. pylori* in an aquatic environment, the organism remains viable in a spiral-shaped form and culturable on solid media for up to 10–20 days after exposure to the environmental conditions. After longer incubation under

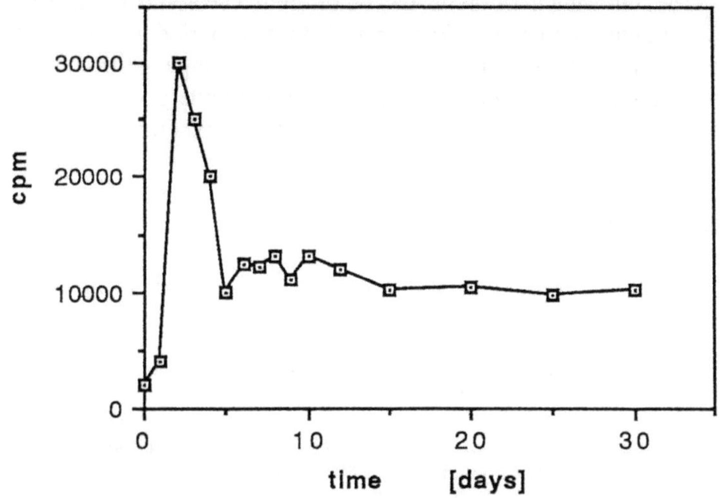

Fig. 2. H. pylori suspended in sterile water for 30 days. Persisting measurable uptake of thymidine indicates that not culturable cells remain metabolically active

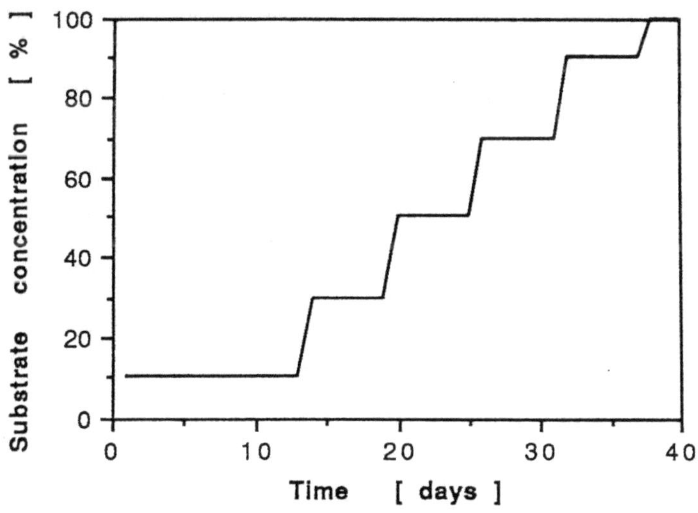

Fig. 3. H. pylori aged in sterile river water for 1 year. Adding of increasing substrate concentrations results in a reappearance of vegetative spiral-shaped urease positive cells at day 30

conditions simulating an oligotrophic aquatic environment, *H. pylori* appeared to enter a viable but dormant stage, exhibiting round-body morphology. Data obtained to date suggest that *H. pylori* can survive under these conditions for at least 1 year, and probably longer. *H. pylori* can undergo transformation to vegetative spiral-shaped cells under conditions of optimal substrate concentration for growth.

The following hypothesis may be offered. The ability of *H. pylori* to persist in the aquatic environment in a dormant state for long periods of time may play an important role in the transmission of this organism. Following ingestion of water containing *H. pylori,* the organism may regain infectivity as it undergoes functional and morphological transformation in vitro, as demonstrated in experiments described in this paper.

References

1. Dooley CR, Cohen M (1988) The clinical significance of *Campylobacter pylori.* Ann Intern Medicine 108:70–79
2. Xu HS, Roberts N, Singleton FL, Attwell RW, Grimes DJ, Colwell RR (1982) Survival and viability of non-culturable *Escherichia coli and Vibrio cholerae* in the estuarine and marine environment. Microb Ecol 8:313–323
3. Stevenson LH (1978) A case for bacterial dormancy in aquatic systems Microb Ecol 4:127–133
4. Roszak DB, Grimes DJ, Colwell RR (1984) Viable but non-recoverable stage of *Salmonella enteritidis* in aquatic systems. Can J Microbiol 30:334–338
5. Kurath G, Morita Y (1983) Starvation-survival physiological studies of a marine *Pseudomonas sp.* Appl Environ Microbiol 45:1206–1211
6. Anderson JIW, Hefernan WP (1965) Isolation and characterization of filterable marine bacteria. J Bacteriol 90:1713–1718
7. Novitsky JA, Morita RY (1976) Morphological characterization of small cells resulting from nutrient starvation of a psychrophilic marine vibrio. Appl Environ Microbiol 32:617–622
8. Meyer-Reil L (1978) Autoradiography and epifluorescence microscopy combined for the determination of numbers and spectrum of actively metabolizing bacteria in natural waters. Appl Environ Microbiol 36:506–512
9. Tabor PS, Neihof RA (1982) Improved microautoradiographic method to determine individual microorganisms active in substrate uptake in natural waters. Appl Environ Microbiol 44:945–950
10. Zimmermann R, Iturriaga R, Becker-Birck J (1978) Simultaneous determination of the total number of aquatic bacteria and the number there of involved in respiration. Appl Environ Microbiol 36:926–935
11. Dutton RJ, Bitton G, Koopman B (1983) Malachite green-INT (MINT) method for determining active bacteria in sewage. Appl Environ Microbiol 46:1263–1267
12. Wade HE, Morgan DM (1954) Differentiation of growing and non-growing bacteria by a staining method. Nature 174:920–921
13. Chrzanowski TH, Crotty RD, Hubbard JG, Welch RP (1984) Applicability of the fluorescein diacetate method of detecting active bacteria in freshwater. Microb Ecol 10:179–185
14. Francisco DE, Mah RA, Rabin AC (1973) Acridine orange epifluorescent technique for counting bacteria in natural waters. Trans Am Microsc Soc 92:416–421

Discussion

McNulty: Can I open the questions by asking you if your hypothesis is that these persisting coccal forms are the source of human infection? Have you inoculated these organisms into an animal model to see if they are infectious?

Mai: We plan to use one of the established animal models for *H. pylori* infection to prove our hypothesis in vivo.

Veldhuyzen van Zanten: Does the organism become urease negative at any of these transformation stages? And if so, do you know at which stage?

Mai: During all our experiments, we monitored the cellbound urease. In general, urease remained positive for the first 15 or 20 days under adverse environmental conditions. On the other hand, in *H. pylori* aged about half a year in river water environments, urease was not detectable any longer though there was evidence for the viability of this population. But under regrowth conditions from this environment, urease became positive again coinciding with retransformation of *H. pylori* into spiralic vegetative bacteria.

Ober: With the reduced metabolism of the cell wall and the inside of the organism one wouldn't expect it, but did you test any influence of antimicrobials on this dormant state?

Mai: We could induce coccoid forms by adding subinhibitoric doses of antibiotics to *H. pylori* cultures, but we haven't tested the antibiotic sensitivity of the coccoid form of *H. pylori.* There could be an unspecific resistance of coccoid *H. pylori* to different antibiotic substances based on the low metabolic activity.

Tytgat: Have some of these coccoid forms ever been found in nature?

Mai: Not for *H. pylori* yet. Coccoid forms of *E. coli* and other gram-negative bacteria could be observed in the natural aquatic environment. From our in vitro experiments up to now we only can expect that *H. pylori* has the ability to withstand simulated aquatic environmental conditions. Experiments to screen natural aquatic environments for coccoid forms of *H. pylori* are in progress.

Westblom: Have you tested the durability of these coccoid forms in different environments? For instance, would they survive drying or other hostile environments?

Mai: In fact we excluded the condition drying, after a preliminary study failed. We investigated on the other hand influence of temperature, salinity, nutrient concentration, etc.

Malfertheiner: Dr. Mai, when you used subinhibitory doses of antibiotics, were you also able to induce coccoid forms? Were these coccoid forms you observed different, and could you discriminate between forms in the process of disintegration and persistent forms and what is the relative proportion. A second question concerning the ultrastructure analysis of the coccoid form, did you find different forms such as big and small coccoid forms, and could you still observe flagella on the coccoid forms or fimbriae?

Mai: Morphologically, the original population of vegetative, spiral-shaped *H. pylori* consisted at the beginning of the experiment of curved rods and changed to closely coiled, horseshoe, and finally coccoid forms. These coccoid forms were in fact heterogenous and only a very low percentage of this population coincided morphologically with intact organisms.

Hazell: Very interesting. It's the first set of data that I've seen that's somewhat convincing about coccoid forms. But what I'd like to bring up is the information that Steve Krakowka produced earlier today indicating the importance of motility in terms of virulence. I think it's very important that you test this in an animal model, or you could be a hero and swallow it yourself, to see whether these forms really are important in terms of transmission. Given that *H. pylori* seems to be viable in water in the spiral form for a short period, is this the most important period in terms of transmission and is the coccoid form a less important stage in terms of transmission from person to person?

Mai: I agree and I think it is very important to find out how relevant our in vitro findings are in vivo. We plan to inoculate all these different forms of *H. pylori* in a suitable animal model to answer the question.

Helicobacter pylori in Human Populations: The Present and Predictions of the Future Based on the Epidemiology of Polio*

D. Y. Graham

Introduction

Helicobacter pylori infections are worldwide; *H. pylori* gastritis has been found in every country where attempts have been made to discover it. Most reports have emphasized *H. pylori* infections in patients presenting for endoscopy and thus provide little information about the frequency in the general population. Current data suggest fecal-oral transmission. Part of the evidence for fecal-oral transmission comes from studies of the prevalence of *H. pylori* infection in different parts of the world. We now know that the prevalence of *H. pylori* and the rate of acquisition varies greatly in different populations [1,5–7, 12, 14–18, 26]. Table 1 shows data from published studies that described the frequency of *H. pylori* infection in the specific populations. Each of these studies included more than 50 individuals and provided tabular data that could be averaged to illustrate relative differences in the prevalence of *H. pylori* infection between countries and populations. There are a number of problems (e.g., selection biases, methodological differences) with those studies [2] and these will be discussed in some detail later. Despite the problems, there are definite patterns that provide fundamental insights into the epidemiology of *H. pylori* infection.

The acquisition of *H. pylori* infection continues in the population throughout life. Availabe data strongly support the notion that the age-specific prevalence of *H. pylori* infections (as measured by acquisition of anti-*H. pylori* IgG) is higher in developing countries than in developed countries. Even within developing countries, there are stratifications such that *H. pylori* infection is more common in those of lower socioeconomic status (reflected by income, housing, sanitation, educational level, etc.).

Gastritis and Gastric Carcinoma as an Index of the Age of Acquisition of *H. pylori* Infection

Helicobacter pylori is the most common cause of type B gastritis. The natural history of type B gastritis is inexorable progression with involvement of more and more stomach, ultimately leading to gastric atrophy. In general, this is a slow process taking between 20 and 40 years to complete. Knowledge of the age-specific frequency of

* This work was supported by the Veterans Affairs; by grant DK39919 from the National Institute of Diabetes and Digestive and Kidney Diseases and by the generous support of Hilda Schwartz

H. Menge et al. (Eds.)
Helicobacter pylori 1990

Table 1. Frequency of *H. pylori* infection in general populations of mixed ages as reflected by the presence of anti-*H-pylori* IgG

Geographic area	No. tested	Percentage positive	Reference number
England	607	21	14
France	1199	28	17
Vietnam	365	61	17
Ivory Coast	374	70	17
Algeria	277	78	17
Finland	500	36	15
New Zealand			18
Whites	483	36	
Maori	192	21	
Cook Island	85	39	
Samoan	129	44	
Togan	56	70	
Australia			4,6
Whites	154	15	
Northern Aborigines	285	50	
Southern Aborigines	274	<1	
Vietnamese	190	18	
El Salvadoreans	75	40	
Ethiopians	74	43	
New Guinea	157	25*	16
White Australians	785	20	16
Saudia Arabia	557	66	1
India	241	79	BCM
United States			BCM
Whites	191	27	
Blacks	145	63	

* If not adsorbed with *C. jejuni,* then this figure is 56% BCM, Baylor College of Medicine *H. pylori* study group

gastritis in a population provides indirect data about the epidemiology of *H. pylori* in that population. Atrophic gastritis/gastric atrophy is thought to be the precursor lesion of gastric carcinoma [3]. Early acquisition of *H. pylori* infection results in a development of the precursor lesion sufficiently early in life that if secondary factors such as intragastric bacterial transformation of potential carcinogens in the diet are present, gastric carcinoma will be at high frequency. Thus, countries or populations with a high frequency of gastric carcinoma are thus expected to exhibit a rapid rate of acquisition of *H. pylori* infection and this is borne out by the available data. The converse, countries with a high early acquisition of *H. pylori,* is not necessarily true as the population may not exhibit the expected large increase in gastric cancer because other factors, such as the absence of carcinogens in diet or the presence or absence of factors that completely or partially nullify the action of the carcinogen (e.g., fresh fruits), modify the overall results [9].

Relation of the Epidemiology of *H. pylori* and Other Fecal-Oral Transmitted Diseases

Hsu et al. reported that the clinical picture of hepatitis A (HAV) was changing in Taiwan coincident with an improved standard of living [13]. The change in age of acquisition was evident by a shift in the acquisition of anti-HAV from infancy to older children and young adults. Clinical hepatitis is much more frequent in older children and adults than infants. Thus, the change in the epidemiology resulted in clinical hepatitis becoming a much more common problem. We postulated that, if both HAV and *H. pylori* were transmitted by the fecal-oral route, a parallel shift in the acquisition of *H. pylori* infection could also be demonstrated in the same population. Unfortunately, the paired sera used to measure anti-HAV in Taiwan were no longer available and we were unable to test that hypothesis. We also postulated that the rate of acquisition of anti-HAV IgG would roughly parallel the rate of acquisition of anti-*H. pylori* IgG and thus one could predict the epidemiology of *H. pylori* if one knew the epidemiology of hepatitis A in a population. We were able to confirm our prediction of prevalence of anti-HAV being a predictor of the prevalence of antibody to *H. pylori* in studies we have done in Saudi Arabia, in India, and in the United States (unpublished observations).

Poliomyelitis as a Model for *H. pylori*

One is immediately struck with the marked similarities between the emerging pattern of the epidemiology of *H. pylori* infection and the epidemiology of poliomyelitis before vaccination became available [19–22, 24]. Like polio virus and hepatitis A virus, humans and nonhuman primates appear to be the only natural hosts of *H. pylori*. The lessons learned from the epidemiology of poliomyelitis predicted the epidemiology of hepatitis A and appear remarkably applicable to *H. pylori*. Paralytic poliomyelitis was a rare disease until the first epidemics in the late 1800s (1860–1880 in Scandinavia, 1880–1890 in northern Europe, and 1890 in northeastern United States). Of interest, this same period saw the beginning of the epidemic of duodenal ulcer disease that only recently has shown signs of waning.

Later, when it was recognized that poliomyelitis was caused by a virus, it was suggested that paralytic poliomyelitis was either a new disease or that a new strain of virus was spreading through the world's population. The ability to test for the presence of antibody against polio viruses rapidly clarified the situation. Ultimately, paralytic poliomyelitis was found to be an indirect consequence of the remarkable improvements in sanitation and the development of clean water supplies that occurred in the latter half of the nineteenth century [21]. These changes resulted in a marked reduction in the frequency of enteric diseases caused by bacterial pathogens but led to the emergence of hitherto unrecognized or rare diseases caused by viruses transmitted by the fecal-oral route.

In retrospect, poliomyelitis had always been a mild or subclinical disease in infants and, as immunity is lifelong, older children and adults were immune. Improvements in the public environment, personal hygiene, sanitation, housing, and education resulted in an increasingly larger portion of the population that escaped exposure during infancy. This resulted in an even larger population of susceptible individuals in whom the disease would manifest as a paralytic poliomyelitis. The change from endemic to epidemic poliomyelitis prompted a number of excellent epidemiology studies proving an inverse relationship between the rate of acquisition of antipolio antibody and standards of hygiene; in populations with poor standards the steepest rise in antibody prevalence occurred in the youngest age group, whereas those with better standards (e.g., directly related to socioeconomic levels) experienced a delay with the steepest point of the curve in children of school age or adolescence. The differences in the prevalence of paralytic poliomyelitis were not based on geography but were related to standards and practices of hygiene and socioeconomic conditions.

The epidemiology of hepatitis A was found to mirror that of poliomyelitis [4, 10, 13, 23]. The change in the average age of onset of polio infection led to the appearance of paralytic poliomyelitis. The delay in acquisition of hepatitis led to epidemic hepatitis. The current data suggest that a similar mechanism is responsible for the appearance of duodenal ulcer disease and the reduction in frequency of gastric carcinoma (i.e., delay in onset of *H. pylori* infection results in the precursor lesion, atrophic gastritis occurring late in life).

Only one remote population has yet been described in whom *H. pylori* infection is almost absent, the northern Australian Aborigines. In contrast, southern Australian Aborigines exhibit a high prevalence of *H. pylori* infection [4]. There is an interesting parallel between the epidemiology of *H. pylori* and poliomyelitis and *H. pylori* as small remote populations were discovered that had escaped polio infection for a prolonged period (e.g., Eskimo communities) [21].

Interpretation of Data from Individual Countries

Currently available studies on the epidemiology of *H. pylori* infection have not been formal epidemiological studies and have often relied on preexisting serum sample collections from uncharacterized populations. Data derived from such studies may not represent the frequency of infection within the population or even within a specific subset of the population of a country. Data obtained from blood donors are difficult to interpret unless one also knows the pattern of giving blood in a particular country. For example, in some countries, blood is typically given by family members or relatives; in others paid donors are used. The recent problem with AIDS has lead to marked restrictions on who can and who will donate blood.

A second problem relates to the details of the assay used to identify the presence of a *H. pylori* infection. The first generation serological tests employing whole bacteria, bacterial sonicates, or extracts of whole bacteria have all suffered from a high frequency of false-positive tests caused by the presence of antibodies directed against antigen of *C. jejuni* or other bacteria that cross-react with *H. pylori* [2]. The presence of cross-reacting antibodies appears to be particularly severe in studies using sera obtained from individuals living in developing countries. Recently, the suggestion was made that serological tests should be restandarized for each population [16].

Second-generation tests using purified antigens such as the high-molecular-weight cell-associated antigens [7], or potentially one using a pool of the different antigenic types of the fibrillar putative colonization factor antigen(s) [8], provide accurate data without the associated problems of cross-reactivity. Using the HM-CAP antigen as a goal standard, we found that ELISAs based on relatively crude *H. pylori* extracts had positive predictive values in the range of 60% and equally poor negative predictive values when used to evaluate the prevalence of *H. pylori* in underdeveloped countries (unpublished observations).

The Future

Although epidemiological data are still largely rudimentary, there are sufficient observations to allow us to predict the general pattern of the epidemiology of *H. pylori* infections and to design experiments to test those hypotheses directly. For example, from experience with polio virus we expect the age-specific prevalence to be inversely related to sanitation, socioeconomic class, education, hygiene, and directly related to the number of children in the family, age, infant mortality, and enteric exposure. The prevalence of *H. pylori* infection has already been shown to be independent of gender. Improvements in the socioeconomic status, sanitation, hygiene, and health of a population are expected to lead to a reduction in the rate of acquisition of *H. pylori* infection in a population. This has already been demonstrated for hepatitis A and we anticipate that studies will subsequently show similar changes for *H. pylori*. An increase in the average age of acquisition of *H. pylori* infection will result in a gradual reduction in epidemic gastric cancer as a cohort phenomenon. Similarly, in countries where duodenal ulcer is prevalent, we will see a gradual increase in the age of onset. Knowledge of the effect of socioeconomic class will cause possible associations of frequency of *H. pylori* infection with specific groups within the same geographic area to be reconsidered [25].

References

1. Al-Moagel MA, Evans DG, Abdulghani ME, Adam E, Evans DJ Jr, Malaty HM, Klein PD, Graham DY (1989) Comparison of the prevalence of *C. pylori* infection in individuals with and without upper gastrointestinal symptoms. Gastroenterology 96:A10
2. Alpert LC, Graham DY, Evans DJ Jr, Yoshimura HH, Hazell SL, Evans DG, Klein PD (1989) Diagnostic possibilities for *Campylobacter pylori* infection. Eur J Gastroenterol Hepatol 1:17–26
3. Correa P, Cuello C, Duque E, Burbano LC, Garcia FT, Bolanos O, Brown C, Haenszel W (1976) Gastric cancer in Colombia. III. Natural history of precursor lesions. JNCI 57:1027–1033
4. Dienstag JL, Szmuness W, Stevens CE, Purcell RH (1978) Hepatitis A virus infection: new insights from seroepidemiologic studies. J Infect Dis 137:328–340
5. Dwyer B, Kaldor J, Tee W, Raios K (1989) The prevalence of *Campylobacter pylori* in human populations. In: Rathbone BJ, Heatley RV (Eds) *Campylobacter pylori* and gastroduodenal disease. Blackwell, Oxford, pp 190–196
6. Dwyer B, Nanxiong S, Kaldor J, Tee W, Lambert J, Luppino M, Flannery G (1988) Antibody response to *Campylobacter pylori* in an ethnic group lacking peptic ulceration. Scand J Infect Dis 20:63–68
7. Evans DJ Jr, Evans DG, Graham DY, Klein PD (1989) A sensitive and specific serologic test for detection of *Campylobacter pylori* infection. Gastroenterology 96:1004–1008
8. Evans DJ Jr, Evans DG, Smith KE, Graham DY (1989) Serum antibody responses to the *N*.acetylneuraminyllactose-binding hemagglutinin of *Campylobacter pylori*. Infect Immun 57:644–647

9. Fontham E, Zavala D, Correa P, Rodriguez E, Hunter F, Haenszel W, Tannenbaum SR (1986) Diet and chronic atrophic gastritis: a case- control study. JNCI 76:621–627
10. Frosner GG, Papaevangelou G, Butler R, Iwarson S, Lindholm A, Courouce-Pauty A, Haas H, Deinhardt F (1979) Antibody against hepatitis A in seven European countries. I. Comparison of prevalence data in different age groups. Am J Epidemiol 110:93–99
11. Graham DY, Adam E, Klein PD, Evans DJ Jr, Evans DG, Hazell SL, Alpert LC, Michaletz PA, Yoshimura HH (1989) Epidemiology of *Campylobacter pylori.* Gastroenterol Clin Biol 13:84B–88B
12. Graham DY, Klein PD, Opekun AR, Boutton TW, et al. (1988) Epidemiology of *Campylobacter pylori* infection: ethnic considerations. Scand J Gastroenterol 23[suppl 142]:9–13
13. Hsu HY, Chang MH, Chen DS, Lee CY, Sung JL (1985) Changing seroepidemiology of hepatitis A virus infection in Taiwan. J Med Virol 17:297–301
14. Jones DM, Eldridge J, Fox AJ, Sethi AJ, Whorwell PJ (1986) Antibody to the gastric campylobacter-like organism *("Campylobacter pyloridis")* – clinical correlations and distribution in the normal population. J Med Microbiol 22:57–62
15. Kosunen TU, Hook J, Rautelin HI, Myllyla G (1989) Age-dependent increase of *Campylobacter pylori* antibodies in blood donors. Scand J Gastroenterol 24:110–114
16. Mitchell HM, Lee A, Berkowicz J, Barody T (1988) The use of serology to diagnose active *Campylobacter pylori* infection. Med J Aust 149:604–609
17. Megraud F, Brassens-Rebbe M-P, Denis F, Belbouri A, Hoa DQ (1989) Seroepidemiology of *C. pylori* infection in various populations. J Clin Microbiol 27:1870–1873
18. Morris A, Nicholson G, Lloyd G, Haines D, Rogers A Taylor D (1986) Seroepidemiology of *Campylobacter pyloridis* NZ Med J (1986) 99:657–659
19. Paul JR (1971) Epidemics in Sweden. Medin and his clinical contributions. In: A history of poliomyelitis. Yale University Press, New Haven pp 71–78
20. Paul JR (1954) Historical and geographical aspects of the epidemiology of poliomyelitis. Yale J Biol Med 27: 101–113
21. Paul JR (1971) Serological surveys and antibody patterns. Endemicity versus epidemicity. In: A history of poliomyelitis. Yale University Press, New Haven pp 357–368
22. Paul JR (1971) The earliest sizable epidemic in the United States. In: A history of poliomyelitis. Yale University Press, New Haven, pp 79–87
23. Szmuness W, Dienstag JL, Purcell RH, Stevens CE, Wong DC, Ikram H, Bar-Shany S, Beasley RP, Desmyter J, Gaon JA (1977) The prevalence of antibody to hepatitis A antigen in various parts of the world: a pilot study. Am J Epidiol 106:392–398
24. Walton M, Melnick JL (1955) Poliomyelitis antibodies in two differing socioeconomic groups within the same city. Yale J Biol Med 27:350–370
25. Vira D, D'Anastasio CD, Holton J, Dowsett JF, Londei M, Bertoni F, Beltrandi E, Grauenfels P, Salmon PR, Gandolfi L (1988) *Campylobacter pylori* in abattoir workers: is it a zoonosis. Lancet II 725–726

Discussion

Newell: I seem to remember that there was a study in Peru comparing the incidence of *H. pylori* infection in patients attending private hospitals as against public hospitals which showed that there was no difference between the two. Does this not indicate that socioeconomic status is not important?

Graham: No, in a country such as Peru, within time adults are 80% infected. What we are asking is age of acquisition. In our studies in Peru, we found that the children, for example, who are 5 years old and live in rural villages are 80% infected. In contrast, by the age of 5 years children from rich families are 30% infected. Interestingly, when one asks whether family size is important, we do have data that increased family size is one of the parameters that shows an increased frequency of *H. pylori* infection.

Tytgat: Is there a correlation between the prevalence of peptic ulcer disease and gastric carcinoma?

Graham: Theoretically, in using the standard I have given you for duodenal ulcer there is an inverse correlation, because if you become infected as a child by the time that you are 20 or 30 years old, you really have pretty much destroyed your stomach. You don't make enough acid to get duodenal ulcers. To get duodenal ulcer, you had to escape becoming infected early and become infected at a later stage. We are now seeing the frequency get less and less. In the United States in our population of white middle-class people, only 50% are infected at the ages of 70 or 80 years. So what we are going to see, and I think we are seeing, is that the onset of duodenal ulcer occurs in an increasingly older population.

Wadström: Could you comment on the situation in Asia. What about rural and urban Japan, Taiwan und mainland China with different socioeconomic situations?

Graham: You don't get cancer because you have *H. pylori* infection. If you believe the epidemic gastric carcinoma story, you get atrophic gastritis and bacterial growth. You have to have carcinogen in the diet, and you need a diet deficient in agents that prevent the carcinogen from working. That is a very complicated situation. But, if you look in Japan today, as I showed you before, by age 20 more than 50% had atrophic gastritis. Today this is 20%. So the frequency of gastritis and the *Helicobacter* is now much less and we are seeing a reduction in frequency of cancer there.

Transmission and Sources of Helicobacter pylori

D. Vaira, J. Holton, G. Oderda, D. Taylor, R. Turner, A. Colecchia
and L. Gandolfi

Introduction

Helicobacter pylori is known to colonize gastric epithelium in human stomachs and duodenum, but little is known about its spread between humans or other possible sources of infection. There are three possible sources for human infection:

a) infection acquired from people by person-to-person spread by some direct route such as faeco-oral,
b) infection from an animal reservoir such as a food source or pets and
c) infection acquired from the environment.

Person-to-Person Spread

Humans can become infected with *H. pylori* by the oral route as demonstrated by Morris [1] and Marshall [2], who ingested a high number of bacteria and subsequently developed gastritis. Also spread of infection from one individual to another has been documented by pH electrodes [3]. Clearly, however, although the source of infection was human, the circumstances of ingestion in these instances were not the usual methods of person-to-person spread and do not account for the human prevalence of the organism. Acquiring *H. pylori* from a human source would be more likely in circumstances of close contact and several studies have advanced this point.

Family Studies

Transmission within the family group has been suggested by Mitchell, who carried out a sero-epidemiological survey and reported an increased level of antibodies against *H. pylori* in nine family contacts of four infected children [4]. This study has been extended to ten families [5], but as the authors indicate the population under study was heterogeneous with respect to ethnic group and as there appear to be differences in colonization rate between different ethnic groups [6, 7] the results should be interpreted with caution.

In another study Langenberg typed the organism isolated from both husband and wife by restriction endonuclease mapping to demonstrate that the separate isolates from different family members had an identical restriction endonuclease pattern [8]. Similar results were obtained by Majewski but in 50% of the cases the restriction endonuclease pattern differed between family members [9]. Jones et al. [10] conduct-

H. Menge et al. (Eds.)
Helicobacter pylori 1990

Children positive for Helicobacter pylori

Age (yrs)	Sex	Endoscopy	Relatives H. pylori status: Parents	Siblings
16	M	DU	●●	●●○
10	M	DU	●○	○
18	M	DU	●○	●
13	M	DU	● DU ○	○
12	M	DU	● DU ●	●●
10	M	DU	● DU ●	○
10	M	GU	●●	●●○
15	M	GU	●●	●

Children negative for Helicobacter pylori

Age (yrs)	Sex	Endoscopy	Relatives H. pylori status: Parents	Siblings
11	M	DU	●●	
8	M	DU	●○	○
12	F	DU	●○	○
4	M	DU	●○	○
14	M	DU	●○	
10	M	GU	●○	
2	M	GU	●○	○

DU : duodenal ulcer
GU : gastric ulcer

● : H. pylori positive
○ : H. pylori negative

Fig. 1. Screening by serum IgG antibody to *H. pylori* in the relatives of 15 children who had either duodenal or gastric ulcers

ed a study of *H. pylori* colonization in family members of 40 adult index cases but could not demonstrate a great incidence of colonization within the family group. We have also conducted a sero-epidemiological survey of family groups and screened the relatives of 15 children who had either duodenal or gastric ulcers. In this study there were no differences in the colonization by *H. pylori* in the relatives of those young people colonized with *H. pylori* compared with those who were not colonized [11] (Fig. 1).

Other Studies

Sero-epidemiological studies of individuals in an institution demonstrated that they become infected at an earlier age than a control population [12]. Similarly one study of gastroenterologists also demonstrated a high incidence of *H. pylori* colonization compared with a group of general practitioners or blood donors [5]. Another study of endoscopists, however, could not demonstrate any difference in seropositivity to *H. pylori* compared with a control population [13]. In any case the family and institutional studies do not prove person-to-person spread as infection could equally well have occurred from some common source other than an infected individual.

Animals as Food Sources

Individuals who come into contact with animals such as abattoir workers would be expected to be colonized more frequently with *H. pylori* than a control population if the animals carried *H. pylori*. A serological study by Morris [6], who compared various animal-associated occupations with normal blood donors, demonstrated a significant association between abattoir workers and positive serology to *H. pylori*.

Similarly, we [14] conducted a sero-epidemiological survey of abattoir workers and demonstrated higher levels of IgG to *H. pylori* even after absorption with *C. jejuni* than in a control population of the same age and sex (Fig. 2). Endoscopy was subsequently performed in those individuals with high IgG levels to *H. pylori* and they were shown to be colonized by *H. pylori* and to have gastritis or ulceration. Clearly this is only indirect evidence that the *H. pylori* may have been acquired from the animals. The organism has been looked for in the animals by serology, culture, and

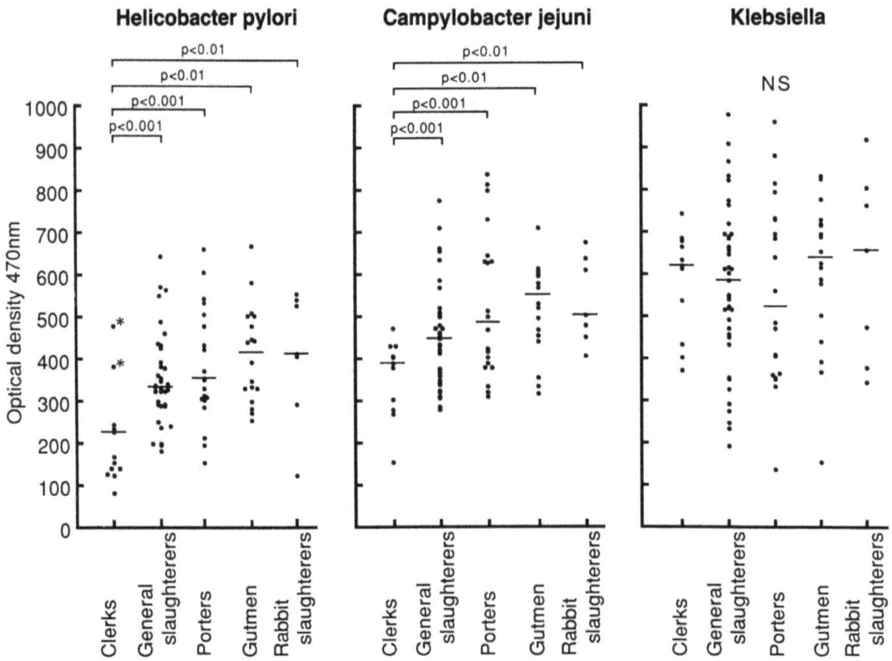

Fig. 2. Serum antibody levels to *H. pylori, C. jejuni,* and *Klebsiella* in abattoir workers. * Two clerical workers had endoscopically proven active duodenal ulcers

histology. *H. pylori* was not isolated from the stomachs of cows, pigs, or rabbits because of excess bacterial overgrowth. Three out of five rabbits and four out of five pigs, however, had high levels of anti *H. pylori* IgG antibodies (times three optical density of control well in an ELISA test) after absorption of the animal sera with *C. jejuni*. Histologically, gastritis was seen in the stomach of the pigs. The sections were also stained by a monoclonal antibody raised against *H. pylori* by Dr. Newell, but organisms were not detected.

As the possibility of animals acting as a source of infection for humans is important, further work is required particularly in attempts to culture *H. pylori* from the animal stomachs.

Zoo Animals as a Source of *H. pylori*

Helicobacter pylori has been detected in the stomach of rhesus monkey [15] and baboons [16] which is indistinguishable from the human-associated *H. pylori*. Also a *H. pylori*-like organism has been isolated from the stomach of ferrets [17]. This organism resembles *H. pylori* in many respects but differs from the human isolates in its protein profile on SDS-polyacrylamide gel electrophoresis, and in fatty acid methyl-ester profiles [18]. Dolphins are known to suffer from peptic ulceration [19]. Four dolphins have been endoscoped and biopsied and blood was taken both from dolphins and killer whales to look for antibodies to *H. pylori*. The organism was not isolated and neither animals had antibodies against *H. pylori*. Additionally, zoo keepers and vets were screened for antibodies to *H. pylori* and compared with a population of clerical workers who did not have contact with zoo animals. Only three out of 22 keepers had evidence of *H. pylori* confirmed by endoscopy and culture. It would seem that zoo animals are no colonized by *H. pylori* but to date there is no evidence that they act as a source of *H. pylori* for humans.

Pets as a Source of *H. pylori*

There is no evidence that pets are a source of *H. pylori*, although it has been reported by McNulty that spiral-shaped bacteria, clearly different from *H. pylori* and provisionally called *Gastrospirillum hominis*, have been detected in human stomachs in association with active gastritis [20]. Morphologically similar organisms have been detected in the stomachs of cats and dogs, and obviously the colonization of the human stomach could have originated from contact with domestic animals. However, none of the individuals colonized with this organism had close contact with pets. Further, any proposed causal relationship between *Gastrospirillum hominis* and gastritis must as yet remain an open question.

Environment as a Source of *H. pylori*

Helicobacter pylori is known to undergo a morphological variation between the familiar vibrio shape and a coccoid shape. The coccoid variety of *H. pylori* is formed spontaneously in older cultures, by subinhibitory levels of antibiotics and adverse environmental pressures such as a nutrient limitation [21]; in this study there was no difference between the two forms with respect to protein profiles by SDS-PAGE but there was a notable decrease in the phospholipid and an increase in the keto-deoctonic acid content of the coccoid variety.

The coccoid variety of *H. pylori* is viable but not culturable and can be induced to revert to the vibrio form. This could provide a means of transmission from person-to-person or acquiring the organism from the environment. Clearly the environment could become contaminated by such coccoid forms from human or animal sewage. This important aspect of *H. pylori* requires further study.

References

1. Morris A, Nicholson G (1987) Ingestion of *Campylobacter pyloridis* causes gastritis and raised fasting gastric pH. Am J Gastroenterol 82:192–199
2. Marshall BJ, Armstrong JA, McGechie DB, Glancy RJ (1985) Attempt to fulfil Koch's postulates for pyloric campylobacter. Med J Australia 142:436–439
3. Ramsey EJ, Carey KV, Peterson WL, et al. (1979) Epidemic gastritis with hypochlorhydria. Gastroenterology 76:1449–1457
4. Mitchell HM, Bohane TD, Berkowicz J, et al. (1987) Antibody to *Campylobacter pylori* in families of index children with gastrointestinal illness due to *Campylobacter pylori*. Lancet ii:681–682
5. Mitchell HM, Lee A, Bohane TD (1989) *Campylobacter pylori* and gastroduodenal disease. In: Rathbone BJ, Heatley RV (eds) Campylobacter pylori and gastroduodenal disease. Evidence for person-to-person spread of Campylobacter pylori. Blackwell Science, Oxford, pp 197–208
6. Morris A, Nicholson G, Lloyd G et al. (1986) Seroepidemiology of *Campylobacter pyloridis*. N Z Med J 99:657–659
7. Lee A, Hazell SL (1988) *Campylobacter pylori* in health and disease: an ecological perspective. Micro Ecol Health Dis i:1–16
8. Langenberg W, Rauws EAJ, Widjojokusumo A, et al. (1986) Identification of *Campylobacter pyloridis* isolates by restriction endonuclease DNA analysis. J Clin Microbiol 24:414–417
9. Majeweski SIH, Goodwin SC (1988) Restriction endonuclease analysis of the genome of *Campylobacter pylori* with a rapid extraction method: evidence for considerable genomic variation. J Infect Dis 157:465–471
10. Jones DM, Eldrige J, Whorwell PJ (1987) Antibodies to *Campylobacter pyloridis* in household contacts of infected patients. Br Med J 294:615
11. Oderda G, Vaira D, Holton J, et al. (1989) *Campylobacter pylori* (CP) in families of children with peptic ulcer. Gut 30:A1472
12. Berkowicz J, Lee A (1987) Person-to-person transmission of *Campylobacter pylori*. Lancet ii:680–681
13. Morris A, Lloyd G, Nicholson G (1986) *Campylobacter pyloridis* serology among gastroendoscopy clinic staff. N Z Med J 99:820–821
14. Vaira D, D'Anastasio C, Holton J, et al. (1988) *Campylobacter pylori* in abattoir workers: is it a zoonosis? Lancet ii:725–726
15. Baskerville A, Newell DG (1988) Naturally occurring chronic gastritis and *C. pylori* infection in the rhesus monkey: a potential model for gastritis in man. Gut 29:465–472
16. Curry A, Jones D, Eldrige J (1987) Spiral organism in the baboon stomach. Lancet ii:634–635
17. Cave DR, Taylor N, Tuczynshi C, Fox JG (1986) *Campylobacter* like organism (CLO) from man and ferret: towards an animal model of CLO induced disease. Gastroenterology 90:1368
18. Goodwin CS, McCulloch RK, Armstrong JA, Wee SH (1985) Unusual cellular fatty acids and distinctive ultrastructure in a new spiral bacterium *(Campylobacter pyloridis)* from the human gastric mucosa. J Med Microbiol 19:257–267

19. Greenwood AG, Taylor DC (1978) Fibreoptic gastroscopy in dolphins. The Vet Record 102:495–497
20. McNulty CAM, Dent JC, Curry A, et al. (1989) New spiral bacterium in gastric mucosa. J Clin Pathol 42:585–591
21. Mai U, Geis G, Leying H, et al. (1988) First European *Campylobacter pylori* study group. Megraud and Lamoulette, Bordeaux, p 10

Discussion

Veldhuyzen van Zanten: Did you do any kind of breath test in the children with duodenal ulcers in whom you did not find *Helicobacter pylori?*

Vaira: No, because the age range of these children, as you saw, was from 2 to 18 years, and first of all there were no facilities available for this test in Turin (Italy). And secondly, Dr. Oderda does not consider it to be a useful technique for testing children.

Veldhuyzen van Zanten: How many biopsies did you take in each child to assess their *Helicobacter pylori* status.

Vaira: We took three biopsies from the antrum and two biopsies from the duodenum. There is another point to make: I think this population is really the most important one because the children with duodenal ulcers or gastric ulcers but without *Helicobacter pylori* have really very low antibody levels to H. pylori. We are therefore following this population because we think maybe this is the key to the *Helicobacter pylori* story.

Lee: Yes, I think basically you can explain your data on the incidence of *Helicobacter pylori* in the abbatoir workers by the fact (as you've already shown) that there is increased contact with animals and therefore an increased level of *C. jejuni* antibodies. I think this is a valid criticism of that conclusion. I think David Graham's point is also well made, that one has to be very careful in any study, particularly in seroepidemiological studies, in terms of age matching and culture matching one's population and as I've already pointed out, socioeconomic matching. I would therefore like to challenge you and say I do not believe your data on abbatoir workers is consistent with increased *Helicobacter pylori* levels and I'd like to hear what you have to say on that.

Vaira: Unfortunately I cannot say any more than what we wrote in the letter in the "Lancet", in which we clearly wrote that we performed absorption with *C. jejuni.*

Lee: But you didn't absorb every serum did you? As I understood it, you absorbed some of the high positive *Helicobacter pylori* sera. If you do not absorb every serum, absorption will have no effect whatsoever, whether or not *C. jejuni* is present.

Vaira: I cannot dispute that there could be a cross-reaction, of course. For this reason when we examined this data we said that we do not believe that the *Helicobacter pylori* reservoir comes from animals. The second point is that we did not absorb more than 45 out of 90 patients' sera. But another point I think we must try not to forget is that when we examined these patients' sera after a 4-week course of treatment with De-Nol, all the patients treated showed a fall in IgG antibody to *Helicobacter pylori.* The levels of IgG antibody to *C. jejuni* were identical! However, we cannot exclude a possible cross-reaction. Regarding Dr. Graham's question, I know that it's hard to believe, but Bologna is one of the richest cities in Italy. The Ferrari factory is 20 km away, the Lamborghini factory is 50 km away. This is the reason why there is not really a big gap between the workers and the clerks. When we looked retrospectively at the socioeconomic status, we discovered that only three members of the clerks' group had secondary school education. The remainder had only primary school education as did all the workers in the abbatoir. Therefore, it doesn't seem that there is really a big gap between the workers and the clerks. I'm sure this situation would be completely different, however, if one looked at an abbatoir in Naples.

McNulty: Dr. Newell, would you like to make any comments about cross-reactions in these serological tests.

Newell: Apart from the antigenic cross-reactivity with *Campylobacter jejuni,* it's also evident from some recent work done using a monoclonal antibody directed against the urease of *Helicobacter pylori* that other organisms have antigenically identical ureases, for example Dr. Lee's cats spiral CSI. It is therefore not impossible to envisage a situation where these humans are being exposed to antigens like urease, from the animal sources and false positives for *Helicobacter pylori* serodiagnosis would be observed.

Graham: I believe the data in your paper, but I don't believe the conclusions. I think the data are perfectly fine, but you need to ask about socioeconomic conditions. I showed you that for blacks and whites in the United States that the lines are parallel, so there's no genetic difference there. What we are seeing, I think, is that 20 years ago or longer, the blacks had a different socioeconomic status and have now moved into the next category. If you look at your Lamborghini and your Ferrari workers, you have to ask what it was like 10, 15, 20, or 30 years ago when all those people were children and Italy was a developing country.

Vaira: Once again I must speak about Bologna's historical background. The people who own the factories today were the farm workers of 20 years ago. So almost the same people with the same way of life, but with more money.

Graham: But that's when they were getting infected and that's maybe when it was different. I can't believe that a clerk in an abbatoir has the same socioeconomic class background as a man who kills rabbits.

Vaira: It's difficult to explain this point. – I'm sorry to bore you by talking again about Bologna. The Bologna abbatoir is not a private one and was built by the same people who now work in it, and one of the workers is also the president.

McNulty: Does anybody have any more comments to make on soil or water as a source of *Helicobacter pylori*. Professor Tytgat, one comment.

Tytgat: If the human stomach is the reservoir, how does the organism spread from the human stomach to the other people? We know from inoculation experiments that you need quite a big inoculum for colonization to occur. How is the organism transmitted in real life?

Vaira: I really ask myself this question a lot of the time, particularly in this last week, but really we don't know.

Graham: We don't know that a large inoculum is needed, but we know that you need a large inoculum if you fast and take it once. But if you live in an environment that's heavily contaminated and with poor sanitation, you may take a small inoculum every time you put something in your mouth. Well, I don't think we can answer the question of real-life transmission. I would suspect that in heavily contaminated environments, your chances of becoming infected are good every day.

Tytgat: You know that we have proven without any doubt that endoscopic transmission is a reality. The most conservative estimates are 2%–3%. In addition there have been several outbreaks of *Helicobacter pylori* infection in endoscopy units. Do you know of other studies which examine the real risk of transmitting *Helicobacter pylori* via endoscopic equipment?

Vaira: There was a study in the journal "Endoscopy" by people from Ferrara near Bologna. They found the same result that you found in Amsterdam and they showed this transmission. But we must remember the previous study which appeared in the "British Medical Journal". These investigators looked just for serology in the endoscopic staff and there were some data in favor of and some against this. Some investigators found a higher level of antibody against *Helicobacter pylori* in the endoscopic staff, some other investigators didn't find it. What you are asking me is whether anyone else carried out the same study as you did in Amsterdam. The answer is yes and they reached exactly the same conclusions.

Chronic Gastritis: Epidemiology and Relationship to Peptic Ulcer Diseases

P. Sipponen

Introduction

Gastritis comprises several types, some of which are specific but relatively rare (granulomatous, eosinophilic, "lymphocytic", etc.). Most commonly, gastritis is a chronic condition and comprises at least three different subtypes which show dissimilarities in the pathogenesis and in the topography of lesions in the stomach.

The significance of gastritis lies in its association to some clinically important gastric diseases, such as gastric cancer and peptic ulcer. The importance of chronic gastritis has been markedly emphasized by recent observations that *Helicobacter pylori* or related organisms might have a causative role in the pathogenesis of chronic gastritis [1], and that both the gastritis and the related diseases can be affected by eradication of these organisms.

Chronic Gastritis

Chronic gastritis is characterized by an infiltration of mononuclear inflammatory cells (plasma cells, lymphocytes) into the lamina propria of gastric antrum or corpus, or of both. In the early stage of gastritis, the inflammation usually affects the upper part of mucosa, in corpus gastritis in particular. Later, the inflammation is followed by a loss of normal glands in the underlying mucosa and by a subsequent growth of intestinal or pseudopyloric metaplastic glands, resulting in atrophy [2–5]. Thus, gastritis is a progressive lesion that begins with a simple inflammation but later leads to destruction and atrophy of the mucous membrane.

Gastritis can be graded arbitrarily into several stages by using the inflammation and the loss of glands as histological criteria (Table 1). In practice, grading into superficial gastritis and further into mild, moderate, or severe atrophic gastritis has been successful. In both antral and body mucosa, this grading correlates well with the function of

Table 1. Histological grading of chronic gastritis using chronic inflammation and loss of normal mucosal glands as criteria

1. Normal
2. Chronic inflammation without atrophy (chronic superficial gastritis)
3. Atrophic gastritis
   a) Slight
   b) Moderate
   c) Severe (total atrophy)

H. Menge et al. (Eds.)
Helicobacter pylori 1990

Table 2. Histological typing of some specific phenotypes of chronic gastritis on the basis of topography of the lesions in stomach

1. Antrum
   a) "B gastritis": moderate or severe antral atrophy, nonatrophic body
2. Body
   a) "A gastritis" or "gastric atrophy": moderate or severe body atrophy, nonatrophic antrum
3. Antrum and body jointly
   a) "Pangastritis": superficial gastritis in both antrum and body
   b) "AB gastritis": moderate or severe atrophy in both antrum and body

gastric mucosa, and also makes sense with regard to their relationship with several gastric diseases [6, 7].

The typing of gastritis is controversial and problematic. The topography of inflammation and atrophy in the stomach probably forms the most reliable basis for this typing. The presence of overt atrophic changes in antral or body mucosa, or in both, represents specific paths in the progression of gastritis: that is, they represent atrophic gastritis of the B, A, or AB type, respectively (Table 2). In regard to epidemiology, biology, and pathogenesis, these types show remarkable dissimilarities (Table 3) [7–9].

Table 3. Short summary of some important associations between gastritis and common gastric disorders

1. Superficial gastritis in the antrum or superficial "pangastritis"
   a) DU or GU disease
2. "B gastritis"
   a) DU or GU disease
   b) Gastric cancer and dysplasia
3. "A gastritis"
   a) Pernicious anemia, hypochlorhydria, achlorhydria, hypergastrinemia
   b) Hyperplastic polyps
   c) Multifocal small carcinoid tumors and hyperplasias of oxyntic endocrine cells
   d) Gastric cancer and dysplasia
4. "AB gastritis"
   a) GU disease in some instances
   b) Gastric cancer and dysplasia

The A type of gastritis is determined genetically, being dependent on one major gene and on autoimmune pathogenesis [10]. The environmental factors may be most significant in the pathogenesis of gastritis of the B or AB type [11, 12]. However, the pathogenesis of gastritis and their progression to overt atrophic stages in particular are obviously multifactorial and complex, and can hardly be explained by any single factor. Prediction of the specific end stages of gastritis is problematic in the early inflammatory phases (superficial gastritis), and confusion certainly occurs in the proper classification of these cases. In the recent literature, gastritis is further considered to be "active" if an acute erosive inflammation accompanies the chronic inflammation [13].

The adoption of this "active" component into the terms of gastritis implies a process that is indeed progressive and continuous.

The bacterial origin of gastritis is strongly proposed in large number of recent independent studies (e.g., see 1). This infective background may particularly concern gastritis that later develop to B or AB type or those that express themselves as a simple superficial inflammation in the antrum or jointly in the antrum and corpus.

Epidemiology

On average, the progression of gastritis is an age-dependent, stepwise phenomenon which occurs roughly similarly in both antrum and corpus [4, 14–16]. The mean prevalence of gastritis, in both antrum and corpus, increases nearly linearly with an increase in the age of the population (Tables 4, 5). As a result, over 60% of people have gastritis of some degree in the age groups above 50 years. A gradual stepwise shift of the subjects occurs from one stage of gastritis to the next, resulting in an increase in the prevalence of atrophic end stages with the increasing age of the cohort [14]. On average, this risk of a subject moving from one gastritis stage to the next is approximately 2%–3% annually [8].

However, some dissimilarities seem to occur in the progression of gastritis between different topographic types of gastritis, as well as between subjects liable to different

Table 4. Prevalence of chronic gastritis in the antral mucosa in population-based samples of subjects and in a series of consecutive outpatient endoscopies

Mucosa: age group (years)	Prevalence (%)	
	Population[a] samples	Outpatient[b] series
Normal Mucosa		
31–50	44	43
51–65	23	26
66–	18	18
Superficial gastritis		
31–50	33	48
51–65	34	51
66–	34	38
Slight or moderate atrophic gastritis		
31–50	23	8
51–65	41	20
66–	48	33
Severe atrophic gastritis		
31–50	0	0.3
51–65	2	3
66–	0	3

[a] Data from ref. [55]; number of subjects around 800
[b] Consecutive series of approximately 1200 patients

Table 5. Prevalence of chronic gastritis in the body mucosa in population-based samples of subjects and in a series of consecutive outpatient endoscopies

Mucosa/ age group (years)	Prevalence (%)	
	Population[a] samples	Outpatient[b] series
Normal mucosa		
31–50	46	54
51–65	24	31
66–	18	22
Superficial gastritis		
31–50	49	40
51–65	48	52
66–	39	43
Slight or moderate atrophic gastritis		
31–50	5	5
51–65	25	13
66–	36	26
Severe atrophic gastritis		
31–50	0	1
51–65	3	5
66–	7	8

[a] Data from ref. [55]; number of subjects around 800
[b] Two consecutive series of approximately 1200 patients

gastric diseases [17, 18]. For instance, in type A gastritis and in pernicious anemia, the transition risk increases in the later phases of progression, and is extremely rapid from the moderate to the severe stage [8, 15]. On the other hand, the progression of gastritis from the stage of superficial gastritis to an atrophic one in the body mucosa seems to be very slow or is totally lacking in patients with peptic ulcer, particularly in those with duodenal ulcer disease [17, 18].

Knowledge of the prevalence of gastritis in different ethnic and cultural populations is scanty. The available data [12, 19, 20] indicate, however, that gastritis obviously is very common in all parts of the world, and that a great proportion of the human adult population has gastritis of some grade. Great differences in the prevalence of gastritis may, however, exist between populations. The greatest differences may concern the prevalence of type A gastritis [19, 20], in the pathogenesis of which the genetic mechanisms obviously are most important.

Influence of Gastritis on Stomach Function

Gastritic and atrophic alterations markedly affect the function of gastric mucosa with regard to for instance, the release of gastrin from the antral (pyloric) glands or the secretion of acid and pepsins from the oxyntic body mucosa [7, 21–23]. In the classification of atrophy into slight, moderate, or severe (total), the atrophy correlates nearly linearly to a decrease in the outputs of acid, pepsins, and gastrin. These influences may understandably influence the physiological homeostasis of the stomach and may also modulate the risk and likelihood of a subject contracting peptic ulcer or other related gastric diseases.

Gastritis may also impair mucosal resistance. Atrophic gastritis affects synthesis, composition, and thickness of the mucous layer at the gastric surface [24]. Although the effects of gastritis or atrophy on the resistance factors are largely unknown and poorly examined, simple diffusion experiments with vital dyes in biopsy specimens from normal or gastritic mucosa indicate a decrease in the integrity of epithelium in gastritis, as well as in the stomach infected by *H. pylori* [25, 26].

Risk of Peptic Ulcer

Cross-sectional studies on gastritis in peptic ulcer patients show a strong relationship between gastritis and coexistent ulcer [27, 29]. Ulcer is rare in patients with a histologically normal stomach, and over 90% of duodenal ulcer (DU) or gastric ulcer (GU) patients seem to have coexistent gastritis, usually in the antrum [27, 28]. B type gastritis shows the strongest links to ulcer diseases. The odds ratio (relative risk) of peptic ulcer (either DU or GU) is approximately 20-fold in subjects with B type gastritis compared with those who have an endoscopically and histologically normal antrum (relative risk = 1).

Gastritis in the body mucosa also determines the ulcer risk, exerting an influence which is opposite to effects of antral gastritis [26, 27]. Irrespective of the presence or grade of antral gastritis, the risk of peptic ulcer is low in patients who show moderate or severe atrophy in the gastric body. In such patients, the relative risk (RR) of peptic ulcer, of DU in particular, is below 1; that is, the risk is even lower than the ulcer risk in subjects with a normal stomach (RR = 1).

Atrophic body gastritis may occur in GU patients in some instances. The progression of body gastritis may modulate the clinical course of the GU disease in these patients. It has been proposed that ulcer may heal spontaneously and recur more infrequently in the presence of atrophic body gastritis and low acid output compared with the behavior of ulcer disease in the presence of nonatrophic body mucosa [29–32].

The intimate association of gastritis with peptic ulcer suggests a causative role of gastritis in ulcer formation. However, the available cross-sectional studies on gastritis in ulcer patients and controls do not justify straightforward conclusions about this causality. The prior role of gastritis in ulcer formation is, however, likely [27, 28]. Our most recent observations support this view: in a follow-up of 388 outpatients without prior evidence of peptic ulcer disease, 31 (8%) patients were recorded to have contracted a symptomatic peptic ulcer within the intervening 10 years. In the initial endoscopy, all except one of these patients showed gastritis in antral biopsies.

The above conclusions mean that some clinically relevant interpretations can be presented with regard to risk and probability of a subject contracting peptic ulcer in gastritis. These interpretations may be based on the presence, type, and grade of gastritis. The development of peptic ulcer can be considered unlikely if the subject has an endoscopically and histologically normal stomach, whereas it may be possible if the subject shows chronic antral gastritis in connection with a nonatrophic body mucosa. This is likely even if the subject has clear-cut B type gastritis (AG in antrum in association with a nonatrophic body mucosa).

Summary

Gastritis is usually a stepwise process that begins as chronic inflammation and gradually progresses to slight, moderate, and severe atrophic gastritis. Gastritis is very common in the general adult population and increases in prevalence with increasing age similarly in males and females. In age groups above 50 years, over 60% of the population shows some degree of gastritis. The atrophic end stages of gastritis in antrum, body, or both, i.e., the B, A, or AB types of gastritis, differ in pathogenesis and relationship to different gastric diseases.

Gastritis is very closely associated with gastric cancer and peptic ulcer diseases. With regard to ulcer diseases, the presence and grade of gastritis can be considered to predict the risk and probability of the subject contracting peptic ulcer. This risk is increased in the presence of gastritis and is estimated to be 20 times higher in subjects with type B gastritis (moderate or severe atrophic gastritis in the antrum in connection with nonatrophic body mucosa) than in persons with a normal stomach.

References

1. Graham DY (1989) *Campylobacter pylori* and peptic ulcer disease. Gastroenterology 96:615–625
2. Schindler R (1947) Gastritis. Grune and Stratton, New York
3. Siurala M, Isokoski M, Varis K, Kekki M (1968) Prevalence of gastritis in a rural population. Scand J Gastroenterol 3:211–223
4. Whitehead R, Truelove SC, Gear MWL (1972) The histological diagnosis of chronic gastritis in fiberoptic biopsy specimens. J Clin Pathol 25:1–11
5. Siurala M, Kivilaakso E, Sipponen P (1984) Gastritis. In: Demling L, Domschke S (eds) Klinische Gastroenterologie, vol I. Thieme, Stuttgart, pp 321–337
6. Ihamäki T, Varis K, Siurala M (1979) Morphological, functional and immunological state of the gastric mucosa in gastric carcinoma families. Comparison with a computer-matched family sample. Scand J Gastroenterol 14:801–812
7. Varis K, Ihamäki T, Härkönen M, Samloff M (1979) Gastric morphology, function and immunology in first-degree relatives of probands with pernicious anaemia and controls. Scand J Gastroenterol 14:129–139
8. Siurala M, Varis K, Kekki M (1980) New aspects on epidemiology, genetics, and dynamics of chronic gastritis. Front Gastrointest Res 6:148–166
9. Kekki M, Siurala M, Varis K, Sipponen P, Sistonen P, Nevanlinna HR (1987) Classification principles and genetics of chronic gastritis. Scand J Gastroenterol 22[Suppl 22]:1–28
10. Varis KA (1971) A family study of chronic gastritis; histological, immunological and functional aspects. Scand J Gastroenterol 6[Suppl 13]:1–70
11. Bonney GE, Elston RC, Correa P, Haenzel W, Zavala DE, Zarama G, Collazos T, Cuello C (1986) Genetic etiology of gastric carcinoma: I. Chronic atrophic gastritis. Genet Epidemiol 3:213–224
12. Correa P (1989) Chronic gastritis. In: Whitehead R (ed) Gastrointestinal and oesophageal pathology. Churchill Livingstone, Edinburgh, pp 402–420

13. Whitehead R (1985) Mucosal biopsy of the gastrointestinal tract. Saunders, London
14. Hovinen E, Kekki M, Kuikka S (1976) A theory of the stochastic dynamic model building for chronic progressive disease process with application to chronic gastritis. J Theor Biol 57:131–152
15. Kekki M, Ihamäki T, Saukkonen M, Varis K (1976) Progression of gastritis at a population level. Scand J Gastroenterol 11:597–601
16. Villako K, Kekki M, Tamm A, Tammur R, Savisaar E, Viirsalu V, Sipponen P (1982) Epidemiology and dynamics of gastritis in a representative sample of an Estonian urban population. Scand J Gastroenterol 17:601–607
17. Tarpila S, Kekki M, Samloff IM, Sipponen P, Siurala M (1983) Morphology and dynamics of gastric mucosa in duodenal ulcer patients and their first-degree relatives. Hepatogastroenterology 30:198–201
18. Kekki M, Sipponen P, Siurala M (1984) Progression of antral and body gastritis in patients with active and healed duodenal ulcer and duodenitis. Scand J Gastroenterol 19:382–388
19. Cheli R, Simon L, Aste H, Figus IA, Nocolo G, Bajtai A, Puntoni R (1980) Atrophic gastritis and intestinal metaplasia in asymptomatic Hungarian and Italian populations. Endoscopy 12:105–108
20. Cabrierés F, Benhamou E, Bigard MA, Bommelaer G, Varannes SB, Colombel F, Florent C, Hostein J, Potet F, Rampel P, Slama A, Tournut R (1989) Study of frequency of clinical, endoscopic, and histological features of chronic gastritis. Gastroenterology 96:A68
21. Siurala M, Sipponen P, Kekki M (1985) Chronic gastritis: dynamic and clinical aspects. Scand J Gastroenterol 20[Suppl 109]:69–79
22. Stadelmann O, Elster K, Stolte M, Miederer SE, Deyhle P, Demling L, Siegenthaler W (1971) The peptic ulcer – histotopographic and functional investigations. Scand J Gastroenterol 6:613–623
23. Jansen JB, Schaardenburg DJ, Lamferts EJ, Boomgaart DM, Lammers CB (1986) Low antral gastrin content and impaired bombesin stimulated gastrin secretion in the intestinal type of gastric cancer. Dig Dis Sci 31[Suppl 10]:4S
24. Domschke W (1981) Normale und gestörte Schleimsekretion des Magens – Therapeutische Maßnahmen. In: Domschke W, Wormsley KG (eds) Magen und Magenkrankheiten, Thieme, Stuttgart, pp 162–174
25. Pristautz H (1984) Evaluation of the epithelial gastric mucosal barrier in gastric diseases using supravital staining of mucosal biopsies. Wien Med Wochenschr 134:1–15
26. Sarosiek J, Slomiany A, Slomiany BL (1988) Evidence for weakening of gastric mucus integrity by *Campylobacter pylori.* Scand J Gastroenterol 23:585–590
27. Sipponen P, Seppälä K, Äärynen M, Kettunen P (1989) Chronic gastritis and gastroduodenal ulcer: a case-control study on risk of coexisting duodenal or gastric ulcer in patients with gastritis. Gut 30:922–929
28. Sipponen P, Äärynen M, Kääriäinen I, Kettunen P, Helske T, Seppälä K (1989) Chronic antral gastritis, Lewis^{a+} phenotype and male sex in predicting coexisting duodenal ulcer. Scand J Gastroenterol 24:581–588
29. Jönsson K-Å, Ström M, Bodemar G, Norrby K (1988) Histologic changes in the gastroduodenal mucosa after long-term medical treatment with cimetidine or parietal cell vagotomy in patients with juxtapyloric ulcer disease. Scand J Gastroenterol 23:433–441
30. Tatsuta M, Iishi H, Ichii M, Noguchi S, Okuda S, Taniguchi H (1985) Chromoendoscopic observations on extension and development of fundal gastritis and intestinal metaplasia. Gastroenterology 88:70–74
31. Maaroos H-I, Salupere V, Uibo R, Kekki M, Sipponen P (1985) Seven-year follow-up of chronic gastritis in gastric ulcer patients. Scand J Gastroenterol 20:198–204
32. Laszewicz W, Gabryelewicz A, Sipponen P, Kekki M, Laxén F, Siurala M (1987) Gastric ulcer and gastritis: results of short term follow-up examinations. Hepatogastroenterology 34:265–268

Gastritis Epidemiology and Natural History

B. J. Marshall

Introduction

Gastritis has been studied intensively over the past 20 years. In older studies, *Helicobacter pylori* was overlooked, the terminology used to describe histological findings was unstandardized, and observations were only occasionally backed up with published illustrations. As a result, it is not always possible to relate new findings to earlier observations, and many of the earlier studies are being duplicated.

Normal Histology

Antrum. The normal gastric antrum has an epithelial cell layer of mucus-secreting cells, folded into glandular structures within a loose lamina propria. Seen under the dissecting microscope, antral mucosa appears similar to the surface of the brain, with "gyri" and "sulci." The mucous epithelial cell layer occupies about one-half the depth of the mucosa, the remaining half being taken up by mucus glands, gastrin cells (G cells), and rare parietal cells. There are few mononuclear cells in the lamina propria and virtually no polymorphonuclear leukocytes.

Body (Corpus). The body mucosa has an epithelial cell layer similar to that of the antrum, but the lamina propria is of course quite different. The mucus epithelial cells are not folded into glands but merely dip into depressions called gastric pits. Several acid-secreting glands connect to each pit. The lamina propria is packed with these glands, so that the only space below the epithelial cell layer is the tissue between the gastric pits. In this region, immediately below the surface epithelium, however, a small amount of loose connective tissue contains room for the migration of inflammatory cells. In the normal body mucosa, as in the antrum, there are few mononuclear cells and virtually no polymorphonuclear leukocytes.

Duodenal Bulb Mucosa. The normal appearance of duodenal bulb mucosa and the transition zone between duodenum and stomach has recently been described by Lawson et al. [1]. The mucosal change between the stomach and duodenum usually occurs at the pylorus where the gastric mucus-secreting epithelium has a scalloped junction with the duodenal intestinal-type mucosa. A 10-mm transition zone exists between gastric- and intestinal-type epithelium. In this zone, microscopic islands of gastric-type epithelium commonly occur within the villous intestinal-type epithelium. Such gastric epithelium has been observed in 90% of duodenal ulcer borders, often in

H. Menge et al. (Eds.)
Helicobacter pylori 1990

association with adherent *H. pylori* [2]. It can therefore be assumed that duodenal ulcers are more likely to occur in this junctional zone than elsewhere in the duodenum. Thus the junction between the stomach and duodenum has three zones:
a) antral-type duodenal mucosa,
b) transitional-type duodenal mucosa, and
c) jejunal-type duodenal mucosa.

Gastritis

Clinical Gastritis and Endoscopic Gastritis. Clinical symptoms and endoscopic findings are mentioned here only to state that they are unreliable indicators of the gastric histology. Clinically apparent gastritis (symptoms) and endoscopic gastritis (red stomach) are often accompanied by histological changes [3], but they may also occur when there is no histological evidence of gastritis. They may be the result of superficial erosion of the epithelium with subsequent bleeding (erosive gastritis) or capillary dilatation (red stomach). The endoscopic appearance may be abnormal if the patient heaves excessively during the endoscopic intubation, if bile refluxes into the stomach, or if undigested food is present. Many investigators have tried to correlate endoscopic findings with the presence of histological gastritis, usually without success [3, 4].

Histologic Gastritis. The histological description of gastritis is by quantification of the various normal and abnormal components of the gastric epithelium. In practice this is done by grading these components for degrees of abnormality, as described by several authors [5–9]. The two major grading systems in use prior to the discovery of *H. pylori* were those of Siurala et al. [7] (Table 1) and Whitehead et al. [14] (Table 2).

Table 1. Histological classification of gastritis – Siurala et al. [7]

Grade 1: normal gastric mucosa	May include a small number of mononuclear cells in the loose connective tissue beneath the epithelial cell layer; may also include small collections of lymphoid cells above the muscularis	
Grade 2: superficial gastritis	Increased plasma cells and lymphocytes just below the surface epithelium but with normal body mucosa glands	Includes specimens with increased mononuclear cells between relatively normal glands and tubules
Grades 3–5: atrophic gastritis	Loss of body mucosa glands, usually with inflammation affecting both superficial and glandular areas of mucosa: – mild, Grade 3 – Moderate, Grade 4 – Severe, Grade 5	This definition is applied regardless of the occurrence of inflammatory changes and metaplasia; in fact, as metaplasia and atrophy increase, inflammation may decrease.

Table 2. Histological classification of gastritis by Whitehead et al. [14]

Mucosal type	Grade of gastritis	Metaplasia
Pyloric (antrum)	Superficial	Pseudopyloric
Body (corpus)	Quiescent	
Cardiac (fundus)	Active	Intestinal
Transitional	Atrophic	
Indeterminate	Mild	
	Moderate	
	Severe	
	Quiescent	
	Active	

The former had the advantage of simplicity, but the classification fitted a model in which gastritis was age related, and intestinal metaplasia was an aspect of the inflammatory process. When the original paper of Siurala et al. [7] is studied carefully, it can be seen that most of the illustrations of gastritis are in fact pictures of *H. pylori*-associated gastritis, mainly of body mucosa, with varying amounts of intestinal metaplasia present. The classification of Whitehead et al. [14] was descriptive and did not assume any progression from one type to another. It correctly separated intestinal metaplasia as a process not always linked to inflammation. Careful examination of the original illustrations of gastritis presented by Whitehead et al. reveals that most of these are also pictures of *H. pylori*-associated gastritis.

The major disadvantage with both of these classification systems is that they do not lend themselves easily to assessment of gastritis healing. This would not be a problem if gastritis were only an accompaniment of aging since reversal would be unlikely. With the discovery of *H. pylori,* however, reversal of at least some components of gastritis are seen to be possible and must be measured. The second disadvantage is that they can not distinguish late type A (pernicious anemia type) gastritis from type B *(H. pylori* type) gastritis. Both systems ignore damage to gastric epithelial cells. Such damage is more likely to be the result of type B *(H. pylori)* gastritis. An additional problem with the classification of Siurala et al. is that it totally ignors the presence or absence of polymorphonuclear leukocytes. Thus, residual mild chronic inflammation from past *H. pylori* infection would be graded only on the amount of atrophy present (see column 2, Table 1) and would receive the same grading as gastritis with epithelial cell damage, polymorphonuclear leukocyte infiltration, and atrophy due to current *H. pylori* infection.

Since the classification of Whitehead et al. [14] distinguished anatomical changes (mucosal type, atrophy, metaplasia) from inflammation, it is more easily modified into a grading scale for gastritis. Warren and Marshall [10] recognized the limitations of the previous methods and adapted Whitehead et al.'s classification. The second column in Whitehead's classification (Table 2) relates to the amount of inflammation in the mucosa. This component can be accurately assessed only when the specimen contains mainly the gastric type of mucosa, either antral or body type. Once this has been replaced by metaplasia, gastritis may no longer be an appropriate term to use, particularly if inflammatory cells are no longer present.

If polymorphonuclear leukocytes, mononuclear cells, and mucus cell damage are graded separately on a scale of 0–3, a combined score of 0 to 9 can be obtained for all biopsies containing gastric epithelium [10]. When graded in this way, any excess of polymorphonuclear leukocytes is likely to be associated with *H. pylori* infection. After the bacterium has been eradicated, past *H. pylori* infection leaves a slight excess of mononuclear cells [11], which may be referred to as inactive or quiescent chronic gastritis [14]. Thus, a grading of 2, 2, and 1 in terms of mononuclear cells, polymorphonuclear leukocytes, and epithelial cell damage (decline in mucin content), respectively, may be followed after therapy by one of 1, 0, and 0; however anatomical changes such as atrophy and intestinal metaplasia remain.

Superficial Gastritis. The location of inflammatory changes may be superficial or spread throughout the mucosa, but there is no clinical difference between the two histological types. In body mucosa, because the lamina propria is already tightly packed with glands, inflammation is superficial, immediately below the luminal epithelial cell layer. Another reason for this superficial distribution may be that the mucus-secreting epithelial cells do not fold down into the lamina propria in the case of body mucosa as they do in that of the antrum. As a result, *H. pylori* attach only to the superficial epithelial cell layer, and the inflammation is located nearby. In antral mucosa the mucus-secreting epithelial cells occupy about 50% of the depth of the mucosa, and *H. pylori* often colonize these deeper areas. Since glandular elements are less prominent in antral mucosa, and there is more space between them, widespread inflammation is less likely to appear as atrophy.

Atrophy and Atrophic Gastritis. Atrophy refers to loss of glandular elements from the mucosa. In body mucosa, atrophy occurs when acid-secreting glands are compressed or destroyed by inflammation within the lamina propria. The terms atrophy and atrophic gastritis were developed as means of describing an appearance seen mainly in body-type acid-secreting mucosa [12]. Studies by Kekki et al. [13] indicate that the usual progression is from superficial gastritis to atrophic gastritis. Examination of the grading system and illustrations of their method [7] indicate that lesser degrees of atrophic gastritis resemble extension of superficial gastritis into the glandular elements. In early biopsy studies blind suction instruments were used which sampled mainly the body of the stomach. In this location any inflammation of the glandular elements must be associated with displacement of glands since there is very little space present between glands. This is perhaps why atrophic gastritis was such an impressive entity to the earlier investigators. Atrophy may also be seen when severe chronic gastritis is present in antral mucosa. According to Whitehead et al. [14], atrophy is best appreciated by reticulin stains which show collapse of glandular supporting elements. Atrophic gastritis is variably associated with intestinal metaplasia (see below).

Intestinal Metaplasia. The replacement of normal gastric epithelium with that of intestinal type (brush border and goblet cell) is referred to as intestinal metaplasia. Although it is often associated with gastritis, this may also occur in the absence of gastritis. Studies by Kekki et al. [13] and Siurala et al. [15] suggest that chronic gastritis, as well as being associated with intestinal metaplasia, may actually hasten its progression. Any process which continually damages normal gastric epithelium may select out an alternate cell type which is resistant to such change. *H. pylori* infection, a disease discriminating against mucus-secreting epithelial cells, may thus favor the growth of intestinal-type epithelium in the stomach.

Confusing Terminology for Gastritis. In some patients intestinal metaplasia of the stomach occurs without apparent inflammation. Intestinal metaplasia may also be present in patchy fashion in patients who have normal histology elsewhere in the stomach, and who also have normal acid secretion (personal observations). In an extreme case, intestinal metaplasia may completely replace the acid-secreting mucosa of the gastric body and thus cause achlorhydria. Such a state is referred to as gastric atrophy. According to Siurala et al. [7], this may also be called severe atrophic gastritis even if inflammation is absent. Such an event is clearly different from the gastric atrophy caused by severe type A (autoimmune) gastritis and from severe long-standing type B *(H. pylori)* gastritis. The term atrophic gastritis should always be further qualified to prevent confusion. In order to assign a probable etiology it is necessary to know the location of the biopsy specimen within the stomach, the proportions of various epithelial cell types present, and the degree of inflammation. If the specimen contains only intestinal epithelium, it may not be possible to determine etiology. In many cases, biopsy specimens from both antrum and body mucosa must be examined to be certain of the type of gastritis.

Type A and Type B Gastritis. Strickland et al. [16] may have been the first to define the two major types of gastritis. They studied 22 patients with histologically established atrophic gastritis and severe hypochlorhydria, 11 of whom had raised serum gastrin and 11 normal serum gastrin. Of those with raised gastrin, nine also had parietal cell antibody. The histological pattern of the hypergastrinemic patients was one of severe body mucosa atrophy in the presence of normal antral histology. In the normogastrinemic patients, the antrum was also abnormal, with at least grade ⅔ gastritis. The authors thus postulated two types of gastritis. Both resulted in atrophic gastritis and gastric atrophy of body mucosa, but in the autoimmune hypergastrinemic type (type A) the antrum remained normal, whereas in the normogastrinemic type (type B) the antrum was severely inflamed (now known to be caused by *H. pylori* infection). Walker et al. [17] examined the prevalence of these two types of gastritis in 1970 in an Australian population and concluded the following.

a) The prevalence of atrophic gastritis was around 25%
b) The prevalence of pernicious anemia was around 1% in a population over the age of 50 years.
c) If the lifetime incidence of gastric carcinoma was 10% for both types of gastritis, type B gastritis was 10–28 times more likely (on a population basis) to cause gastric carcinoma than type A gastritis.

Relationship Between Chronic Gastritis and Intestinal Metaplasia

Before the discovery of *H. pylori,* the topography of gastritis was measured by Hebbel in Minnesota (1949) [18]. By studying the gastric mucosa of persons who died from sudden death he was able to determine the background frequency of the disease in normal persons. Hebbel studied all ages and found that below the age of 50 years, 55% of adults had gastritis whereas above the age of 50 years the prevalence was 87%. Hebbel also noted that 5% of young persons showed intestinal metaplasia of the body or greater curve mucosa in the stomach. In persons over the age of 15 years, 23% showed metaplasia. He concluded that metaplasia is more common in persons with gastritis and is probably the result of long-standing inflammation.

Kreuning et al. in 1978 [19] studied the gastric mucosa of 50 healthy volunteers with a mean age of 33 years and found gastritis to be present in 18 (33%). Antral gastritis was usually confirmed when fundic gastritis was present (16/18). These authors found severe atrophic gastritis in one patient but did not state exactly what definition of this term was used; they may have been describing intestinal metaplasia. In this study, as in most others, antral and fundic gastritis were usually found to coexist if the fundus was abnormal.

In Japan, Tatsuta et al. [20] studied the topography of the gastric mucosa with a chromoendoscopic technique. Their method [21] consisted of filling the patient's stomach with 20000 units of pronase administered orally to digest the mucus layer; the patient was then given an anticholinergic subcutaneously. At endoscopy 20 min later, the mucosa was sprayed with methylene blue to indicate intestinal-type mucosa (unstained by the dye); the stomach was then sprayed with bicarbonate and Congo red, and, finally, pentagastrin was given to make the stomach secrete acid. At this stage, intestinal metaplasia appeared white, gastric, antral type mucosa blue, and acid-secreting mucosa black. Biopsies confirmed the method to be an excellent indicator of epithelial cell type.

After an observation period of 1–3 years, Tatsuta et al. repeated the studies and found that progression of the lesion occurred mainly in subjects with gastritis. In 6.8% of patients extension from antral to fundic gastritis occurred. In subjects with gastric ulcer or merely gastritis, 25% worsened during the study period. In healthy subjects without gastritis, there was little intestinal metaplasia in the initial biopsies, and only two of 44 normal subjects developed metaplasia during the observation period. However, in the groups with gastritis or gastric ulcer, 44.5% developed extension of metaplasia during the study period. In addition, of persons with gastric ulcer who did not have metaplasia initially, 35% developed it by the time of the second examination. The authors concluded that intestinal metaplasia was related to gastritis, and that aging was a less important cause.

Relationship Between Chronic Gastritis and Gastric Metaplasia in the Duodenum

In a study directed more at the lower stomach, Shousha et al. [22] looked at 120 patients with the nonulcer dyspepsia syndrome. Most of the patients were males. The mean age was 50 years. Intestinal metaplasia of the antrum was present in 25% of the males and 34% of the females (not statistically significant). Notably, 89% of those with intestinal metaplasia also had gastritis – 100% of 17 males and 83% of 15 females. Paneth's cells (which secrete lysozyme) were present in the intestinal metaplasia tissue of one-third of the patients. Gastric metaplasia of the duodenal mucosa was present in 54% of males and 21% of the females. If this difference is also present in normal persons, it could explain why duodenal ulcers are more common in males. There was no statistically significant relationship between gastric metaplasia in the duodenum and gastritis or intestinal metaplasia in the stomach. Both types of metaplasia were present in 11 patients, representing 9% of all patients and 16% of those with metaplasia. Thus, a duodenal ulcer type of appearance in the duodenal bulb (gastric metaplasia) was no guarantee that there would not also be a gastric ulcer type of appearance (gastritis and gastric metaplasia) in the stomach. Duodenitis was seen only in patients with gastric metaplasia.

Overview

From the available literature it can be concluded that there are two types of gastritis (Fig. 1), which together account for at least 90% of the abnormalities seen in the gastric mucosa. Type A gastritis is uncommon, affects the body (acid-secreting) mucosa, and is associated with antibodies to parietal cells. This type spares the antrum but may lead to atrophy and metaplasia in the body mucosa. The endpoint of type A gastritis may be gastric atrophy with either intestinal-type mucosa or antral-type

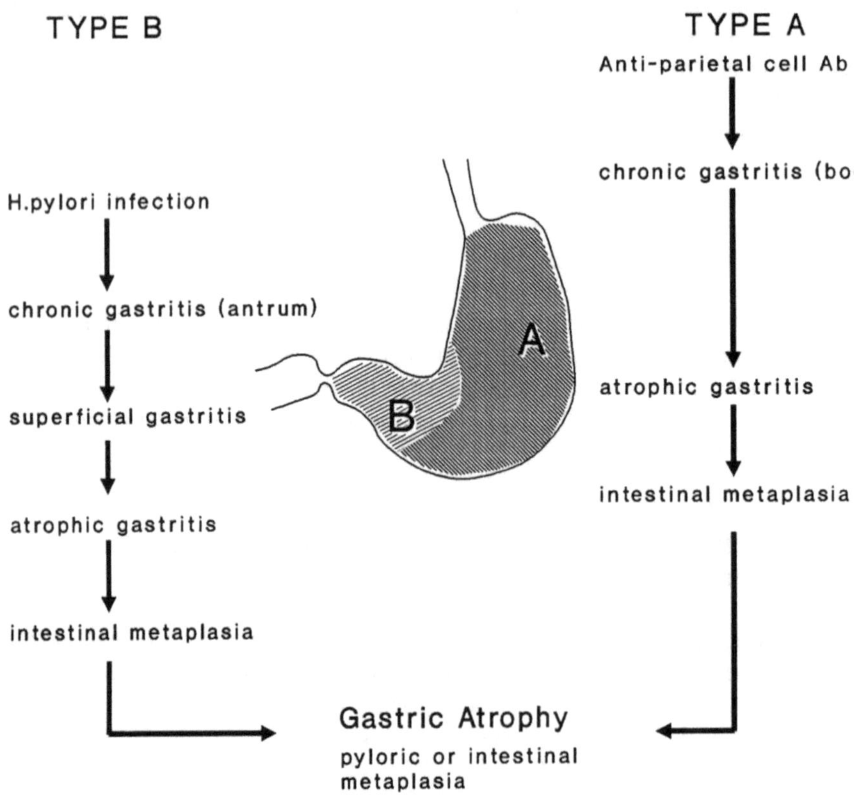

Fig. 1. Natural history of gastritis

mucosa (pyloric metaplasia). Type A gastritis is underrepresented in patients attending gastroenterologists because acid secretion is very low or absent and dyspeptic symptoms are uncommon. The endstage of type A gastritis is gastric atrophy. When gastric atrophy is present, it can be assumed to be type A gastritis when the antrum is relatively uninflamed, parietal cell antibody is present, and serum gastrin is raised.

Type B gastritis is caused by *H. pylori* or in rare cases by other spiral bacteria [23]. Type B gastritis commences as a pangastritis with achlorhydria. At some time, probably 3–12 months after initial infection, acid secretion returns, and gastritis becomes milder and very superficial in the fundus, but remains more extensive in the antrum. The lower density of *H. pylori* in the fundus may result from mucus-secreting epithelial cells being less numerous in the fundus or differing in their ability to attract the organism [24]. With time, type B gastritis extends to involve deeper layers of the antral mucosa and more of the body mucosa. As this occurs, glandular elements are replaced with inflammatory cells. In many cases, mucus-secreting epithelium is replaced by epithelium of the intestinal type. These changes result in the appearance of atrophic gastritis or atrophic gastritis with intestinal metaplasia. Severe, widespread replacement with intestinal epithelium may cause hypochlorhydria and a decreased tendency to form peptic ulcers. The endstage of type B gastritis in body mucosa is very similar to that of type A gastritis, with an appearance of gastric atrophy both endoscopically and histologically.

Type B gastritis is 10–20 times more common than type A gastritis. Both types may predispose to gastric carcinoma. Other types of gastritis are far less common and have not been discussed here. Types A and B gastritis make up 80%–90% of all histological abnormalities seen in gastric mucosa.

References

1. Lawson HH (1988) Definition of gastroduodenal junction in healthy subjects. J Clin Pathol 41:393–396
2. Marshall BJ, Goodwin CS, Warren JR et al. (1988) Prospective double-blind trial of duodenal ulcer relapse after eradication of *Campylobacter pylori*. Lancet 2:1439–1442
3. Goldner FH, Boyce HW (1976) Relationship of bile in the stomach to gastritis. Gastrointestinal endosc 22:197–199
4. Fung WP, Papadimitriou JM, Matz LR (1979) Endoscopic, histological and ultrastructural correlations in chronic gastritis. Am J Gastroenterol 71:269–279
5. Schindler R (1947) Gastritis. Grune and Stratton, New York
6. Magnus HA (1952) Gastritis. In: Jones FH (ed) Modern trends in gastroenterology. Butterworth, London, pp 323–351
7. Siurala M, Isokoski M, Varis K, Kekki M (1968) Prevalence of gastritis in a rural population: bioptic study of patients selected at random. Scand J Gastroenterol 3:211–223
8. McNulty CA, Gearty JC, Crump B, Davis M, Donovan IA, Melikian V, Lister DM, Wise R (1986) *Campylobacter pyloridis* and associated gastritis: investigator blind, placebo controlled trial of bismuth salicylate and erythromycin ethylsuccinate. Br Med J 293(6548):645–649
9. Marshall BJ, Armstrong JA, Francis GJ, Nokes NT, Wee SH (1987) Antibacterial action of bismuth in relation to *Campylobacter pyloridis* colonization and gastritis. Digestion 37:16–30
10. Marshall BJ, Warren JR (1984) Unidentified curved bacilli in the stomach of patients with gastritis and peptic ulceration. Lancet i:1311–1315
11. Borody TJ, Cole P, Noonan S et al. (1989) Recurrence of duodenal ulcer and *Campylobacter pylori* infection after eradication. Med J Aust 151:431–435

12. Joske RA, Finckh ES, Wood IJ (1955) Gastric biopsy: a study of 1000 consecutive successful gastric biopsies. Quart Med J 24:269–294
13. Kekki M, Villako K, Tamm A, Siurala M (1977) Dynamics of antral and fundal gastritis in an Estonian rural population sample. Scand J Gastroenterol 12:321–324
14. Whitehead R, Truelove SC, Gear MWL (1972) The histological diagnosis of chronic gastritis in fibreoptic gastroscope biopsy specimens. J Clin Pathol 25:1–11
15. Siurala M, Sipponen P, Kekki M (1988) *Campylobacter pylori* in a sample of Finnish population: relations to morphology and functions of the gastric mucosa. Gut 29:909–915
16. Strickland RG, Bhathal PS, Korman MG, Hansky J (1971) Serum gastrin and the antral mucosa in atrophic gastritis. Br Med J 4:451–453
17. Walker IR, Strickland RG, Ungar B, Mackay IR (1971) Simple atrophic gastritis and gastric carcinoma. Gut 12:906–911
18. Hebbel R (1949) The topography of chronic gastritis in otherwise normal stomachs. Am J Pathol 25:125
19. Kreuning J, Bosman FT, Kuiper G, vdWal AM, Lindeman J (1978) Gastric and duodenal mucosa in "healthy" individuals: an endoscopic and histopathological study of 50 volunteers. J Clin Pathol 31:69–77
20. Tatsuta M, Iishi H, Okuda S (1986) Location of peptic ulcers in relation to antral and fundal gastritis by chromoendoscopic follow-up examinations. Dig Dis Sci 31:7–11
21. Tatsuta M, Okuda S, Taniguchi H, Tanura H (1979) Relation of intestinal metaplasia to the acid secreting area. Endoscopy 11:166–171
22. Shousha S, Barrison IG, Wafaa E-S, Khan S, Parkins RA (1984) A study of incidence and relationship of intestinal metaplasia of gastric antrum and gastric metaplasia of duodenum in patients with non-ulcer dyspepsia. Dig Dis Sci 29:311–316
23. Dye KR, Marshall BJ, Frierson HF, Guerrant RL, McCallum RW (1990) Ultrastructure of a new spiral organism associated with human gastritis. Am J Pathol (in proof)
24. Lingwood CA, Law H, Pellizzari A, Sherman P, Drumm B (1989) Gastric glycerolipid as a receptor for *Campylobacter pylori*. Lancet 2:238–241

Discussion

Tytgat: Dr. Sipponen, could you clarify the slide on the evolution of gastritis in duodenal ulcer disease? The gastritis score in duodenal ulcer disease was very low. Was that the overall gastritis score or only the score for the body mucosa?

Sipponen: It was the mean score of gastritis in the body mucosa. Duodenal ulcer patients nearly always have gastritis in antrum, but not so often in the gastric body. That is the reason why the mean score was so low.

Graham: Dr. Sipponen, I loved your talk. I am pleased actually to see you present after reading your data all these years. I have one question, or maybe a comment relating to your slide about what happens when each kind of mucosa is compared. I think this still needs modification because a certain percentage of the patients with normal mucosa, say 1% per year will move into the next group and so that group does not remain zero with respect to the development of gastritis. Over 10 years, 10% of these patients will then get the next type of gastritis. This makes the concept a bit more dynamic and the numbers will change only slightly.

Sipponen: We have to remember that gastritis is an age-related disease. The data I showed are from cross-section analysis of an adult population. When a patient gets older he moves from one box to the next.

Talley: I enjoyed your talk. I do have a comment and a question. The comment concerns the Minnesota data. We have recently looked in a small study at the epidemiology of *H. pylori* in asymptomatic volunteers. In contrast to Hebbel in 1949, we found that the prevalence of *H. pylori* gastritis was actually very low even in older persons. Overall only 11% were infected. This is really quite different to some of the other epidemiology studies reported from different parts of the United States. The question I have relates to eosinophils. You did not mention eosinophils in your discussion of gastritis classifications. I am wondering if you think that eosinophils play any role in gastritis.

Marshall: There is evidence in the literature. I believe, that eosinophils were prominent in acute infection and I think in Dr. Graham's description of an acute infection there was a prominent eosinophil infiltration. But I am not sure that there is any new information on it.

Talley: The reason I ask is the following: we have an immunofluorescent technique that measures antibody to eosinophilic major basic protein, which is one of the cationic proteins. We observed that in *H. pylori* gastritis there was a significant increase in eosinophilic infiltration and degranulation compared with all other types of gastritis including specific gastritis and what appears to be the rare *H. pylori*-negative non-specific gastritis.

Veldhuyzen van Zanten: I would like to ask Dr. Sipponen whether he has stratified his data for aspirin, nonsteroidals and smoking, and if so, whether he found any differences.

Sipponen: Unfortunately, we have no data concerning smoking and dietary habits in relation to gastritis, but as far as I have understood from the literature, smoking is not related to gastritis. It is related to peptic ulcer disease and is a very heavy risk factor in this connection, but it is unrelated to gastritis.

Stadelmann: Dr. Sipponen, in your material, patients with AB gastritis had a high degree of atrophy. We examined by stepwise biopsies more than 50 patients with gastric carcinoma of the intestinal type related to the definition of *Lauren* and found in more than 50% AB gastritis, mostly with a low degree of atrophy. Only one patient presented the pernicious type of gastritis. Can you give any comment on this?

Sipponen: In our grading and in our classification, we call gastritis AB type if there is at least a moderate degree of it in both antrum and body.

Stadelmann: I think that in the 1960s and 1970s atrophic gastritis was overdiagnosed because we mostly grouped together all degrees of atrophy.

Tytgat: Dr. Sipponen, did you have a chance to restudy all that material looking for the prevalence of *Helicobacter* organisms according to the various stages of gastritis and atrophy.

Sipponen: Yes, we did do this. The data were published in "Gut" last year. We analyzed the frequency of *Helicobacter* as stained by the Giemsa method. The frequency of *Helicobacter pylori* in our population was very, very high and it went hand by hand with gastritis.

Marshall: Dr. Sipponen, in your recent paper published in "Gut", you found that when there was atrophic gastritis in the body, not as much *H. pylori* was seen. But from reading the paper, I could not tell whether the atrophic gastritis patients had intestinal metaplasia. If you sampled intestinal I-type mucosa in the biopsy, the sensitivity of your biopsy for *H. pylori* would be decreased.

Sipponen: Yes, you are right. Usually the patients also have intestinal metaplasia. And you are also right about the sensitivity.

Petersen: Tomorrow I am going to show you my slides which suggest not only that acute gastritis may heal but also that chronic gastritis may heal. A question to both speakers: Do you consider healing possible?

Marshall: I have observed that chronic gastritis can virtually heal but atrophic gastritis does not heal.

Sipponen: Yes, I agree. We have performed studies with bismuth compounds where we have morphometrically counted the cells in the mucosa. The acute gastritis component disappears immediately when the bacteria have been eradicated. There seems to be also some effect on chronic gastritis, but the effect is very small as Prof. Tytgat has shown.

Epidemiology of Gastric Metaplasia

J.I. Wyatt

Introduction

The presence of abnormally located gastric-type epithelium in the duodenum was first described in experimental animals during healing of surgically induced mucosal defects [1] and subsequently in response to acid injury [2]. In 1962 James [3] reported the important observation of extensive gastric metaplasia in a patient with hyperacidity, subsequently confirmed in another report from Parrish and Rawlins [4]. Like instances of metaplastic change in general, this gastric metaplasia was attributed to chronic damage to the mucosa of the duodenum, and appeared to have little significance beyond that as a histological marker of mucosal injury.

The specificity of the attachment of *Helicobacter pylori* to gastric epithelial cells [5–8] gives a new significance to gastric metaplasia. We have shown that peptic duodenitis – the pattern of inflammation seen at ulcer margins and in a proportion of patients with non-ulcer dyspepsia – occurs specifically in those patients with two risk factors: gastric metaplasia of more than a minimal degree, and *Helicobacter*-associated gastritis [8]. We hypothesized that this is due to duodenal infection by *H. pylori* and that the impairment of mucosal defences associated with the consequent active inflammation would render the mucosa susceptible to ulceration [9]. On the basis of this model, factors involved with duodenal ulcer pathogenesis may act at one or more of three points: (a) influence the development of gastric metaplasia, (b) affect a person's susceptibility to chronic *H. pylori* infection, or (c) further damage the already inflamed duodenal mucosa to cause ulceration. As yet we know little of the factors determining susceptibility to *H. pylori,* but only a minority of patients with *H. pylori* ever develop duodenal ulcers. In this review, the factors which have been associated with gastric metaplasia in the duodenum are described.

Gastric Metaplasia and Heterotopia

Gastric epithelium is easily recognized in the duodenum (Fig. 1); it ranges in extent from small foci of a few adjacent cells up to extensive areas which may cover the whole of the biopsy surface. The terms "metaplasia" and "heterotopia" have both been used to describe gastric epithelium in the duodenum, "heterotopia" where the change in mucosal histology affects glandular cells as well as the surface epithelium [7, 10–13]. These two terms have become confused, but have different implications. "Heterotopia" refers to the presence of fully developed but abnormally located tissue, and is now generally used by pathologists to imply a developmental origin of the abnormally

H. Menge et al. (Eds.)
Helicobacter pylori 1990

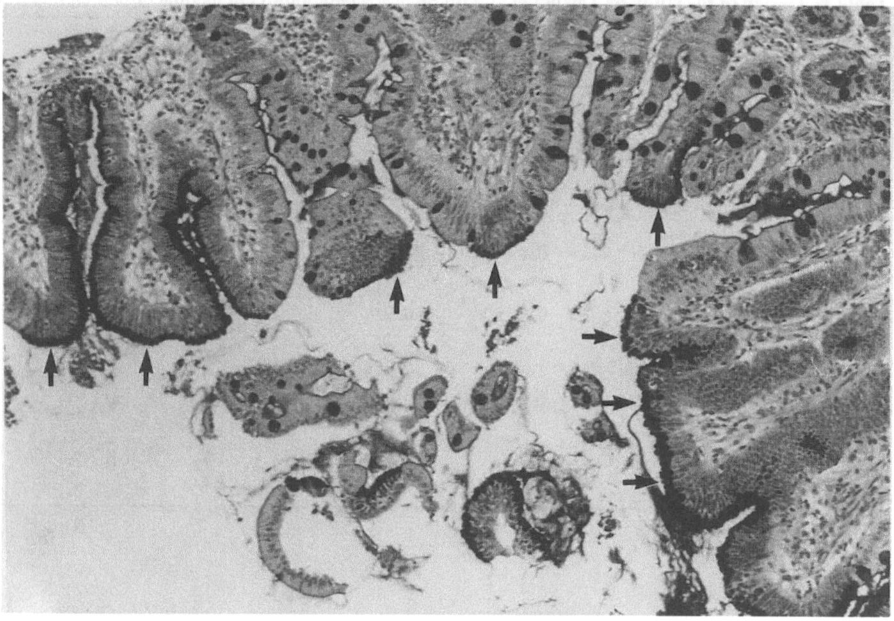

Fig. 1. Duodenal mucosa showing foci of gastric metaplasia, mainly on the tips of the villi. Alcian blue/PAS stain

located tissue, e.g., heterotopic pancreatic and gastric tissue in Meckel's diverticula, and adrenal or splenic tissue in the gonad [14]. Metaplasia on the other hand defines an acquired change from one fully differentiated tissue to another due to the divergent differentiation of proliferating adult tissues [14]. The metaplastic process, for example intestinal metaplasia in the stomach, or metaplastic gastric and intestinal mucosa in Barrett's oesophagus, results in the presence of all cell lineages normally present in the prototype tissue, e.g. absorptive, goblet and Paneth's cells in intestinal metaplasia in the stomach, implying an early change in differentiation pathways, perhaps at the stem cell level. Carrick et al. [13] found that parietal and chief cells may be present in biopsies in which the surface epithelial change to gastric epithelium was most extensive, and Hara et al. [15] have shown that the neuroendocrine cells in gastric metaplasia contain gastrin and somatostatin, i.e. are of a type associated with gastric mucosa. We therefore consider that "metaplasia" is synonymous with "acquired heterotopia". We suggest that the term "heterotopia" should not be used unqualified, but be restricted to examples of congenital heterotopia of developmental origin, which in the duodenum form a rare cause of endoscopic nodularity not associated with duodenal ulceration or inflammation [8, 16]. Areas of metaplasia may contain foveolar type cells only or more rarely fundic gland cells [7] and we agree with Wolff [17] that a partial replication of fundic mucosa distinguishes an acquired (i.e. metaplastic) change in the duodenum from a congenital heterotopia.

Table 1. Design of the study by Tatsuta et al. [19] on gastric metaplasia in healing duodenal mucosa

Group	1	2	3	4
n	35	40	40	40
Gastric installation	0.9% NaCl	5% NaOH	5% NaOH	5% NaOH
Operation	Sham	Sham	Sham	Truncal vagotomy
Postoperative	Placebo	Placebo	Tetragastrin	–
Week 10				
Percentage rats with gastric metaplasia	0	23	59	0
Mean % villi with gastric metaplasia	0	0.6	2.4	0
Week 35				
Percentage rats with gastric metaplasia	0	0	15	0
Mean % villi with gastric metaplasia	0	0	1.5	0

Animal Models of Gastric Metaplasia

Gastric metaplasia develops in the duodenum of experimental animals following mechanical trauma [1] or in response to hyperacidity [2, 18]. Brunner's glands appear to be necessary for the metaplasia to occur [18], and their presence gives some protection to the mucosa against ulceration. In a recent detailed study by Tatsuta, chemical injury was applied to the mucosa of rats treated with tetragastrin and vagotomy (study design shown in Table 1). The extent and duration of gastric metaplasia was increased in the tetragastrin-treated group, and metaplasia was apparently prevented by vagotomy [19]; metaplasia was a feature of mucosal healing in the presence of acid.

Prevalence and Distribution

Gastric metaplasia occurs as a patchy change in the duodenum; it is not identifiable by endoscopy, and its frequency in biopsies is therefore subject to sampling error. There is little information on the frequency of gastric metaplasia in the normal population, since most surveys of duodenal histology have inevitably been on patients with upper gastrointestinal symptoms. The two exceptions to this are the study of Fitzgibbons et al., who found gastric metaplasia in single biopsies from 22% of 116 volunteers [20] and that by Kreuning et al. [21], who examined 6 duodenal biopsies from each of 50 healthy volunteers, and found gastric metaplasia in 64% of subjects. We have studied 4 circumferential biopsies from 62 dyspeptic patients and found a similar overall prevalence of gastric metaplasia of 56% [22]. There was no significant difference in frequency of gastric metaplasia in any particular site in the proximal duodenum, and 63% of the patients with gastric metaplasia would have been detected by a single anterior biopsy. Not surprisingly, the more extensive the gastric metaplasia was in individual biopsies, the more likely it was to be present at several sites. One biopsy detected about two-thirds of subjects who had gastric metaplasia by multiple biopsy, and the position of the biopsy did not significantly affect these results. A single random biopsy can therefore justifiably be used to study the epidemiological associations of gastric metaplasia.

Age

We found gastric metaplasia in a single duodenal biopsy from 7% of 58 children (age < 20 years), compared with 33% of adults [22]. This significant difference confirms that gastric metaplasia is indeed a metaplastic process, and does not reflect a congenitally more distal location of the gastroduodenal junction as suggested by Marshall et al. [23]. Among adult subjects, there is no evidence that gastric metaplasia varies with age [22, 24].

Sex

Studies have found gastric metaplasia to be more common in males [16, 22], females [25], or similar between the two sexes [11, 24]. In general, a male predominance was found in the larger studies, including our own [22].

Smoking, Non-steroidal Anti-inflammatory agents (NSAIDs) and Alcohol Consumption

All of these factors have been linked with duodenal ulceration. As potentially injurious to the mucosa, they may theoretically be associated with gastric metaplasia. However, no group has been able to find any association between smoking [13, 16, 22] or NSAIDs [13, 22] and gastric metaplasia. A high usage of NSAIDs has been reported in duodenal ulcer patients who are *H. pylori* negative [22, 26], suggesting these agents may induce mucosal ulceration directly by a mechanism distinct from any interaction with *H. pylori* and gastric metaplasia. Smoking appears to delay healing or cause early relapse of duodenal ulcer, and therefore may affect the integrity of already damaged mucosa.

Whether or not alcohol increases gastric metaplasia is controversial – an association has been found by some groups [16, 27], but not recently by ourselves or Carrick [13]. The dose of alcohol may be a factor, since the series studied by Lev included very heavy drinkers.

Duodenal Bulb Acidity

There is strong experimental evidence from animal studies of gastric metaplasia, most notably that of Tatsuta [19], that acid may promote and perpetuate gastric metaplasia.

The relationship between acidity and gastric metaplasia in humans is less clearly established, and accurate methods for measuring the pH at the duodenal surface [28, 29] have not been used in any study related to mucosal histology. Some studies have found a qualitative (but not quantitative) association between acid output and gastric metaplasia [11, 24, 30]. Acid output tends to be greater in males than females [31], and logistic regression analysis has suggested that the significant association of gastric metaplasia with male sex was dependent on differences in fasting gastric juice pH between the sexes [22].

Gastritis and *H. pylori*

Shousha et al. [32] found an inverse relationship between the presence of intestinal metaplasia in the stomach and gastric metaplasia in the duodenum. We have not observed gastric metaplasia in the duodenum of any patients with intestinal metaplasia in the body mucosa [22] – an observation attributable to the reduced acid output associated with such atrophic gastritis. Apart from this, the overall prevalence of gastric metaplasia is the same in patients with or without gastritis or *H. pylori* [20] (32% vs. 34%) [22]. However, when the extent of the gastric metaplasia was estimated, we found that the proportion of the biopsy surface showing gastric metaplasia was significantly greater in duodenal specimens from patients who were *H. pylori* positive, with a compensatory reduction in number of biopsies showing only slight degrees of gastric metaplasia. This suggests that while gastritis is not related to the "initiation" of the metaplasia, it is associated with a progression of the change to involve a greater area. This observation is further considered in the next section in the light of duodenal inflammation itself as a cause of metaplasia.

Duodenal Inflammation and Ulceration

Gastric metaplasia occurs both as an isolated change in otherwise normal duodenal mucosa [21] and in association with active duodenitis [32, 33]. Several groups have found a quantitative relationship between the extent of gastric metaplasia and the degree of inflammation [16, 22, 34]. In a detailed quantitative study, Jenkins et al. [34] demonstrated a significant association between gastric metaplasia and both mucosal polymorph infiltration and villous blunting; there was no association with the degree of mononuclear cell infiltration. This suggests that epithelial damage associated with active inflammation heals by gastric metaplasia. Either *Helicobacter*-associated duodenal inflammation, or duodenal acidity, or a combination of both factors could be the chronic insult leading to persistence of the metaplasia. Functional acid secretion by parietal cells in the duodenum in patients with more extensive gastric metaplasia, recently demonstrated by Carrick et al. [13], would be a further local stimulus to increasing metaplasia. Follow-up of the changes in gastric metaplasia in patients treated by acid-reducing measures or *H. pylori* eradication will clarify the contribution of each factor to the dynamics of gastric metaplasia.

The most widespread gastric metaplasia is encountered in duodenal ulcer patients, particularly at the margin of the ulcer [35–37], suggesting that duodenal ulcer occurs when there is breakdown of the inflamed mucosa. After healing of the ulcer, the gastric metaplasia and duodenitis persist at the site of the ulcer scar [35], which may therefore explain the tendency for ulcer recurrence to occur at the same site. That the gastric metaplasia is reversible is shown by its reduced frequency after duodenal ulcer surgery [8].

Summary

The evidence currently available suggests that there are two stages in the development of gastric metaplasia in the duodenum. Factors which are qualitatively associated with the presence but not the extent of gastric metaplasia are adulthood, male sex, and gastric acid secretion. These factors may influence the "initiation" of the switch to gastric-type differentiation by cells in the duodenal mucosa. Other factors – the presence of *H. pylori* in the stomach, of active inflammation in the duodenum, rare cases of severe hyperchlorhydria in patients with Zollinger-Ellison syndrome, and possibly heavy alcohol consumption – show a quantitative association with the extent of the gastric metaplasia, indicating their involvement in the progression to a more widespread metaplastic change. Duodenal ulcer may then develop on this background of duodenitis, resulting from a progressive increase in the severity of inflammation at this site.

References

1. Florey HW, Harding HE (1935) The healing of artificial defects of the duodenal mucosa. J Pathol 40:211–218
2. Florey HW, Jennings MA, Jennings DA et al. (1939) The reactions of the intestine of the pig to gastric juice. J Pathol Bacteriol 49:105–123
3. James AH (1963) Gastric epithelium in the duodenum of a patient with gastric hyperacidity. 2nd World Congress of Gastroenterology, Munich, 1962, II:540–543
4. Parrish JA, Rawlins DC (1965) Intestinal mucosa in Zollinger-Ellison syndrome. Gut 6:286–289
5. Thomas JM, Poynter D, Gooding C et al. (1984) Gastric spiral bacteria. Lancet II:100
6. Blaser MJ (1987) Gastric *Campylobacter*-like organisms, gastritis, and peptic ulcer disease. Gastroenterology 93:371–383
7. Graham DY (1989) *Campylobacter pylori* and peptic ulcer disease. Gastroenterol 96:615–625
8. Wyatt JI, Rathbone BJ, Dixon MF et al. (1987) *Campylobacter pyloridis* and acid-induced gastric metaplasia in the pathogenesis of duodenitis. J Clin Pathol 40:841–848
9. Wyatt JI, Rathbone BJ, Dixon MF et al. *Campylobacter pylori* and development of duodenal ulcer. Lancet I:118–119
10. Hoedemaker PJ (1970) Heterotopic gastric mucosa in the duodenum. Digestion 3:165–173
11. Johansen AA, Hansen OH (1973) Heterotopic gastric epithelium in the duodenum and its correlation to gastric disease an acid level. Acta Pathol Microbiol Immunol Scand [A]81:676–680
12. Johansen A (1974) Enzyme histochemical investigation of heterotopic gastric epithelium in the duodenum. Acta Pathol Microbiol Immunol Scand [A] 82:613–617
13. Carrick J, Lee A, Hazell S, Ralston M, Daskalopoulos G (1989) *Campylobacter pylori*, duodenal ulcer, and gastric metaplasia: possible role of functional heterotopic tissue in ulcerogenesis. Gut 30:790–797
14. Willis RA (1968) Some unusual heterotopias. Br Med J 3:267–272
15. Hara M, Harasawa S, Tani N, Miwa T, Tsutsumi Y (1988) Gastric metaplasia in duodenal ulcer; histochemical considerations of its pathophysiological significance. Acta Pathol Jpn 38:1011–1018

16. Shousha S, Spiller RC, Parkins RA (1983) The endoscopically abnormal duodenum in patients with dyspepsia: biopsy findings in 60 cases. Histopathology 7:23–34
17. Wolff M (1971) Heterotopic gastric epithelium in the rectum. A report of three new cases with a review of 87 cases of gastric heterotopia in the alimentary canal. Am J Clin Pathol 55:604–616
18. Rhodes J (1964) Experimental production of gastric epithelium in the duodenum. Gut 5:454–458
19. Tatsuta M, Ishii H, Yamamura H, Yamamoto R, Taniguchi H (1989) Enhancement by tetragastrin of experimental induction of gastric epithelium in the duodenum. Gut 30:311–315
20. Fitzgibbons PL, Dooley CP, Cohen H, Appleman MD (1988) Prevalence of gastric metaplasia, inflammation, and *Campylobacter pylori* in the duodenum of members of a normal population. Am J Clin Pathol 90:711–714
21. Kreuning J, Bosman FT, Kuiper G et al. (1978) Gastric and duodenal mucosa in 'healthy' individuals. An endoscopic and histopathological study of 50 volunteers. J. Clin Pathol 31:69–77
22. Wyatt JI, Rathbone BJ, Sobala G et al. The prevalence and distribution of gastric epithelium in the duodenum and its relationship to *Campylobacter pylori* and inflammation. J Chifathol (in press)
23. Marshall BJ, McGechie DB, Rogers PA, Glancy RJ (1985) Pyloric campylobacter infection and gastroduodenal disease. Med J Aust 142:439–444
24. Patrick WJA, Denham D, Forrest APM (1974) Mucous change in the human duodenum; a light and electron microscopic study and correlation. Gut 15:767–776
25. James AH (1964) Gastric epithelium in the duodenum. Gut 5:285
26. Johnson BJ, Reed PI, Ali MH (1986) *Campylobacter* like organisms in duodenal and antral endoscopic biopsies; relationship to inflammation. Gut 27:1132–1137
27. Lev R, Thomas E, Paul FF (1980) Pathological and histomorphometric study of the effects of alcohol on the human duodenum. Digestion 20:207–213
28. McCloy RF, Greenberg GR, Baron JH (1984) Duodenal pH in health and duodenal ulcer disease: effect of a meal, Coca-Cola, smoking and cimetidine. Gut 25:386–392
29. Quigley AMM, Turnberg LA (1987) pH of the microclimate lining human gastric and duodenal mucosa in vivo. Gastroenterology 92:1876–1884
30. Rodes J, Evans KT, Lawrie JH et al. (1968) Coarse mucosal folds in the duodenum. Q J Med 37:151–169
31. Feldman M, Richardson G (1986) Total 24 hour gastric acid secretion in patients with duodenal ulcer. Gastroenterology 90:540–544
32. Shousha S, Harrison IG, El-Sayeed W et al. (1984) A study of incidence and relationship of intestinal metaplasia of gastric antrum and gastric metaplasia of duodenum in patients with non ulcer dyspepsia. Dig Dis Sci 29:311–316
33. Whitehead R (1985) Mucosal biopsy of the gastrointestinal tract. 3rd edn. Saunders, Philadelphia, pp 128–135
34. Jenkins D, Goodall A, Gillett FR et al. (1985) Defining duodenitis; quantitative histological study of mucosal responses and their correlations. J Clin Pathol 38:1119–1126
35. Fullman H, Van Deventer G, Schneidman D et al. (1985) 'Healed' duodenal ulcers are histologically ill. Gastroenterology 88:1390A
36. Caselli M Bovolenta MER, Aleotti A et al. (1988) Epithelial morphology of duodenal bulb and *Campylobacter*-like organisms. J Submicrosc Cytol 20:237–242
37. Marshall BJ, Waren JR, Blincow ED et al. (1988) Prospective double-blind trial of duodenal ulcer relapse after eradication of *Campylobacter pylori*. Lancet II: 1437–1441

Discussion

Graham: As always it was a lovely presentation. I do worry about your single biopsies. As one who looks in duodenums every day, I think, there is a tremendous opportunity for selection bias, as when the abnormal duodenum with duodenitis is to be biopsied. If high magnification videoendoscopy is used I think probably 100% of people show gastric metaplasia as little bumps of metaplastic or heterotopic mucosa.

Wyatt: I agree with you, unfortunately we can't examine the whole duodenum of all these patients histologically, which might well show metaplasia in a high proportion. By taking one uniformly positioned duodenal biopsy from a group of patients who fall in the different clinical groups and different epidemiological categories we are comparing the "point prevalence" of metaplasia in a representative site in the duodenum. This is clearly sufficient to show changes between the groups, which are meaningful and which are statistically significant.

Malfertheiner: I was going to ask Dr. Wyatt, but after Dr. Graham's comment, I would rather ask him about the endoscopic magnification and detection of gastric metaplasia. I think, there is a difference in what we are talking about. Dr. Wyatt presented data on gastric metaplasia and Dr. Graham is now talking about gastric heterotopia. Dr. Wyatt, how often do you really find gastric heterotopia in your specimen? I would never agree that by endoscopic magnification we could see gastric metaplasia. By using more specific techniques including histochemistry we see that there is quite a range of metaplastic cells including transitional cells where you only have the loss of alkaline phosphatase. Dr. Wyatt, could you clarify the ideas about gastric metaplasia?

Wyatt: I will give you my ideas about it, it is a very confusing area because the terminology is confused. The term "heterotopia" is used to indicate the presence of parietal and chief cells in the duodenal mucosa. This covers two different situations. One is a congenital heterotopia, which is a congenitally misplaced group of parietal and chief gastric body cells. This occurs in various places in the gastrointestinal tract, the best example, of course, is Meckel's diverticulum. Congenital heterotopia may be a rare cause of duodenal nodularity, which in my experience is seen in less than 2% of duodenal biopsies while this figure may be higher if we had Dr. Graham's high magnification videoendoscopy. Our data are similar to other published studies of duodenal biopsies. "Acquired heterotopia" is synonymous with metaplasia, which may contain other elements of gastric mucosa (endocrine cells, parietal cells) in addition to surface foveolar cells. Such acquired heterotopia or metaplasia is seen adjacent to duodenal ulcers and histologically it rarely has the regular, organized appearance of the glandular components that characterize congenital heterotopia.

Epidemiology of Duodenal Ulcer Disease

D. G. Colin-Jones

Introduction

It is clear from the literature that many factors contribute to peptic ulcer disease. Whilst it would be convenient to attribute the aetiology of duodenal ulcer (DU) to a single factor, there can be little doubt that this is a multifactorial disease, not only for a given population, but also probably for the majority of individual sufferers. This makes it particularly difficult to unravel the different factors, so that the aetiology of peptic ulcer disease is still unknown. It follows that, although treatments are improving dramatically, ignorance of its aetiology has meant that it is still impossible to cure peptic ulcer disease.

Helicobacter pylori is a good example of this problem. There is overwhelming evidence from the literature that *H. pylori* is found in almost all cases of duodenal ulcer disease [1], and this holds true around the world wherever the association has been tested. However, there is a steady increase with age in the prevalence of *H. pylori* in the population as a whole, rising to over 50% after middle age in the West. Since the point prevalence of peptic ulcer disease is well below this figure, clearly the two are not simply related.

If *H. pylori* has a major role in peptic ulcer disease it has to fit with a number of observed features in the epidemiology of DU. It is, for example, known that DU was relatively uncommon in the last century in Britain, with gastric ulcer being the dominant peptic ulcer lesion and occurring especially in young women [2]. In the twentieth century the incidence of DU has been steadily rising, especially between the wars, but now the evidence is pointing towards a steady fall over the past 20 years or so. There is, of course, no information about the prevalence of *H. pylori* during these past two centuries, but its widespread distribution throughout the human population makes it relatively unlikely to have changed greatly in its prevalence over the past two centuries.

Problems with Epidemiological Data on Peptic Ulcer Disease

Accurate Diagnosis of Duodenal Ulcer

The only accurate means of diagnosing DU is by endoscopy. Although a barium meal can show changes in the duodenal cap, it is unable to distinguish scarring from active ulceration in the majority of cases. It is therefore much less accurate than endoscopy. However, upper gastrointestinal endoscopy is an invasive procedure, carrying a low

H. Menge et al. (Eds.)
Helicobacter pylori 1990

but appreciable morbidity. Widespread use as a screening tool is therefore not feasible, although in special situations such as in Japan, where screening for gastric cancer is commonplace, there is some information [3]. Sadly, symptomatic questionnaires are notoriously unreliable. Nonulcer dyspepsia, which in many cases can mimic DU and is much more common than ulcer disease, probably results in an overestimate of the prevalence of the DU, despite some ulcers being asymptomatic.

Asymptomatic Duodenal Ulcer

There is a significant number of cases of duodenal ulcer which are virtually asymptomatic. This has been demonstrated in Japan [4], where 456 cases of DU were found out of a population of 10605 male office workers over the age of 40 years (4.3%), who were being screened for gastric cancer. These cases were subsequently followed up every 6 months for 2 years, 276 completing the study, of which 169 had ulcer craters and 107 had scars. After 2 years of follow-up, 21% of the ulcers had healed whilst 29% of the scars had relapsed. Overall, about two-thirds of the cases showed no change over the period of the study, that is to say that either the ulcer crater remained or the scar did not break down. The remaining one-third clearly demonstrated waxing and waning, with the ulcer spontaneously healing and relapsing. Cigarette smoking was a particularly adverse feature in the behaviour of the DU. It is worth noting that 6 patients of the 276 had a GI haemorrhage from their ulcer during the 2-year period under study. With such figures it is clear that a significant number of ulcers will be overlooked if an epidemiological survey uses symptoms as one of its main criteria for study.

Complications

Several studies have used complication and hospitalization rates to study the disease [5–8]. It is largely based on these figures that the stated overall fall in the incidence of ulcer disease is based. This, however, is not without its dangers in interpretation. Treatments have changed, which have resulted in a substantial reduction in hospitalization for uncomplicated ulcer disease, and very probably a reduction in referral for specialist opinion, with self-medication and General Practitioner treatment without a firm diagnosis always being made. Furthermore, it seems unlikely that the percentage of ulcers which develop a complication will remain uniform and fixed over years. It may well be higher for certain subgroups (such as the very elderly), and we have no idea whether it has changed over the decades. Maintenance treatment with H2-receptor antagonists may well reduce the complication rate appreciably, which will further complicate assessment of ulcer prevalence if this treatment pattern becomes widespread. Nonetheless, that having been said, the most important aspect of ulcer disease is any complication, as it may lead to death, and so it is essential that such epidemiological work is undertaken.

Factors Related to Prevalence of Duodenal Ulcer

Age

In the western world there is evidence of a steady rise in the prevalence of ulcer disease with age, peaking for DU at around 45–55 years of age in men. The same holds true for the Japanese [3] and northern India [9]. However, breaking the age groups down by age, Walt et al. [6] have shown a steady rise in the DU perforation rates amongst women, with a low rise for the 65–74 age group but a dramatic one for the over 75s. For men there is the expected steady fall in DU perforations under the age of 74 but there is a rise in elderly men over the age of 75. These workers attribute such a change to a striking rise in the prescription of non-steroidal anti-inflammatory drugs (NSAIDs) in recent years. Data in the undeveloped world are less clear cut, but there is evidence that the peak age for DU is mid-thirties in West Africa and also large parts of India, about a decade earlier than in the West [10]. The peak may be below 30 in Ethopia [11].

Race

Much information on the prevalence of DU in different racial groups has to be qualified by the limitations of the data – as discussed above. Nonetheless, important clues regarding aetiology might well come from such information. The high prevalence of DU in Scotland and of GU in Japan [3] are well documented, but these are very different populations. In Singapore, a small island country, there are wide differences in the prevalence of DU and GU, with both being much more common in the Chinese than the Malay population, the Indian population coming in between [12]. This does not seem to be due to smoking, NSAID use or alcohol.

Sex Ratio

As mentioned above, in the western world there seems to be a steady decline in the ratio of male to female. Formerly this was greater than 2 to 1, but in the older population this approaches unity – notably in the United States [8]. In northern India the ratio is 2 to 1 [9].

Smoking

Smoking is a major factor in peptic ulcer disease, being strongly correlated with incidence. Kurata has produced impressive data correlating the male DU deaths with the percentage of the adult male population smoking [8]. This relationship holds true for female smokers although less dramatically. This must provide a major clue but as yet it is uncertain as to how smoking produces its adverse effects.

Diet

The general population has always held dear that diet has been crucial in the development of their ulcer. In recent years, however, only a few lone researchers have followed up that belief, but their efforts are increasingly being rewarded by data suggesting that diet is indeed relevant. Epidemiological data collected by Tovey in both Africa and India show that there is a low prevalence of ulcer disease where there is a low rainfall and the population tends to eat unrefined foods, especially unrefined wheat or maize [10, 13]. This has been supported by clinical trial, where, although a high-fibre diet did not heal ulcers more effectively than a low-fibre diet, it did reduce the relapse rate [14]. A lipid-soluble factor has been derived from a number of foods, which experimentally confers protection against peptic ulcer. This lipid factor could well be linoleic acid, which is a precursor for arachidonic acid, itself important in the prostaglandin synthetic chain. Linoleic acid has been shown to increase the prostaglandin content of the mucosa and to diminish acid secretion [15]. Diet therefore seems to be highly relevant to DU prevalence, but, bearing in mind the infinite variety of diets eaten around the world, makes evaluation all the more difficult [16].

Aspirin and NSAIDs

There is convincing evidence that aspirin is associated with the development of GU, and that NSAIDs have a number of adverse gastrointestinal effects, including an increased frequency of haemorrhage [17]. A rise in prescription rate for these drugs has been held responsible for the rise in perforation and haemorrhage rates from ulcers in elderly women. Many of them have powerful effects on prostaglandin metabolism, which could interfere with mucosal protection.

Other factors

A number of factors such as alcohol, stress and caffeine consumption have all been incriminated but have been insufficiently investigated to allow a firm opinion to be formed. In addition there are internal factors such as gastric acid and pepsin secretion which may have both acquired and inherited components.

Helicobacter pylori

As mentioned in the introduction, *H. pylori* is found in the gastric antrum of almost all DU patients. But its high prevalence in many populations makes determination of its role very difficult – one method of evaluation might be to look at the prevalence of *H. pylori* and DU in parallel, both for the whole population and for different age groups. Studies in the third world suggest that it is commonly found through all populations, although the Australian aborigine seems to have a low prevalence of both *H. pylori* and, interestingly, of DU as well [18]. In central Africa [19], which appears to have a high prevalence of DU, there is also a high prevalence of *H. pylori* (75% of a group of patients investigated for dyspeptic symptoms); similar results have been observed in Kenya [20]. In Ghana, where there is probably a high prevalence of DU [10], almost all the dyspeptic patients were found to have been infected with *H. pylori* [21]. Other reports from Africa (to be published) are consistent in demonstrating a high prevalence of histological gastritis and carriage of *H. pylori* in areas where DU is common and at a much younger age than in the West. Studies from China also give similar, if less dramatic, figures – in a population with an average age of 41 there was a 59% positivity of *H. pylori* [22]. It would appear that *H. pylori* colonization occurs at an earlier age in some populations (notably Africa) and bearing in mind that such epidemiological studies as we do have on the peak incidence of DU, the occurrence of both *H. pylori* and DU in a younger age group in parts of Africa and India is of great importance.

Conclusion

Duodenal ulcer disease results from a number of factors, not all of which are known, and probably with different emphases in each individual. *H. pylori* appears to be found in almost all populations studied and may well be more common in some groups (for example parts of Africa) which have a greater than average prevalence of DU. This supports the concept that *H. pylori* has a role in DU but may well do so by enabling other factors to exert their influence.

Acknowledgement. I am indebted to Mr. Frank Tovey, Basingstoke, UK for advice and much recent data, especially from Africa.

References

1. Graham DY (1989) *Campylobacter pylori* and peptic ulcer disease. Gastroenterology 96:615–625
2. Bonnevie O (1985) Changing demographics of peptic ulcer disease. Dig Dis Sci 30:(11) 85–145
3. Kawai K, Shirakawa K, Misaki F, Hayashi K, Watanabe Y (1989) Natural history and epidemiologic studies of peptic ulcer disease in Japan. Gastroenterology 96:581–585
4. Kaneko E, Ooi S, Ito G, Honda N (1989) Natural history of duodenal ulcer detected by the gastric mass surveys in men over 40 years of age. Scand J Gastroenterol 24:165–170
5. Somerville K, Faulkner G, Langman M (1986) Non-steroidal anti-inflammatory drugs and bleeding peptic ulcer. Lancet I:462–464
6. Walt R, Katschinski B, Logan R, Ashley J, Langman M (1986) Rising frequency of ulcer perforation in elderly people in the United Kingdom. Lancet I: 489–492
7. Kurata JH, Honda GD, Frankl H (1982) Hospitalization and mortality rates for peptic ulcers: a comparison of a large health maintenance organization and United States data. Gastroenterology 83:1008–1016
8. Kurata JH (1989) Ulcer epidemiology: an overview and proposed research framework. Gastroenterology 96:569–580
9. Khuroo MS, Mahajan R, Zargar SA, Javid G, Munshi S (1989) Prevalence of peptic ulcer in India: an endoscopic and epidemiological study in urban Kashmir. Gut 30:930–934
10. Tovey FI, Tunstall M (1975) Duodenal ulcer in black populations in Africa south of the Sahara. Gut 16:564–576
11. Mengistu M (1983) The diagnosis of duodenal ulcer and non-ulcer dyspepsia on the basis of symptomatology. In: Tsega E (ed) Non-ulcer dyspepsia and gastritis in Ethiopia. Addis Ababa, Research and Publications Office, Addis Ababa University

12. Kang JY, Labrooy SJ, Yap I, Guan R, Lim K, Math V, Tay HH (1987) Racial differences in peptic ulcer frequency in Singapore. J Gastroent Hepatology 2:239–244
13. Tovey FI (1979) Peptic ulcer in India and Bangladesh. Gut 20:329–347
14. Rydning A, Berstad A (1986) Dietary fibre and peptic ulcer. Scand J Gastroenterol 21:1–5
15. Grant HW, Palmer KR, Kelly RW, Wilson NH (1988) Dietary linoleic acid, gastric acid, and prostaglandin secretion. Gastroenterology 94:955–959
16. Tovey FI, Jayaraj AP, Lewin MR, Clark CG (1989) Diet: its role in the genesis of peptic ulceration. Dig Dis 7:309–323
17. Langman MJS (1987) The changing face of peptic ulceration. Scand J Gastroenterol 22 [Suppl. 136]:37–40
18. Dwyer B, Nanxiong S, Kaldor J et al (1988) Antibody response to *Campylobacter pylori* in an ethnic group lacking peptic ulceration. Scand J Infect Dis 20:63–68
19. Rouvroy D, Bogaerts J, Nsengium O, Omar M (1987) *Campylobacter pylori,* gastritis and peptic ulcer disease in central Africa. Br Med J 295:1174
20. Lachlan GW, Gilmour H, Jass JJ (1988) *Campylobacter* in Central Africa. Br Med J 296:66
21. Wyatt JI, De Caestecker J, Rathbone BJ, Heatley RV (1987) *Campylobacter pyloridis* in tropical Africa. Gut 28:A1409
22. Yong-yi Feng, Ya Wang (1988) *Campylobacter pylori* in patients with gastritis, peptic ulcer, and carcinoma of the stomach in Lanzhou, China. Lancet I:1055–1056

Discussion

Mégraud: May I ask you what you think about the cohort phenomenon to explain the variation of prevalence of ulcers in developed countries.

Colin-Jones: I must say I am not persuaded by this theory. The concept is of a cohort born around the turn of the century the members of which were particularly vulnerable. If they were perhaps especially exposed to *H. pylori* at an early age, would that make them more vulnerable? We really don't know the answer. I must say, I am not persuaded that a cohort phenomenon is convincing. I think if you look around the world, the varying prevalence of ulcer disease means that there must be other factors coming in. So, I am not persuaded.

Tytgat: On which arguments did you base your summary slide? Can you explain that?

Colin-Jones: I was trying to draw together the several threads that I had tried to highlight in my talk, the influence of different factors, such as smoking, anti-inflammatory drugs, and diet. I was not trying to conclude that *H. pylori* has no place in ulcer disease but rather to draw attention to one or two aspects to explain the work particularly in relation to the third world.

Tytgat: I accept that there are many confounding factors, for example the world consumption of antibiotics which you did not plot on the screen. There are a lot of other factors involved. On which arguments did you base your statement that there was no correlation between *H. pylori* and the prevalence of peptic ulcer disease?

Colin-Jones: I will accept entirely that there is no positive or strong negative information. I was taking from the data that I presented, if you like, a lack of influence that I was able to see in terms of what we know about the epidemiology of ulcer disease and *H. pylori.*

Petersen: There are a lot of things which influence the prevalence of peptic ulcer disease apart from *H. pylori.* You mentioned a North-South problem, and from my knowledge about conditions in the Northern part in Norway, it is a really tough environment there. One must only consider the light situation: the long dark period may explain a lot.

Colin-Jones: Speaking as an Englishman, the high prevalence of ulcer disease in Scotland is entirely due to whisky, but truly that is an incomplete assessment!

Section 3

Theoretical Site of *Helicobacter pylori* Therapy

In Vitro Sensitivity of *Helicobacter pylori*

C. A. M. McNulty

Initial results indicate that long-term eradication of this *Helicobacter pylori* will be difficult. The first step in the search for a suitable antimicrobial to treat any infection is to determine the in vitro susceptibility of the causative organism to suitable therapeutic agents. The activity of a range of antimicrobial agents against *H. pylori* was first determined at neutral pH (Table 1) [1, 2]. *H. pylori* is highly sensitive to most of the β-lactams except cefsulodin. Penicillin, ampicillin, cefuroxime, cefoxitin and cephalexin have minimum inhibitory concentrations for 90% of organisms (MIC 90s) of less than 0.5 mg/litre; flucloxacillin and aztreonam are moderately active with MIC 90s of 2 mg/litre. The macrolides and quinolones except amifloxacin (MIC 90, 4 mg/litre) also have good activity with MIC 90s of less than 0.5 mg/litre. Other agents that have good in vitro activity include nitrofurantoin (MIC 90, 0.5 mg/litre), gentamicin (MIC 90, 0.25 mg/litre), tetracycline (MIC 90, 0.25 mg/litre) and rifampicin (MIC 90, 1 mg/litre). Metronidazole has moderate activity but about 25% of strains are less sensitive [3]. *H. pylori* is resistant to vancomycin, cefsulodin, trimethoprim and the sulphonamides.

Table 1. Minimum inhibitory concentration values of 21 antimicrobial agents for isolates of *Helicobacter pylori*

Antimicrobial agents	No. of isolates tested	MIC 50	MIC (mg/litre) MIC 90	Range
Penicillin	70	0.015	0.03	0.002 - 0.06
Ampicillin	97	0.015	0.03	≤ 0.008 - 0.12
Flucloxacillin	50	1	2	0.12 - 8
Cefuroxime	97	≤ 0.12	≤ 0.12	≤ 0.12 - 0.25
Cefoxitin	70	0.12	0.12	0.015 - 0.5
Cephalexin	97	≤ 0.25	0.5	≤ 0.25 - 2
Cefsulodin	97	16	> 16	8 > - 16
Aztreonam	97	1	2	0.06 - 8
Erythromycin	97	0.12	0.25	≤ 0.008 - 0.25
Azithromycin	97	0.12	0.25	0.03 - 0.5
Ciprofloxacin	97	0.25	0.5	≤ 0.06 - 0.5
Ofloxacin	21	0.12	0.25	0.12 - 0.25
Amifloxacin	97	4	4	1 - 8
Nitrofurantoin	96	0.5	0.5	≤ 0.03 - 0.5
Furazolidone	96	0.12	0.25	≤ 0.03 - 0.5
Gentamicin	70	0.12	0.25	0.06 - 0.5
Tetracycline	70	0.25	0.25	0.12 - 1
Rifampicin	21	0.5	1	0.12 - 2

H. Menge et al. (Eds.)
Helicobacter pylori 1990

Many of the antimicrobial agents with in vitro activity have now been used in clinical trials. Amoxycillin and nitrofurantoin give short-term clearance in over 80% of patients [4, 5]. However, erythromycin ethyl succinate [6], josamycin [7], cephalexin, ofloxacin [8] and ciprofloxacin [9, 10] are usually ineffective. The differences in clinical success may be related to reduced activity in the acid environs of the gastric mucosa or subinhibitory concentrations attained by the antimicrobials in the gastric crypts and mucus where *H. pylori* is found. To investigate this, McNulty et al. have performed MICs at different pH values [11] and have determined antimicrobial gastric mucosal concentrations [12].

In the pH study the activities of various antimicrobial agents were determined over the range of pH 5–8, at which *H. pylori* survives (Table 2). Penicillin was tenfold less active at the most acidic pH than at neutral pH, with an MIC 90 of 0.5 mg/litre at pH 5–6, and 0.03 mg/litre at pH 7.5. There was a tenfold change in the activity of ampicillin and a 16-fold change in the activity of cephalexin between pH 5.5 and 7.5 (ampicillin 0.5–0.06 mg/litre, cephalexin 32–2 mg/litre). Cephalexin was 50-fold less active than ampicillin. The erythromycin base was 100-fold less active at pH 5.5 (MIC 90, 8 mg/litre) than at pH 7.5 (MIC 90, 0.12 mg/litre). Ciprofloxacin was more than tenfold less active at pH 5 (MIC 90, 2 mg/litre) than at pH 7.5 (MIC 90, 0.12 mg/litre). There was little change in the activity of tetracycline and nitrofurantoin; metronidazole and bismuth were unaffected by pH.

Table 2. Effect of pH on the activity of antimicrobial agents against *H. pylori*

Agent	No. of isolates	MIC 90 mg/litre		
		pH 7.5	pH 6.0	pH 5.5
Penicillin	20	0.03	0.5	0.5
Ampicillin	20	0.06	0.25	0.5
Cephalexin	17	2	16	32
Erythromycin	20	0.06	2	8
Ciprofloxacin	20	0.12	0.5	2
Tetracycline	17	0.12	0.25	0.5
Nitrofurantoin	17	1	2	2
Metronidazole[a]	15	2	2	2
Bismuth subcitrate	17	16	8	–

[a] Sensitive isolates

In the gastric mucosal concentration study 500 mg amoxycillin (Bencard), pivampicillin (Leo), erythromycin ethylsuccinate suspension (Abbott), erythromycin stearate (Abbott) and ciprofloxacin (Bayer) were administered orally with 30 ml water. During the endoscopic examination biopsy specimens were taken from the pyloric area for mucosal concentrations. Except in one patient who received erythromycin stearate, all the antimicrobials attained gastric mucosal concentrations above their MIC 90 values at neutral pH for *Helicobacter pylori* (Table 3). Excluding three high results (21.7, 36.7, 40.9 mg/litre) the two macrolide preparations attained consistent concentrations in the range 1.2–5.2 mg/kg; these concentrations are subinhibitory at pH 5.5. The range of concentrations with amoxycillin was great: from 15 mg/kg at 91

Table 3. Antimicrobial concentrations in the gastric mucosa after a 500-mg oral dose

Agent	No. of patients	Range of concentrations in the gastric mucosa in mg/kg (time)			
Erythromycin ethylsuccinate	8	1.8	(85 min)	-	40.9 (53 min)
Erythromycin stearate	10	< 0.7	(60 min)	-	36.7 (42 min)
Amoxycillin	7	15	(91 min)	-	322 (100 min)
Pivampicillin	5	47.5	(120 min)	-	209 (49 min)
Ciprofloxacin	14	35	(357 min)	-	1239 (84 min)

min to > 322 mg/kg at 100 min; the lowest concentration was still 30 times the MIC 90 of ampicillin at pH 5.5 (0.5 mg/litre). Pivampicillin attained ampicillin gastric mucosal concentrations of between 47.5 and 209 mg/kg; the lowest gastric mucosal concentration attained at 2 h (47.5 mg/kg) was 100 times the MIC 90 at pH 5.5. Ciprofloxacin attained the highest concentration (range < 1.5–1762 mg/kg); the concentrations were more than 15 times the MIC 90 at pH 5.5 (2 mg/ml) until 6 h after the dose.

These two studies help to explain why some antimicrobial agents are ineffective in vivo. The pH of the stomach contents, and mucus and crypts where *H. pylori* colonizes, is probably the most important factor that affects drug activity. A significant pH gradient was observed by Quigley and Turnberg [13] from the gastric lumen (body pH 1.82, antral pH 3.52). through the gastric mucus to the mucosa (body pH 5.5, antral pH 5.42). *H. pylori* also produces urease that releases high concentrations of ammonium ions, which may raise the pH in the immediate environs of the bacterium that survives between pH 5 and 8 [14].

The theoretical attainable concentration of drugs in an area such as the gastric mucus with a different pH to serum may be calculated from a modification of the Henderson-Hasselbalch equation.

$$\text{Ratio } \frac{\text{tissue conc}}{\text{plasma conc}} \text{ (basic drug)} = \frac{1 + 10^{\text{pKa} - \text{pH (tissue)}}}{1 + 10^{\text{pKa} - \text{pH (plasma)}}}$$

The un-ionized portion of basic drugs such as erythromycin and ciprofloxacin will diffuse into the acidic gastric secretions. At the lower pH of the gastric mucus "trapping" in the ionized form occurs and concentrations in excess of those in the serum are achieved. Although active concentration may occur because of this increasing ionization, this will result in decreased activity – as confirmed by the pH studies.

Erythromycin activity was affected more than any of the other antimicrobials tested by the reduction in pH; the inhibitory concentrations required below pH 6 were not attained in the gastric mucosal study and would explain the lack of clinical efficacy. Cephalexin was also much less active, with an MIC 90 of 32 mg/litre at pH 6.5; although gastric mucosal concentrations have not been measured its lack of clinical efficacy is probably also due to subinhibitory concentrations in the gastric crypts.

Although the MIC of ciprofloxacin was much higher at pH 5 (2 mg/litre) than at neutral pH, gastric mucosal concentrations were inhibitory up to 6 h after the oral dose. Thus decreased activity at more acidic pH cannot completely explain the lack of clinical efficacy of the quinolones.

The activity of metronidazole was unaffected by pH but acquired resistance has been reported with this and the other nitroimidazoles. Nitroimidazoles are therefore unsuitable single agents for the treatment of *H. pylori* infection and although combination with a bismuth salt reduces the development of resistance there are probably better alternative agents available.

Amoxycillin and ampicillin are probably more successful in vivo because, although they achieved lower gastric mucus concentrations than ciprofloxacin, they are less ionized at low pH and retain good activity at acidic pH. They are both amphoteric drugs and at pH 3–6 are present as zwitterions, which have a lower partition coefficient than the other ionic species. This may decrease tissue penetration, but may increase penetration into mucus, which is 90% water [15]. Acquired resistance of *H. pylori* to ampicillin or amoxycillin has so far not been described.

The presence of other drugs in the stomach may alter the pH, or bind to the preparation. Fleming et al. [16] showed that ciprofloxacin binds to polyvalent cations, and therefore absorption is reduced by antacids containing Mg^{2+} and Al^{3+}; this could be problematical in dyspeptic patients, who often take these medications. This drug interaction must also be taken into account for any other antimicrobial that forms complexes with divalent or trivalent cations (e.g., tetracycline). The addition of an acid-reducing drug to a treatment regimen would increase the gastric mucus pH and may lead to greater activity of the antimicrobial. In a small study involving 25 patients, Unge et al. found that a combination of omeprazole and amoxycillin was much more effective than either agent given alone [17]. This combination may be very useful in the treatment of duodenal ulcers.

In conclusion, despite good in vitro activity many antimicrobials are unsuitable for the treatment of *H. pylori* infection. The activity of the macrolides, aminoglycosides, quinolones and cephalexin are greatly affected by pH and the quinolones and imidazoles are subject to acquired resistance; these agents are usually ineffective in vivo. The bismuth salts, penicillins, nitrofurantoin and tetracycline retain good activity at acid pH, and in vivo bismuth subcitrate [5], bismuth subsalicylate [6], amoxycillin [18] and nitrofurantoin [4] give good short-term results. Relapse is a major problem and combination treatment with drugs exhibiting different modes of action, especially three rather than two antimicrobial agents, achieve much better long-term results. Current triple therapy is probably an interim solution for patients with severe symptoms until the "ideal" antimicrobial is found – however, this may take some time.

References

1. Goodwin CS, Blake P, Blincow E (1986) The minimum inhibitory and bactericidal concentrations of antibiotics and anti-ulcer agents against *Campylobacter pyloridis*. J Antimicrob Chemother 17:309–314
2. McNulty CAM, Dent JC (1988) Susceptibility of *Campylobacter pylori* to twenty-one antimicrobial agents. Eur J Clin Microbiol 7:566–569
3. McNulty CAM, Dent JC, Wise R (1985) Susceptibility of clinical isolates of *Campylobacter pyloridis* to 11 antimicrobial agents. Antimicrob Agents Chemother 28:837–838
4. Gilman R, Leon-Barua R, Ramirez-Ramos A et al. (1986) Efficacy of nitrofurantoin in the treatment of antral gastritis associated with *Campylobacter pyloridis*. Gastroenterology 92:1405

5. Rauws EAJ, Langenberg W, Houthoff HJ, Zanen HC, Tytgat GNJ (1988) *Campylobacter pyloridis*-associated chronic active antral gastritis. A prospective study of its prevalence and the effects of antibacterial and antiulcer treatment. Gastroenterology 94:33–40
6. McNulty CAM, Gearty JC, Crump B, Davis M, Donovan IA, Melikian V et al. (1986) *Campylobacter pyloridis* and associated gastritis: investigator blind, placebo controlled trial of bismuth salicylate and erythromycin ethylsuccinate. Br J Med 293:645–649
7. Lamouliatte H, Megraud F, De Mascarel A et al. (1987) Placebo-controlled trial of josamycin in *Campylobacter pyloridis* associated gastritis. In: Kaijser B, Falsen E (eds) Campylobacter IV. Goterna, Goteborg, Sweden, pp 388–389
8. Glupczynski Y, Labbe M, Burette A et al. (1987) Treatment failure of ofloxacin in *Campylobacter pylori* infection. Lancet I:1096
9. Hirschl AM, Stanek G, Rotter ML et al. (1988) *Campylobacter pyloridis:* frequency of occurrence, serology and susceptibility to antibiotics and ulcer-drugs. In: Kaijser B, Falsen E (eds) Campylobacter IV. Goterna, Goteborg, Sweden, pp 363–364
10. Stone JW, Wise R, Donovan IA et al. (1988) Failure of ciprofloxacin to eradicate *Campylobacter pylori* from the stomach. J Antimicrob Chemother 22:92–93
11. McNulty CAM (1989) Bacteriological and pharmacological basis for the treatment of *Campylobacter pylori* infection. In: Rathbone BJ, Heatley RV (eds) *Campylobacter pylori* and gastroduodenal disease. Blackwell, Oxford, pp 209–216
12. McNulty CAM, Dent JC, Ford GA et al. (1989) Inhibitory antimicrobial concentrations against *Campylobacter pylori* in gastric mucosa. J Antimicrob Chemother 22:729–738
13. Quigley EMM, Turnberg LA (1987) pH of the microclimate lining human gastric and duodenal mucosa in vivo. Gastroenterology 92:1876–1884
14. Hazell SL, Lee A (1985) The adaption of motile strains of *Campylobacter pyloridis* in gastric mucus and their association with gastric epithelial intercellular spaces abstract. Proceedings of the Third International Workshop on *Campylobacter* infections Ottawa, July 1985, Abstract No. 115:189–191
15. Allen A (1981) Structure and function of gastrointestinal mucus. In: Johnson LR (ed) Physiology of the gastrointestinal tract. Raven, New York, 617–639
16. Fleming LW, Moreland TA, Stewart WK et al. (1986) Ciprofloxacin and antacids. Lancet II:294
17. Unge P, Gad A, Gnarpe H, Olsson J (1989) Does omeprazole improve antimicrobial therapy directed towards gastric *Campylobacter pylori* in patients with enteral gastritis. Proceedings of the Vth international workshop on *Campylobacter* infections. Mexico, Fuerta Vallarta, Febr 1989
18. Glupczynski Y, Burette A, Labbe M et al. (1988) *Campylobacter pylori*-associated gastritis: a double blind placebo-controlled trial with amoxycillin. Am J Gastroenterol 83:265–372

Discussion

Marshall: From the data you showed for erythromycin, it seems possible to treat a patient with omeprazole and then achieve satisfactory levels of erythromycin in the gastric mucosa without it being effected by an acid pH. Have you tried that? I think David Graham was the first one to suggest this therapy.

McNulty: I have not used a combination of omeprazole and erythromycin, but its use is nonsensical to me as erythromycin is so easily inactivated by acid. Further details from Jury Glupczynski later on resistance to erythromycin and the use of omeprazole will stress my point. I think that it is reasonable to give omeprazole with one of the β-lactams that achieve higher mucosal concentrations as used by Unge.

Glupczynski: It's more of a comment than a question about your determination of metronidazole in gastric mucus. You have to take into account that there are several metabolites of metronidazole. Some of them have high antibacterial activity. Did you measure the concentration of these metabolites when reporting the levels of metronidazole in gastric mucus?

McNulty: We measured the metronidazole concentrations by HPLC. Unfortunately I do not know whether the metabolites were looked at. I will need to check on this.

Graham: I agree that this type of experiment is important because it tells us which antibiotics not to use, but they are not going to tell us which ones to use. Your statement that pH 5.5 is the lowest pH is quite arbitrary since it holds true only for the mucus of the body of the stomach. As you know the mean pH in a duodenal ulcer patient throughout the day is 1.4. We give all of our drugs with meals, as this greatly prolongs the antibiotic's or other drug's residence in the stomach and probably changes the amount of drug in the gastric mucus. All your studies are done in fasting patients and may give us entirely different results. We all know that today the research has been what I call brute force, i. e., you give your patients drugs and you see what happens. The best combinations may or may not ultimately be predicted by your experiments. These experiments may be important later to help us refine the combinations that someone discovers by the brute force method.

McNulty: I'll agree with that comment in general that these studies are not the ideal method but I do think the results give you a pointer and explain why certain antimicrobials do not work. For example, I think the metronidazole results are particularly interesting as the low concentrations attained may facilitate the production of acquired resistance. I agree that our studies were in fasting patients and that food does alter the pH. However, *H. pylori* does not divide rapidly below pH 5. Although many of these antimicrobials are stable at a lower pH in the stomach, it is their activity where *H. pylori* is found that is important.

Graham: Maybe. But it has clearly been shown that in nutrient media *H. pylori* does survive for more than an hour at pH 3. I honestly do not know what environment it tries to escape into, or which ones it can live in. You know our results have been relatively good with antibiotics that are not the highest ones on your list.

Tytgat: Dr. McNulty, is there good evidence, and if so, for which antimicrobials, that there is indeed absorption in humans through the stomach mucosa or secretion via the stomach mucosa into the gastric lumen?

McNulty: The absorption of radio labelled pivampicillin through the gastric mucosa has been looked at in animals and shown to be 30%.

Graham: What about secretion?

McNulty: I do not know of any work on this but radio labelling of an antimicrobial may help this.

Tytgat: Is the rumour true that metronidazole is actively secreted via the gastric mucosa, as was mentioned in the literature?

McNulty: The results from our metronidazole data suggest that secretion may take place. Less than 1 hour after the dose, the concentrations were initially high. Between 2 and 4 h they dropped to between 2 and 8 mg/kg. Between 2 and 4 h later they rose again. This suggested that there was penetration or secretion from the systemic circulation.

Veldhuyzen van Zanten: Did you find interference with your HPLC measurement of metronidazole by bile, which is a problem that we have encountered? And secondly, have you looked at gradients between the systemic circulation and the mucosa level that you found?

McNulty: We did look at serum concentrations. For most of the antimicrobials, the gastric mucosal concentrations were higher than serum concentrations, they then reached a balance and then the gastric mucosal concentrations decreased.

Veldhuyzen van Zanten: Can you comment on the HPLC measurements of metronidazole?

McNulty: I can't comment on that, I'm sorry.

Ober: Dr. McNulty, you suggested that bismuth salts act by chelating antimicrobials and that the kinetic behaviour in the mucus or in the mucosa is therefore changed in a way that their therapeutic effect is increased.

McNulty: Yes, I think it is a possibility, with some antimicrobials.

Ober: But bismuth salts act by themselves even without antimicrobials.

McNulty: Oh yes.

Ober: So this could just be part of the mechanism of action.

McNulty: Oh absolutely, I am not saying that bismuth salts do not have in vitro activity against the antimicrobial. All I am saying is that the reason why a combination of a bismuth salt and tetracycline may be more effective is that the tetracycline may be targeted to the site of *H. pylori* colonisation.

Tytgat: Is there any evidence that, if you combine bismuth and tetracycline, the tetracycline concentration within the mucus gel or within the biopsy is higher than when you administer tetracycline alone?

McNulty: No, we haven't done that specific study. However when given with a bismuth salt, the absorption of doxycycline was decreased by 50%, suggesting chelation in the gastric mucosa.

Tytgat: Was this perhaps because you thereby create an insoluble complex which cannot be absorbed?

McNulty: Yes, it's a possibility. I am putting forward a hypothesis. That needs to be proven.

Slomiany: It seems to me in your considerations of the ideal drug for eradication of *Helicobacter pylori* that you are missing one important element, that is the measurement of the drug hydrophobicity. Considering the fact that the surface of the gastric mucosa is quite hydrophobic, it would be appropriate to look for the agents which are easily permeable through the mucus blanket. Therefore, one should look for drugs which display hydrophobic, lipophilic properties.

McNulty: I would agree. That's why I said that the physiochemical properties of the drug are important.

Antibiotic Concentrations in Gastric Mucosa: The Guinea Pig Model

T. U. Westblom and D. E. Duriex

Introduction

The discovery of *Helicobacter pylori* has initiated a new approach to the treatment of gastritis and peptic ulcer disease. Effective therapy may need the inclusion of an antimicrobial agent aimed at eradicating the organism. However, several clinical studies have shown poor outcome of antibiotics in spite of good in vitro susceptibilities [1–7]. It has become clear that one can not extrapolate known pharmacokinetics and in vitro data of antibiotics and apply them directly to the treatment of *H. pylori* infection. The stomach represents a unique environment in the host. The presence of hydrochloric acid in the stomach necessitates the use of antibiotics that can retain activity at a pH much lower than what is seen in other parts of the body. They would also have to be secreted back into the stomach in order to achieve sustained tissue levels. In order to investigate which antibiotics might fulfill these criteria, an animal model for antibiotic concentrations in gastric mucosa has been developed [8].

Description of the Model

Adult Hilltop guinea pigs, weighing 700–800 g, are fasted overnight before being injected with the antibiotic to be tested. All antibiotics are given IM in the thigh using a volume that does not exceed 1 ml. The animals are subsequently sacrificed at fixed intervals of 1, 2, 4, 6, and 8 h using IP nembutal. At the time of sacrifice, blood is collected for serum antibiotic levels. The sample is allowed to clot and the serum is separated by centrifugation. The stomach is then removed and cut through a plane going through larger and lesser curvatures. Sterile phosphate-buffered saline (PBS) is used to gently rinse the stomach should any remaining food particles be observed. One half of the stomach is then pinned to a wax plate and the mucosa removed for measurement of antibiotic concentrations. A glass slide is used to gently scrape the mucosal surface, separating its top layer from the deeper mucosal and muscularis layer. All mucosa removed in this fashion is weighed before being mixed with 3 cc PBS in a glass tissue grinder. The homogenate produced is centrifuged in a refrigerated ultracentrifuge at 3000 rpm for 10 min. The supernatant is finally filtered through a 0.2 μm filter for sterility. Antibiotic concentrations are measured on both serum and tissue samples using HPLC technique.

H. Menge et al. (Eds.)
Helicobacter pylori 1990

Clindamycin

The first antibiotic to be evaluated with this model was clindamycin. On theoretical grounds it seemed that this antibiotic had the potential for obtaining high tissue levels. It is known to be stable at low pH and is able to concentrate down a pH gradient [9]. The closely related antibiotic lincomycin has been studied by Saggers and Lawson with regard to its penetration into hog gastric mucus [10]. Not only did it have excellent in vitro penetration into mucus, but it remained biologically active in the mucus, in contrast to other antibiotics such as the tetracyclines, which were inactivated through chelation. Furthermore, in vitro studies had shown good susceptibility data, clindamycin having a MIC_{50} of 0.5 µg/ml and a MIC_{90} of 2.0 µg/ml against *H. pylori* [11].

We found that clindamycin was indeed transported into the gastric mucosa in vivo and that tissue concentrations exceeded serum levels [12]. This was most apparent in the period 6–8 h after injection when serum levels fell to subtherapeutic levels, but the corresponding mucosal levels were almost 100-fold higher (Fig. 1). At all times the MIC_{90} against *H. pylori* was exceeded in the mucosa.

Ciprofloxacin

A dose of 20 mg/kg ciprofloxacin IM produced serum levels which peaked at 0.57 µg/ml at 1 h after injection [13]. These levels were slightly lower than what is commonly seen in human volunteers following a 500 mg dose [14]. Ciprofloxacin did not show the

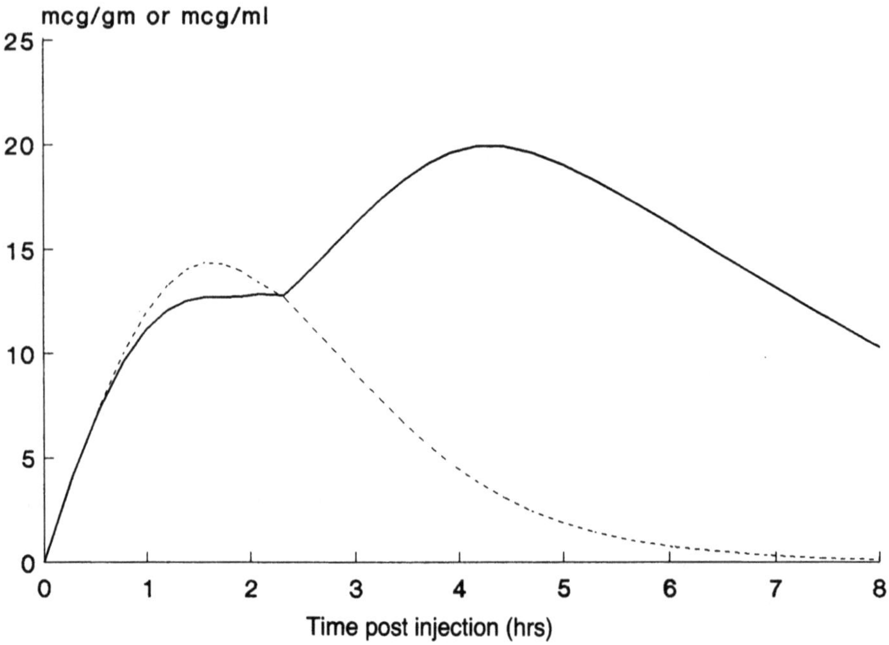

Fig. 1. Serum *(dotted line)* and gastric tissue *(continuous line)* concentrations of clindamycin following 100 mg/kg IM injection. Mucosal levels show a characteristic bimodal curve

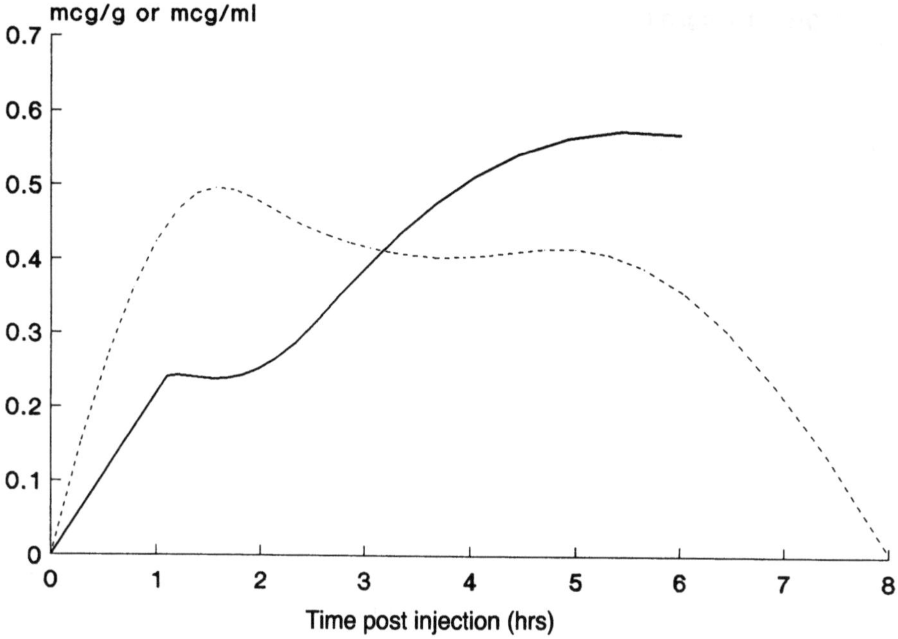

Fig. 2. Serum *(dotted line)* and gastric tissue *(continuous line)* concentrations of ciprofloxacin following 20 mg/kg IM injection. Mucosal levels show a bimodal curve

same pharmacokinetic features as clindamycin. Where clindamycin had shown mucosa levels to be higher than serum levels, ciprofloxacin tissue levels seemed to follow serum levels fairly closely (Fig. 2). However, the concentration curve in gastric mucosa had a bimodal shape, identical to that seen with clindamycin. After an initial peak at 1 h, there was a drop in levels at 2 h, followed by a second peak at 4 h.

Cefuroxime

Cefuroxime is a second generation cephalosporin which has recently become available as an oral preparation. It was given in a dose of 30 mg/kg which produced high serum levels of 25.45 µg/ml at 1 h. Corresponding gastric mucosa levels were, however, considerably lower, peaking at 2.97 µg/g (Fig. 3). Tissue levels fell at 2 h, as had been seen with the other antibiotics, but remained low for a much longer period of time. Only after 8 h was a second peak seen. This gave the tissue concentration curve for cefuroxime the same characteristic bimodal shape as seen with the other antibiotics, but overall levels were low.

Clinical Implications

The results of the first three antibiotics to be tested show that pharmacokinetics in the gastric mucosa differ markedly among antibiotics. This information is important in

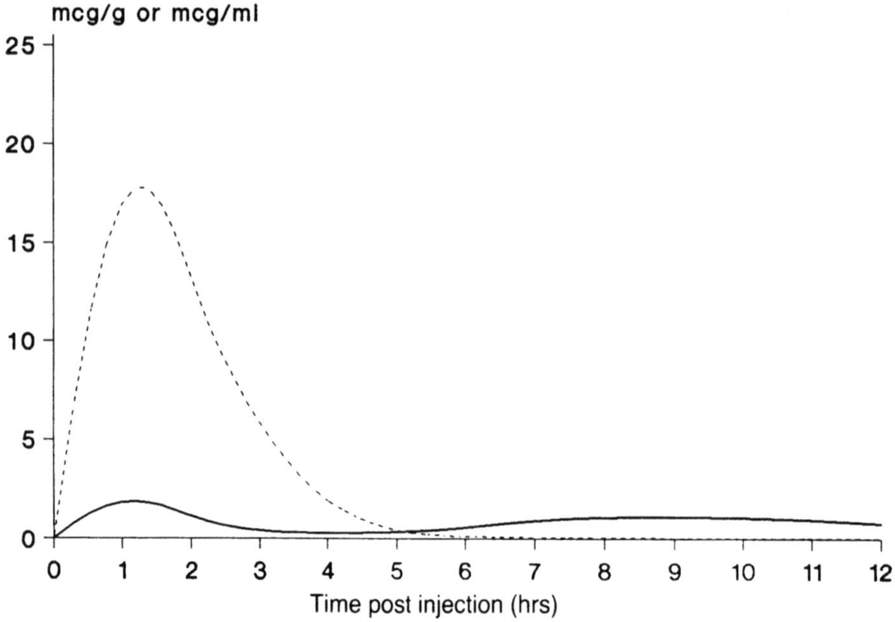

Fig. 3. Serum *(dotted line)* and gastric tissue *(continuous line)* concentrations of cefuroxime following 30 mg/kg IM injection

selecting future therapeutic agents suitable for clinical trials. The poor results reported in a trial with ciprofloxacin [6] can in retrospect be partially explained by relatively low tissue concentrations of the drug. In a similar way it can be predicted that cefuroxime most likely would not eradicate *H. pylori.* In spite of differences in tissue concentrations between the drugs, they all showed concentration curves with a bimodal shape. This indicates that two separate transport mechanisms may be responsible for gastric mucosa levels. The first peak follows the serum peak and may therefore be due to a passive transport driven by the serum concentration. The second peak occurs when serum levels have fallen to low concentrations and may therefore involve an active transport mechanism. The nature of such a transport system is unknown at this time, but it would be important to investigate this. Such knowledge could potentially result in ways of improving gastric secretion of antibiotics through pharmacologic manipulation.

References

1. Glupczynski Y, Labbe M, Burette A, Delmee M, Avesani V, Bruck C (1987) Treatment failure of ofloxacin in Campylobacter pylori infection. Lancet I:1096
2. Hirschl AM, Stanek G, Rotter M, Pötzi R, Gangl A, Hentschel E, Schütze K, Holzner HJ, Nemec H (1987) Campylobacter pylori, gastritis und ulcus pepticum. Wien Klin Wochenschr 99:493–497
3. McNulty CAM, Gearty JC, Crump B, Davis M, Donovan IA, Melikian V, Lister DM, Wise R (1986) Campylobacter pyloridis and associated gastritis: investigator blind, placebo controlled trial of bismuth salicylate and erythromycin ethylsuccinate. Br Med J 293:645–649

4. Unge P, Gnarpe H (1988) Pharmacokinetic, bacteriological and clinical aspects on the use of doxycycline in patients with active duodenal ulcer associated with Campylobacter pylori. Scand J Infect Dis [Suppl] 53:70–73
5. Glupczynski Y, Burette A, Labbe M, Deprez C, DeReuck M, Deltenre M (1988) Campylobacter pylori-associated gastritis: a double-blind placebo-controlled trial with amoxycillin. Am J Gastroenterol 83:365–372
6. Hirschl AM, Stanek G, Rotter M, Hentschel E, Schütze K (1987) Ulcus duodeni und Antibiotika-Therapie. Dtsch Med Wochenschr 112:781
7. Schaub N, Stalder H, Vischer W, Stalder GA, Affolter H, Wegmann W (1987) Versagen von doxycyclin bei Campylobacter-pylori-positiver gastritis. Dtsch Med Wochenschr 112:117–118
8. Westblom TU, Belshe RB (1989) Antibiotic transport across gastric mucosa: a guinea pig model for Campylobacter pylori mediated gastritis. 5th International Workshop on Campylobacter Infections, Puerto Vallarta, Mexico, Feb 25–March 1, 1989
9. Klempner MS, Styrt B (1981) Clindamycin uptake by human neutrophils. J Infect Dis 144:472–479
10. Saggers BA, Lawson D (1966) Some observations on the penetration of antibiotics through mucus in vitro. J Clin Pathol 19:313–317
11. Goodwin CS, Blake P, Blincow E (1986) The minimum inhibitory and bactericidal concentrations of antibiotics and anti-ulcer agents against Campylobacter pyloridis. J Antimicrob Chemother 17:309–314
12. Duriex D, Westblom TU (1989) Mucosal concentrations of clindamycin in a guinea pig model: therapeutic implications for Campylobacter pylori mediated gastritis. 5th International Workshop on Campylobacter Infections, Puerto Vallarta, Mexico, Feb 25–March 1, 1989
13. Duriex D, Westblom TU, Madan E, Midkiff BR, Subik M (1989) Gastric mucosa concentrations of ciprofloxacin in a guinea pig model: a comparison to in vitro susceptibilities in human isolates of Campylobacter pylori. Gastroenterology 96:A133
14. Borner K, Höffken G, Lode H et al. (1986) Pharmacokinetics of ciprofloxacin in healthy volunteers after oral and intravenous administration. Eur J Clin Microbiol Infect Dis 5:179–186

Discussion

Lee: It seems to me that you really do need to validate the model more with the antibiotics that are being used for example by Dr. McNulty because then you can correlate that with what she is finding. It seems to me that this is extremely important before screening newer antimicrobials. So I wonder whether you have started and have been doing anything with beta-lactams for example.

Westblom: We are planning to test beta-lactams next, particularly amoxicillin. With all the clinical experience that exist, I think it is important to test that antibiotic. One way of validating the model has been done with clindamycin in clinical patients. These patients were in the intensive care unit, and were getting intravenous clindamycin. We put down a nasogastric tube and suctioned up the gastric juice from these patients, and we compared serum levels to gastric juice levels. We found a concentration of the drug in the gastric juice. We had serum levels almost identical to the Guinea pig serum levels. The gastric juice concentrations were almost twice the serum levels. Therefore, in humans, at least as measured in the gastric juice, we have a similar concentration of clindamycin. Since the antibiotic has to go across the mucosa to get into the gastric juice, I think this validates the animal model.

Petersen: Have you tried to change the basic conditions by for example giving acid inhibitory drugs or Pentagastrin to see if that influences the gastric mucosa.

Westblom: Those very experiments are going on right now and I hope to have the results of those shortly.

Slomiany: Since the scraping of the mucosal surface may cause the elimination of the topical vasculature, it would be appropriate for you to measure the hemoglobin content in your mucosal scrapings. Have you performed such measurements.

Westblom: No, we did not. We visually inspected all the samples. There was no visual evidence of any bleeding.

Slomiany: But that might not be enough.

Westblom: True, but if you recall the concentration curve of clindamycin the serum levels were almost non-detectable at 8 hours while we had concentrations in mucosa almost a hundred times higher. Even if we had complete mixture with blood it would still not explain the high levels.

Acquired Resistance to Antibiotics: An Underestimated Cause of Failure in the Treatment of *Helicobacter pylori* Infection

Y. Glupczynski and A. Burette

Introduction

There is now overwhelming evidence that *Helicobacter pylori* is the major etiological agent of chronic active (type B) gastritis and that it may further predispose to peptic ulceration. Challenge studies in gnotobiotic piglets and in two human volunteers have reproduced the typical features of gastritis [16, 17, 21, 29]. Clearance of the organism with amoxycillin, furazolidone, or bismuth salts leads to improvement or even total resolution of gastritis [7, 25, 28, 32]. Moreover, several studies have shown that patients with healed peptic ulcer who remain persistently infected with *H. pylori* relapse much more frequently than patients cleared of the organism [3, 22].

In vitro studies of the susceptibility of *H. pylori* have shown that it is sensitive to most antibiotics (penicillin, ampicillin, cephalosporins, macrolides, quinolones, aminoglycosides, tetracylines, and nitroimidazoles) except vancomycin, trimethoprim, and sulfonamides [10, 15, 19, 24]. However, the clinical experience with various antimicrobials has been particularly disappointing especially when these were administered as a single agent.

Amoxycillin – the most extensively studied antibiotic – has been shown to be effective in clearing *H. pylori* in 70%–90% of the patients, but the relapse rate shortly after treatment has been very high and long-term eradication has not been achieved in more than 20% of individuals [1, 32]. In one study, furazolidone has resulted in encouraging results, with an initial clearance rate of 93% and a 6-week eradication rate of about 40% [28]. Monotherapy with other agents has been almost totally ineffective, with clearance rates ranging between 0% and 30% [1, 9, 14].

Different factors have been suggested as being responsible for the lack of clinical efficacy: insufficient drug concentration in gastric mucus and crypts due to poor penetration, local inactivation of the drug, decreased antibacterial activity of some antibiotics at low pH, inappropriate formulation, modality of administration or duration of treatment, or poor compliance to treatment [8, 13, 23, 26]. Although acquired resistance of *H. pylori* has been previously reported [6, 11], its exact role in the treatment failures of *H. pylori* infection has not been thoroughly discussed.

In this paper we will review the different antibiotics which proved ineffective for eradication of *H. pylori* possibly because of the development of acquired resistance during treatment.

H. Menge et al. (Eds.)
Helicobacter pylori 1990

Nitroimidazoles

Several early studies performed before the knowledge of *H. pylori* have demonstrated some efficacy of metronidazole in the treatment of peptic ulcer [31, 34]. However, these studies essentially focused on the initial ulcer-healing rate and did not mention the frequency with which relapses occurred after initial healing. Moreover, in some of these reports the investigators did not differentiate their results between duodenal and gastric ulcer so that their results cannot be further evaluated concerning a pathogenic role of *H. pylori* in either gastric or duodenal ulcer.

In vitro, *H. pylori* is moderately sensitive to metronidazole and to tinidazole (MIC range 0.5–32 mg/liter) and according to different studies [10, 11, 15] between 15% and 50% of strains tested have been found primarily resistant to metronidazole or tinidazole (MIC > 8 mg/liter). Both compounds have proved unsuccessful in clearing *H. pylori* from the gastric mucosa when they have been used as single agent (clearance rate, 3%–20%) [3, 20, 22]. In a double-blind placebo-controlled prospective study in patients with duodenal ulceration, Goodwin et al. [11] found that isolates from 19/27 (70%) patients after a combined treatment of cimetidine and tinidazole had become resistant to tinidazole. By contrast, when colloidal bismuth subcitrate (CBS) was given with tinidazole, acquired resistance associated with failure to eradicate *H. pylori* was observed in only 2/22 patients.

Spontaneous resistance to the nitroimidazoles could be induced in vitro in 3 of 22 sensitive cultures after overnight subculture in liquid medium and plating on agar containing 8 mg/liter metronidazole. In a recent yet unpublished study, we have treated 41 dyspeptic patients with *H. pylori* gastritis with amoxycillin and tinidazole during 7 days. An overall eradication rate of *H. pylori* was found in 60% of the patients (6 weeks after the end of treatment). However, significantly different results were observed according to the sensitivity of *H. pylori* to tinidazole before therapy. All 10 patients originally infected with a *H. pylori* strain naturally resistant to tinidazole failed to respond whereas 25/31 (81%) patients with an initial isolate sensitive to tinidazole responded to treatment ($\chi^2 = 17.4, p < 3.10^{-5}$).

In this subgroup of patients, five of six patients not cleared from *H. pylori* had an isolate resistant to tinidazole at the control endoscopy. Emergence of resistance to tinidazole occurred in only 5/31 (18%) patients under the double amoxycillin/tinidazole combination therapy. It seems thus clear from these two studies that the combination of tinidazole or metronidazole with another anti-*H. pylori* active agent (either CBS or amoxycillin) may be clinically effective and reduce the risk of development of resistance. Moreover, when considering a combination therapy with a nitroimidazole compound, the sensitivity of the *H. pylori* strains before treatment may efficiently predict the outcome of the patient. As far as the mechanisms of resistance are concerned, it is hypothesized that a small subpopulation of resistant mutants may be selected by metronidazole or may preexist and that the association of a second active agent will lower the inoculum size of the infecting organisms, hence preventing the emergence of resistant mutants.

Resistance to metronidazole has not been extensively investigated and the genetic modifications by which bacteria acquire resistance to this drug remain poorly understood. It is usually ascribed to decreased uptake through the bacterial cell wall and/or to decreased nitro reduction by bacterial enzymes inside the bacteria [33] (see Table 1).

Fluoroquinolones

Despite good in vitro activity, several clinical studies with fluoroquinolones (ciprofloxacin, ofloxacin, and norfloxacin) have proved so far unsuccessful at eradication of *H. pylori* from gastric mucosa [6, 14, 27, 35]. In most instances (up to 100% in one study [6] when the susceptibility of the infecting strains has been monitored, the rapid development of resistance has been noted [6, 14, 27, 35]. A 16- to 64-fold increase in the MIC (from 0.25–1 mg/liter before treatment up to 16–32 mg/liter after treatment) of ofloxacin or ciprofloxacin was reported in two studies after the failures observed with these agents [6, 14]. This resistance extended to other 4-quinolone derivatives but not to amoxycillin or to other antibiotics (tetracycline, metronidazole) [6]. Besides this, it has been stated that the lack of clinical efficacy of quinolones may be due to decreased activity at low pH [13, 26].

However, despite a 4- to 16-fold decrease in antibacterial activity against *H. pylori* at pH 5 (MIC, 2 mg/liter) as compared with neutral pH (MIC, 0.12 mg/liter), ciprofloxacin achieves gastric mucosal concentration largely above the MIC even 6 h after a 500-mg single oral dose [26]. This observation and the fact that emergence of resistance frequently occurred in patients receiving concomitant treatment with H2-antagonists indicate that decreased activity at a more acidic pH cannot completely explain the lack of clinical efficacy of the quinolones. In vitro, it is possible to select the development of resistant mutants (at a frequency of about 10^{-8}) after several passages of organisms in the presence of low concentration of various quinolones [13]. The so-selected resistant mutants are 32- to 64-fold less susceptible to quinolones (MIC, 32–64 mg/liter) than their sensitive counterparts (0.25–0.5 mg/liter). As for *Campylobacter* species, two different mechanisms may account for this resistance. It may either involve a modification in the DNA gyrase – the target enzyme of quinolones – or it may be due to a modification in the bacterial outer membrane proteins, rendering the drug unable to penetrate inside the bacteria [36] (see Table 1). It is thus probable that, despite the low frequency of spontaneous mutation, this event may be of clinical significance in patients heavily infected with *H. pylori* (> 10^9 colonies at some sites of infection). Quinolones would thus eliminate most organisms from the gastric mucosa and select for the few resistant mutants which would subsequently replace the susceptible population of bacteria. Additionally, this selection of resistant organisms may be further facilitated by low concentrations of drug in some areas of the colonized stomach and by reduced antibacterial activity in the presence of a low pH.

As for nitroimidazoles, there is some indirect evidence that combination with a second anti-*H. pylori* active agent (a bismuth salt) may perhaps increase the efficacy and reduce the risk of resistance development. Bayerdörffer et al. [2] reported a 78% clearance rate and a eradication rate of 33% (4 weeks after end of treatment) in 14 patients with duodenal ulcer who had received bismuth subsalicylate and ofloxacin for 1 month. After treatment, 3/14 (21%) isolates from these patients were resistant to ofloxacin (MIC > 4 mg/liter). However, this study compared the efficacy of bismuth and ofloxacin versus ranitidine on ulcer healing and *H. pylori* eradication so that no patients received ofloxacin alone.

Another point strongly arguing against the use of quinolones in *H. pylori* gastritis is the fact that these compounds bind to cations and form inactive chelate complexes in the intestinal lumen, and hence have a reduced absorption in the presence of antacids containing Al^{3+} and Mg^{2+} [30]. Such a situation is likely to occur frequently in dyspeptic patients who often take these medications.

In summary, the decreased activity of quinolones at low pH combined with the development of rapid resistance makes these agents unsuitable for the treatment of *H. pylori* infection even in association with bismuth salts because better alternative agents are available.

Macrolides

In vitro, macrolides have excellent activity against *H. pylori* (as active as amoxycillin), the MICs of erythromycin being in the range of 0.06–0.5 mg/liter [4, 13, 18]. In a placebo-controlled trial, however, erythromycin ethylsuccinate has been found ineffective in clearing *H. pylori* from the gastric mucosa of patients with gastritis (1/15 [7%] patients cleared) [25]. Similar studies with other macrolides or related agents such as josamycin, spiramycin, or clindamycin have not been more successful [9, 19, 20].

Since the activity of erythromycin is markedly affected by the reduction in pH (about 100 times less active at pH 5 than at pH 7.5) [23], it can be expected to be even less active in vivo at the pH of gastric mucosa and crypts. Moreover, comparative measurement of gastric mucosal concentrations after a single 500-mg oral dose of erythromycin ethylsuccinate has shown lower levels than after a similar dose of other antibiotics (amoxycillin, pivampicillin, and ciprofloxacin) [26]. Although these local concentrations of erythromycin were above the MIC_{90} value for *H. pylori* at pH 7.5 (0.12 mg/liter) in 17/18 assessed patients, they were found insufficient to achieve inhibitory concentrations at a pH < 6 and would have thus explained the lack of clinical efficacy.

In a recent small pilot study in dyspeptic patients with *H. pylori* gastritis, we have evaluated the efficacy of azythromycin. This new macrolide antibiotic has similar activity as erythromycin against *H. pylori* [4], but better acid stability, and it achieves 10- to 40-fold higher tissue levels than erythromycin following oral dosing [5].

Nevertheless, azythromycin did not prove more effective than other macrolides; only 2/12 [16%] patients were cleared from *H. pylori* after a 1-week course of treatment and the two patients temporarily cleared relapsed again 4 weeks after the end of treatment. Studies of the susceptibility of *H. pylori* after treatment showed that in 10/12 patients the *H. pylori* strain isolated at the second endoscopy (immediately after treatment) was resistant to azythromycin (MIC $>$ 64 mg/liter) and that it showed cross-resistance to erythromycin and also to clindamycin but not to amoxycillin, tetracyclines, and metronidazole. The development of resistance was documented in four patients in whom both the pre- and posttreatment matching isolates were available (pretreatment strain, MIC 0.25 mg/liter; posttreatment, MIC $>$ 64 mg/liter).

This resistance was stable and persisted for up to 3 months in three patients followed up after treatment.

Although more acid stable than erythromycin, the in vitro activity of azythromycin is also significantly decreased when the pH drops from 8 (MIC, 0.25 mg/liter) to 5.5 (MIC, 1 mg/liter) [13]. It is, however, improbable that this factor accounted on its own for the failures since the clinical efficacy of azythromycin was not enhanced by the coadministration of ranitidine in two patients.

Acquired resistance to erythromycin and related agents has not been reported previously in *H. pylori* most probably because no determination of sensitivity was performed in the earlier clinical trials in which these antibiotics have been used.

Resistance to erythromycin and to other macrolides – usually associated with cross-resistance to clindamycin – is, however, well known in *Campylobacter* species *(C. jejuni* and *C. coli)*. Although the mechanisms of resistance in these bacteria have not been fully elucidated, it seems unrelated to the presence of a plasmid but rather to be constitutive and chromosomally mediated [36] (Table 1). As with the quinolones, spontaneous mutants of *H. pylori* resistant to macrolides may be selected in vitro at low frequency (10^{-8}) after successive exposure of *H. pylori* to increasing concentrations of erythromycin [13].

Table 1. Acquired antibiotic resistance in *H. pylori*

Antibiotic	MIC (mg/liter)	Gene	Probable location	Proposed mechanisms
Quinolones	> 32	?	Chromosome (mutation)	• Modification of DNA gyrase • Decreased permeability
Nitroimidazole	> 32	?	Chromosome (mutation)	• Deficient nitrate reductase? • Decreased uptake
Macrolides[a]	> 64	?	Chromosome	• Modification of ribosome

[a] Accompanied by cross-resistance to clindamycin

Other Factors Implicated in the Treatment Failure of *H. pylori* Infection

Among other antimicrobials that have been used for the treatment of *H. pylori* infection, no acquired resistance of *H. pylori* to ampicillin, amoxycillin, furazolidone, or tetracyclines has yet been described. Moreover, no resistance or increase in the MIC to bismuth salts was observed in a group of 15 patients who relapsed their infection after having received CBS [12]. The fact that recrudescence of infection rapidly takes place after single therapy with amoxycillin or CBS without the development of resistance to these compounds clearly indicates that other factors may be important to explain the treatment failures of *H. pylori* infection observed with these agents. Besides gastric mucus concentrations and stability of the drugs to a wide range of pH, the physicochemical properties of a molecule (lipid solubility, degree of ionization) probably have crucial importance on the drug's activity at the site of infection. The respective importance of the local and systemic effects of drugs are still poorly determined and will probably need experimental animal models in order to gain a more comprehensive approach of the treatment in humans. The optimal drug formulation (syrup versus powder, capsules, or tablets) remains unknown as no direct comparative studies with the same agent under different forms have been conducted. However, such studies also need to be performed since different formulations could achieve different local or systemic concentrations and a more or less homogeneous coating of the whole gastric mucosa. It is indeed possible that patchy distribution of a locally active antimicrobial over the gastric mucosa may cause wide variation in concentration in the esophagus, stomach, or duodenum, and hence subsequently lead to relapse or to the development of resistance. Similarly, the best modality of administration (time of administration, number of daily doses) as well as the optimal duration of treatment will have to be determined in the future and adapted individually for each suitable therapeutic agent. Finally, poor compliance of the patients to treatment is not to be overlooked and may account for a significant proportion of failures especially with prolonged antibiotic treatment.

Conclusion

This paper summarizes the clinical trials in which failures possibly occurred because of the development of resistance during treatment. It confirms that the in vitro activity of antibiotics is absolutely not predictive of the in vivo eradication rates of *H. pylori*. There is reasonable evidence from in vitro data that resistance to antibiotics may have occurred because of the selection of naturally resistant mutants [13]. Such an event which occurs at low frequency (about 1 colony out of 10^8) may be avoided by the association of a second anti-*H. pylori* active agent (either a bismuth salt or another antibiotic) (see Table 2). Indeed, almost all reports dealing with acquired resistance in *H. pylori* have been in patients who had received a single antibiotic or association therapy with H2 antagonists. This last observation casts some doubts about the hypothesis that the clinical efficacy of some antimicrobials (quinolones, macrolides, ampicillin) would be enhanced at higher pH by the association with an H2-antagonist.

Table 2. Effect of combination therapy on the emergence of acquired resistance in *H. pylori*

Therapy	*n*	Eradication rate (%)	Time after therapy	Acquired resistance	Reference
Tinidazole (H2-blocker)	29	3	12 months	19/27	11
Tinidazole (+ CBS)	28	75	12 months	2/22	11
Tinidazole (+ amoxycillin)	41	61	6 weeks	5/31	[Burette][a]
Ofloxacin (+ H2-blocker)	6	0	–	6/ 6	6
Ofloxacin (+ BSS)	14	33	4 weeks	3/14	1

[a] Unpublished data

On the contrary, treatment with anti-H2 might increase the degree of stomach colonization of *H. pylori* and subsequently facilitate the selection of resistant mutants. Furthermore, by increasing the colonization of the stomach with a mouth or intestinal flora, there is a theoretical risk that antibiotic-resistance-encoding plasmids might be transferred to *H. pylori* from other bacteria, although this has not yet been described.

On the other hand, combination therapy associating two different antibiotics alone or one or two antimicrobial agents and a bismuth salt will both improve the eradication rate of *H. pylori* and reduce the risk of resistance development. Until the "optimal" drug is found, monotherapy should not be recommended for the treatment of patients with *H. pylori* infection. Whatever the therapeutic combination used, it is also strongly advisable to monitor the susceptibility of *H. pylori* to antimicrobials for possible emergence of resistance during treatment.

References

1. Bayerdörffer E, Ottenjann R (1988) The role of antibiotics in *Campylobacter pylori* associated peptic ulcer disease. Scand J Gastroenterol 23 [Suppl 142]:93–100
2. Bayerdörffer E, Simon T, Bästlein C, Ottenjann R, Kasper G (1987) Bismuth/ofloxacin combination for duodenal ulcer. Lancet II:1467–1468
3. Coghlan JG, Gilligan D, Humphries H, McKenna D, Dooley C, Sweeney E, Keane C, O'Morain C (1987) *Campylobacter pylori* and recurrence of duodenal ulcers – a 12 month follow up study. Lancet II:1109–1111
4. Czinn S, Carr H, Aronoff S (1986) Susceptibility of *Campylobacter pylori* to three macrolide antibiotics (erythromycin, roxithromycin [RU 28,965], and CP 62,993) and rifampin. Antimicrob Agents Chemother 30:328–329
5. Girard AE, Girard D, English AR, English AR, Gootz TD, Cimochowski CR, Faiella JA, Haskell SL, Retsema JA (1987) Pharmacokinetic and in vivo studies with azythromycin (CP-62,993), a new macrolide with extended half-life and excellent tissue distribution. Antimicrob Agents Chemother 31:1948–1954
6. Glupczynski Y, Labbé M, Burette A, Delmée M, Avesani V, Brück C (1987) Treatment failure of ofloxacin in *Campylobacter pyloridis* infection. Lancet I:1096
7. Glupczynski Y, Burette A, Labbé M, Deprez C, Dercuck M, Deltenre M (1988) *Campylobacter pylori* associated-gastritis: a double-blind placebo controlled trial with amoxycillin. Am J Gastroenterol 83:365–372
8. Glupczynski Y, Labbé M, Van der Linden MP, Nyst JF, Burette A (1989) Lack of antibiotic compliance in patients treated for *Campylobacter pylori* associated gastritis. Am J Gastroenterol 84:1126
9. Glupczynski Y, Burette A, Nyst JF, De Prez C, De Koster E, Deltenre M (1988) *Campylobacter pylori*-associated gastritis: attempts to eradicate the bacteria by various antibiotics and anti-ulcer regimens. Acta Gastroenterol Belg 52:329–337
10. Goodwin CS, Blake P, Blincow E (1986) The minimum inhibitory and bactericidal concentrations of antibiotics and anti-ulcer agents against *Campylobacter pyloridis*. J Antimicrob Chemother 17:309–314
11. Goodwin CS, Marshall BJ, Blincow ED, Wilson DH, Blackbourn S, Phillips M (1988) Prevention of nitroimidazole resistance in *Campylobacter pylori* by coadministration of colloidal bismuth subcitrate: clinical and in vitro studies. J Clin Pathol 41:207–210
12. Goodwin CS, Bell B, McCullough C, Turner M (1989) Sensitivity of *Campylobacter pylori* to colloidal bismuth subcitrate. J Clin Pathol 42:216–219
13. Hardy DJ, Hanson CW, Hensey DM, Beyer JM, Fernandes PB (1988) Susceptibility of *Campylobacter pylori* to macrolides and fluoroquinolones. J Antimicrob Chemother 22:631–636
14. Hirschl AM, Hentschel E, Schütze K, Nemec H, Pötzi R, Gangl A, Weiss W, Pletschette M, Stanek G, Rotter ML (1988) The efficacy of antimicrobial treatment in *Campylobacter pylori*-associated gastritis and duodenal ulcer. Scand J Gastroenterol 23 [Suppl 142]:76–81

15. Kasper G, Dickgiesser N (1984) Antibiotic sensitivity of *Campylobacter pylori.* Eur J Clin Microbiol 3:444
16. Krakowka S, Morgan DR, Kraft WG, Leunk RD (1987) Establishment of gastric *Campylobacter pylori* infection in the neonatal gnotobiotic piglet. Infect Immun 55:2789–2796
17. Lambert JR, Borromeo M, Pinkard KJ, Turner H, Chapman CB, Smith ML (1987) Colonization of gnotobiotics piglets with *Campylobacter pyloridis,* an animal model? J Inf Dis 155:1344
18. Lambert T, Mégraud F, Gerbaud G, Courvalin P (1986) Susceptibility of *Campylobacter pyloridis* to 20 antimicrobial agents. Antimicrob Agents Chemother 30:510–511
19. Lamouliatte H, Megraud F, DeMascarel A, Quinton A (1988) Etude controlée de la josamycine dans les gastrites associées au *Campylobacter pylori* (abstract). Gastroenterol Clin Biol 12:A156
20. Langenberg ML, Rauws EAJ, Schipper MEI, Widjojokosumo A, Tytgat GNJ (1985) The pathogenic role of *Campylobacter pyloridis* studied by attempts to eliminate these organisms (Abst. 098, pp 162–163) III Int Workshop on *Campylobacter* infections, June 1985, Ottawa
21. Marshall BJ, Armstrong JA, McGechie DB, Glancy RJ (1985) Attempts to fulfil Koch's postulates for pyloric *Campylobacter.* Med J Aust 142:436–439
22. Marshall BJ, Goodwin CS, Warren JR, Murray R, Blincow ED, Blackbourn SJ, Phillips M, Waters TE, Sanderson CR (1988) Prospective double-blind trial of duodenal relapse after eradication of *Campylobacter pylori.* Lancet II:1437–1441
23. McNulty CAM (1989) Bacteriological and pharmacological basis for the treatment of *Campylobacter pylori* infection. Gastroenterol Clin Biol 13:96B–100B
24. McNulty CAM, Dent JC (1988) Susceptibility of clinical isolates of *Campylobacter pylori* to twenty-one antimicrobial agents. Eur J Clin Microbiol 7:566–569
25. McNulty CAM, Gearty JC, Crump B, Davis M, Donovan IA, Melikian V, Lister DM, Wise R (1986) *Campylobacter pyloridis* and associated gastritis: investigator blind, placebo controlled trial of bismuth salicylate and erythromycin ethylsuccinate. Br Med J 293:645–649
26. McNulty CAM, Dent JC, Ford GA, Wilkinson SP (1988) Inhibitory antimicrobial concentrations against *Campylobacter pylori* in gastric mucosa. J Antimicrob Chemother 22:729–738
27. Mertens JCC, Dekker W, Ligtvoet EEJ, Blok P (1989) Treatment failure of norfloxacin against *Campylobacter pylori* and chronic gastritis in patients with non ulcerative dyspepsia. Antimicrob Agents Chemother 33:256–257
28. Morgan D, Kraft W, Bender M, Pearson A, The Gastrointestinal Physiology Working Group of Cayetano Heredia and the John Hopkins Universities (1988) Nitrofurans in the treatment of gastritis associated with *Campylobacter pylori.* Gastroenterology 95:1178–1184
29. Morris A, Nicholson G (1987) Ingestion of *Campylobacter pyloridis* causes gastritis and raised fasting gastric pH. Am J Gastroenterol 82:192–199
30. Preheim LC, Cuevas TA, Roccaforte JS, Mellencamp MA, Bittner MJ (1986) Ciprofloxacin and antacids. Lancet II:46
31. Quintero Diaz M, Diaz, Sotto Escobar A (1986) Metronidazole versus cimetidine in treatment of gastroduodenal ulcer. Lancet I:907
32. Rauws EAJ, Langenberg W, Houthoff HJ, Zanen HC, Tytgat GNJ (1988) *Campylobacter pyloridis* – associated chronic active antral gastritis – a prospective study of its prevalence and the effects of antiulcer treatment. Gastroenterology 94:33–40
33. Rosenblatt JE, Edson RS (1987) Symposium on antimicrobial agents. Metronidazole. Mayo Clin Proc 62:1013–1017
34. Shirokova KI, Filomonov RM, Polkova LV (1981) Metronidazole in the treatment of peptic ulcer. Klin Med (Mosk) 59:48–50
35. Stone JW, Wise R, Donovan IA, Gearty J (1988) Failure of ciprofloxacin to eradicate *Campylobacter pylori* from the stomach. J Antimicrob Chemother 22:92–93
36. Taylor DE, Courvalin P (1988) Mechanisms of antibiotic resistance in *Campylobacter* species. Antimicrob Agents Chemother 32:1107–1112

Discussion

Tytgat: Dr. Glupczynski: 1) what do we have to do in the future with all these resistant organisms, 2) do you see the same problems of resistance formation with other microorganisms as we see with *Helicobacter pylori,* and 3) what are the prospects that microbiologists will come up with efficacious antibiotics against this organism?

Glupczynski: To answer the second question first, I think that perhaps we see more problems of resistance in the field of *Helicobacter pylori* because of the peculiar location of the organism and the fact that most of the agents achieve low, let us say subinhibitory concentrations and that could be an important factor in facilitating the selection of resistance. Resistance in bacteriology is an old story and it happens with different organisms. I think that the main thing is now to avoid monotherapy. Everyone will agree that we shouldn't use monotherapy anymore, because it doesn't work in the clinic and because it selects resistance to different antibiotics. One important thing for the future in the light of all this resistance would be before treating patients with new agents to see in vitro whether the selection of resistant mutants is possible. I think, this is also very important.

McNulty: Did you check for cross-resistance between the quinolones, nitroimidazoles, and macrolides?

Glupczynski: There was no cross-resistance. We have looked at that for all three classes of antibiotics, in which we described resistance. So, for quinolone-resistant organisms, all the other quinolones proved ineffective. Similarly, when looking at tinidazole-resistant strains this resistance extended to metronidazole, but not to other agents. The resistance to azythromycin included also other macrolides and clindamycin.

McNulty: So, do you think this makes decreased permeability to antimicrobials a less likely mechanism of resistance?

Glupczynski: Not necessarily, because as you know, there are several different ways by which antibiotics can get through the cell wall of bacteria, so different antibiotics do not necessarily cross the bacterial cell wall through the same channels.

Demling: You spoke about eradication, I think this is a big claim and you compared eradications after 4 and 6 weeks and 12 months. Can you compare those results?

Glupczynski: You know there is one large scale study from the Amsterdam group which has shown well that when the patients are cleared after 4 or 6 weeks or more, the risk of relapse seems to decrease markedly. Most of the patients were considered to be cleared of the bacteria if they were *H. pylori*-negative 4–6 weeks after therapy.

Börsch: You had very interesting new data on amoxicillin and tinidazole. From looking at the literature, one learns that the frequency of dosing of the nitroimidazoles might be important. If you administer it three times a day, it might be more effective than administering two doses per day. You had a result of 60% eradication, how often did you dose?

Glupczynski: 1 g, twice a day.

Marshall: In a double-blind study using tinidazole with bismuth, we dosed patients twice a day with 500 mg tinidazole. You said there is no cross-resistance between the quinolones, nitroimidazoles and macrolides. Because the quinolones give such good levels, do you think we would have some success using a quinolone with a nitroimidazole, or a quinolone, a nitroimidazole and a macrolide in triple therapy?

Glupczynski: You know, personally I would not recommend using a combination of two agents for which you know that some problems of acquired resistance might arise, so my view would be to combine agents for which you are sure that there is no or rarely any evidence of resistance. I would not recommend combining quinolones and macrolides.

Graham: A question to Prof. Tytgat: You have been given the right of gold standard here, 4 weeks is the time frame for assessing eradication. Is that the current concept in Amsterdam? We think that is not long enough.

Tytgat: I think it is still sufficient to wait for 4 weeks after the end of therapy. If at that point meticulous cultures are negative, then the chances of recurrence are very low. That holds up in our study, at least. And now I would like to ask Dr. Glupczynski a question: Looking at the data that you show, it seems to me that the combination with bismuth somehow decreases or prevents resistance formation. Does that hold up for all combinations of bismuth and other antibiotics and, if so, what is the mechanism of prevention of resistance formation?

Glupczynski: My view is that for antibiotics, which alone prove ineffective and lead to acquired resistance, the coadministration of bismuth or a second antibiotic would lower the infecting inoculum and hence prevent the emergence of resistant mutants. If you grow one resistant mutant out of 10^8 colonies, by administering a second agent, whether bismuth of amoxicillin, you will lower the density of the inoculum and so reduce the risk of emergence of resistant mutants.

Tytgat: But should bismuth than not be an essential part of any therapeutic regimen?

Glupczynski: You know, from the review of non-comparative open studies I made, it is not quite clear whether bismuth plus another agent achieves better eradication than two antibiotics. The two amoxicillin/tinidazole studies I mentioned, achieved almost the same eradication of *Helicobacter pylori* as the bismuth/tinidazole combination. The problem is that when giving tinidazole or metronidazole, you will lose 20% of your patients because 20% of the *Helicobacter pylori* strains are initially resistant to tinidazole and if you treat such patients with tinidazole, there is no chance of eradicating the organism. So perhaps we have to find alternative antibiotics to metronidazole.

McNulty: In our triple treatment study with bismuth, metronidazole and tetracycline, resistance to metronidazole still ocurred.

Glupczynski: It was not a comparative study. If you compare the emergence of resistance to metronidazole or tinidazole when these agents are given alone, double or triple therapy surely will reduce the emergence of resistance. The question that should be answered is: Is triple therapy better than double therapy for preventing the emergence of resistance and this might perhaps not be the case.

Graham: There is some bias here. I have an antimicrobial that is safe, it is not systemic, no-one ever has trouble with it, it is very effective and eradicates, at least kills most of the organisms with the first dose: it is bismuth. I agree with Dr. Tytgat, it should be part of the program, at least in our experience, which is with triple therapy with tetracycline, metronidazole and bismuth. We don't see emergence of strains that are resistant, because more than 95% of our patients have the infection eradicated, and when their disease has been eradicated, there is not much chance for emergence of resistance.

Börsch: One comment to Dr. McNulty. The statement that triple therapy does not prevent resistance is valid only if you show that there is good compliance by your patients. Your results of 65% eradication may suggest that the compliance might have been quite low.

McNulty: I can comment on this. Our triple treatment study did highlight some problems in comparing treatment studies. We were treating nonulcer dyspepsia patients and we found that the patients with more severe gastritis responded to treatment better than those patients with less severe gastritis. It has been shown that patients with duodenal ulcer often have more severe gastritis or more widespread gastritis than patients with nonulcer dyspepsia. This is a different patient group, which, I think, may be an important point as well.

Graham: Dyspepsia patients are very difficult to deal with and not terribly reliable. Ulcer patients take their drugs because they get benefit from it. We have done both kinds of study: I can tell an ulcer patient to take this incredible combination of drugs and he will take them. No matter what I tell nonulcer dyspepsic patients, they do what they want.

McNulty: Compliance may be an important factor for the failure of triple therapy but the comment still stands that triple therapy does not prevent the development of resistance.

Graham: Continuing that, it may depend when therapy is administered. We give all of our drugs with meals, and so therefore the antibiotics and the bismuth stay in the stomach for a long time and you give them at times when the bismuth is rapidly emptied from the stomach. The bismuth is therefore treating things in the colon.

Tytgat: Mr. Chairman, I think this is an extremely important point. We all were told to administer the drugs before meals in order not to lose too much of the active drug fixed to food residues, etc., and Dr. Graham tells us that the best way is to give the drugs with meals. What is the evidence that it is better with meals than before meals?

Marshall: Dr. Graham has not done a randomized study to show that dosing with meals is better. Somebody obviously needs to do this. Dr. Borody tells his patients to take the medication whenever convenient (qid), so dosing patients with meals or not does not seem to make much difference. In Borody's studies, 94% of infections were still eradicated.

Tytgat: Dr. O'Morain from Ireland stressed the point that it was essential to give bismuth preparations at least 1 h before meals on an empty stomach. We all believed him because he was so meticulous in stressing that point. I am sure a lot of our patients took the medicine only 15 min before meals which may not be optimal. Now Dr. Graham, advises us to give bismuth with meals to prolong intragastric retention.

Clinical Pharmacology of Bismuth – Studies from the Royal Free Hospital

C. U. Nwokolo and R. E. Pounder

Introduction

The Royal Free Hospital in London has a long-standing interest in the use of bismuth for the management of peptic ulceration. Almost 1½ centuries ago Dr. William Brinton, who was a physician to the Royal Free Hospital, reported his experience in the management of a large number of patients with gastric ulceration [1]. His clinical observations were sometimes supported by the results of postmortem analysis, but he remarked in 1855 that he found "the trisnitrate of bismuth to be the most useful agent in allaying symptoms associated with stomach ulcers".

Over the years, bismuth salts remained popular for the management of a range of gastrointestinal problems – although epidemics of bismuth toxicity in France and Australia restricted the availability of some bismuth salts [2].

Bismuth subsalicylate (Pepto-Bismol) and bismuth subnitrate (the active principle in Roter tablets) remained available in many countries, and tripotassium dicitrato bismuthate (De-Nol) has been introduced in progressively more countries since its development in South Africa in the early 1970s [3].

There is now an extensive literature concerning the application of tripotassium dicitrato bismuthate for the management of peptic ulceration, in particular duodenal ulceration [4]. Clinical trials have demonstrated that not only does a short course of treatment with tripotassium dicitrato bismuthate speed duodenal ulcer healing, but also the compound appears to delay the return of ulceration [5–11]. Tripotassium dicitrato bismuthate's exact mode of action has remained unclear, although the identification of *Helicobacter pylori* as an important factor in the pathogenesis of duodenal ulceration has raised the attractive hypothesis that bismuth salts exert their action by an effect on the bacterium [12–14]. However, most of the important studies which demonstrate the clinical effectiveness of tripotassium dicitrato bismuthate have used the drug as a single agent, yet when used alone this bismuth salt eradicates *H. pylori* in the mucosa of only a minority of subjects [15].

If bismuth salts do not generally exert their beneficial effect by eradication of *H. pylori*, an alternative hypothesis has to be developed to explain the persisting beneficial action of a short course of treatment with tripotassium dicitrato bismuthate. Early studies suggested that bismuth is absorbed during oral dosing with tripotassium dicitrato bismuthate [16, 17], and it was suggested that the compound may continue to act for some months because of an accumulation of bismuth in the body [18].

Recent research at the Royal Free Hospital has explored different aspects of bismuth absorption from the three bismuth compounds that are available for oral dosing in the United Kingdom – De-Noltabs [19, 22], Pepto-Bismol liquid [21] and

H. Menge et al. (Eds.)
Helicobacter pylori 1990

Roter Tablets. Bismuth analysis has always been performed by Rooney Laboratories Ltd. (Basingstoke, Hampshire), who were blind to the nature and design of our experiments. The bismuth concentrations were measured by atomic absorption spectrophotometry, following generation of bismuth hydride from a wet oxidized sample [19].

Bismuth Accumulation During Treatment with Tripotassium Dicitrato Bismuthate (De-Noltabs) [19]

Bismuth concentration was measured in plasma, dried leucocytes and urine in nine patients before, during and after treatment with tripotassium dicitrato bismuthate (De-Noltab 2 bd) for 6 weeks. The median plasma bismuth concentration rose significantly during treatment at 3 and 6 weeks to 12 and 17 ng/ml respectively, compared with before treatment (2 ng/ml; $P < 0.01$; Fig. 1). At 3, 6, 9 and 12 weeks after treatment there were non-significant changes in the median plasma bismuth concentration (5, 4, 2 and 4 ng/ml, respectively), compared with before treatment.

The median 24-h urinary bismuth excretion before treatment (2.9 μg/24 h) rose significantly during treatment at 3 and 6 weeks to 698.4 and 1012.2 μg/24 h respectively ($P < 0.01$, Fig. 2). At 3, 6, 9 and 12 weeks after treatment there was a persistent significant elevation of the median 24-h urinary bismuth excretion compared with before treatment (110, 30.4, 11.6 and 9.5 μg/24 h, respectively, $P < 0.01$).

There was a non-significant change of the median bismuth concentration of dry leucocyte pellets during and after treatment with tripotassium dicitrato bismuthate.

This study demonstrated a 349-fold rise in median 24-h urinary bismuth excretion on the 42nd day of treatment with the drug, with a persistent significant 3.3-fold

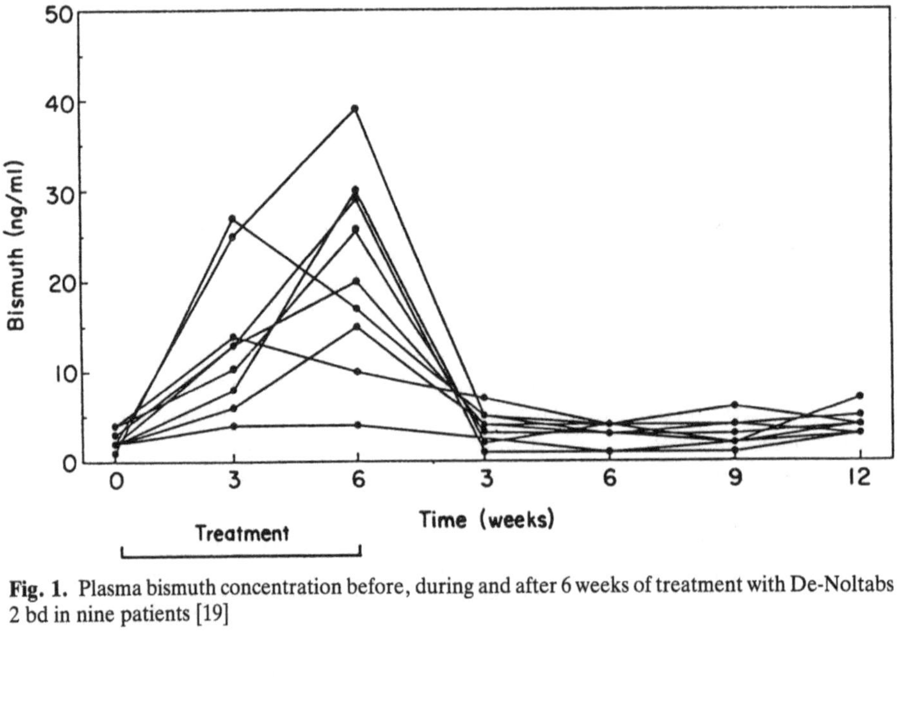

Fig. 1. Plasma bismuth concentration before, during and after 6 weeks of treatment with De-Noltabs 2 bd in nine patients [19]

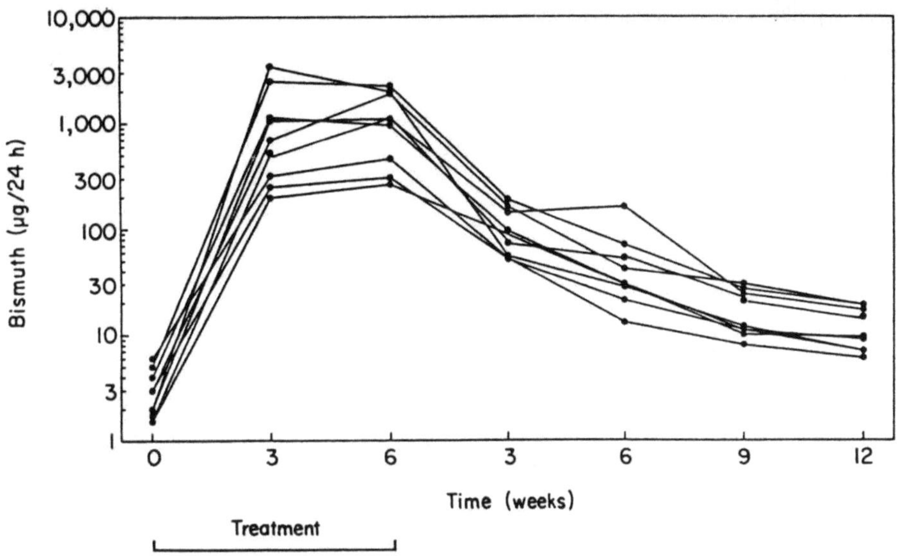

Fig. 2. Twenty-four-hour urinary bismuth excretion before, during and after 6 weeks of treatment with De-Noltabs 2 bd in nine patients [19]

elevation of excretion 3 months after cessation of treatment. A depot of bismuth accumulates during treatment in every patient given De-Noltabs, and bismuth is slowly excreted via the urine over the following months. Unless the depot is exclusively in the kidney, the bismuth must pass from its site of sequestration via the plasma before renal clearance. While in the plasma the bismuth may be available as a trace element for the rapidly dividing enterocytes of the duodenal mucosa, thereby assisting long-term ulcer remission.

Absorption of Bismuth from Oral Doses of Tripotassium Dicitrato Bismuthate (De-Noltabs) [20]

Two additional studies measured plasma concentrations of bismuth during dosing with tripotassium dicitrato bismuthate (De-Noltab). The first study compared 24-h plasma bismuth concentration and urinary bismuth excretion in six patients who had already received 29–131 days (median 47 days) treatment with De-Noltab 2 bd, and six healthy subjects who only received De-Noltab 2 bd on the day of the study. There was a prompt rise in plasma bismuth concentration after each dose of De-Noltabs (Fig. 3). The median 24-h integrated plasma bismuth concentration was similar in both groups – healthy subjects receiving their first doses of bismuth (126.5 ng.h/ml), and the patients during treatment with bismuth (145.3 ng.h/ml).However, there was a significant difference in the 24-h urinary bismuth excretion between the two groups: the median value for the healthy subjects was 326 µg/24 h, compared with 1173 µg/24 h for the patients during treatment. These results demonstrate a reduced urinary clearance of bismuth on the 1st day of dosing with tripotassium dicitrato bismuthate

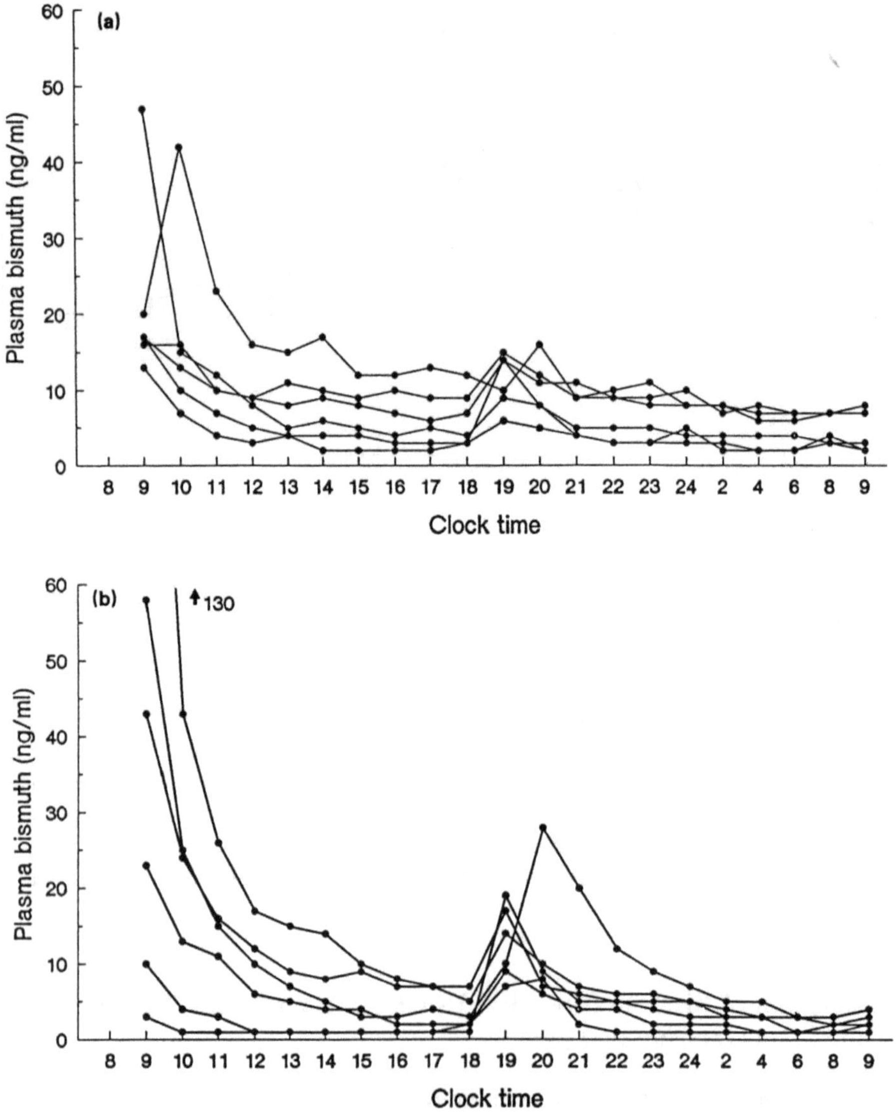

Fig. 3a, b. Twenty-four-hour plasma bismuth concentration in six patients during treatment with De-Noltab 2 bd for 29–131 days (De-Noltab 2 taken at 08.45 h and 18.45 h [20]. **b** Twenty-four-hour plasma bismuth concentration in six healthy subjects during their 1st day of dosing with De-Noltab 2 bd (taken at 08.45 h and 18.45 h [20]

compared with prolonged dosing, which could be explained by sequestration of bismuth within the body.

A second study compared plasma bismuth concentrations after the first and third doses of De-Noltab 2 bd in 16 healthy subjects. The De-Noltabs were taken when fasting, and the median peak plasma bismuth concentration occurred 30 min (range

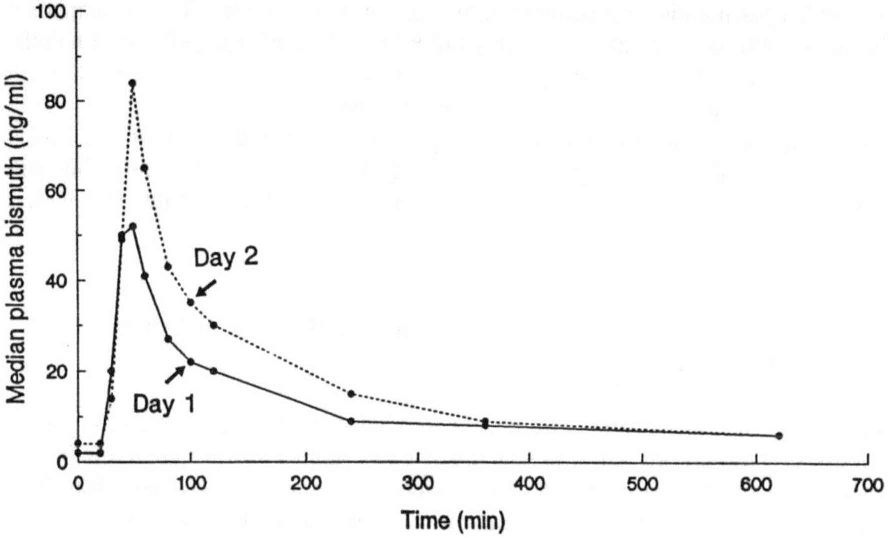

Fig. 4. Median plasma bismuth concentrations in 16 healthy subjects after oral dosing with their first and third doses of De-Noltab 2 on successive mornings [20]

15–105 min) postdosing (Fig. 4). The peak plasma bismuth concentration was greater than 50 ng/ml in 14 of the 16 subjects, and it was greater than 100 ng/ml in 9 of the subjects.

For the first time this study published detailed bismuth pharmacokinetics after oral dosing with tripotassium dicitrato bismuthate, and it revealed not only extremely rapid absorption of bismuth after oral dosing, but also surprisingly high peak plasma bismuth concentrations. These high peak plasma bismuth concentrations raised the possibility of potential neurotoxicity, as the existing literature had identified the threshhold for concern about neurotoxicity as a blood concentration of between 50 and 100 ng/ml [2, 21, 22]. It is probable that these recommendations concerning the toxic levels of blood bismuth relate to through concentrations rather than peak concentrations of the trace metal [20]. De-Nol has been available in three different formulations – liquid, chew tablets and swallow tablets, but their relative bioavailability has not been published. We believe that prospective studies of CNS function and structure are needed in patients before, during and after receiving a full course of treatment with tripotassium dicitrato bismuthate.

Absorption of Bismuth and Salicylate from Oral Doses of Bismuth Subsalicylate (Pepto-Bismol Liquid) [23]

Plasma bismuth and plasma salicylate concentrations were measured before and after three 30 ml oral doses of bismuth subsalicylate (Pepto-Bismol liquid) in ten fasting healthy subjects. From 0–120 min following the first dose of bismuth subsalicylate, the median plasma bismuth concentration was less than 1 ng/ml. The peak median plasma bismuth concentration was at +240 min (1.7 ng/ml; range 0.8–5.3 ng/ml). Salicylate appeared in the plasma [24] of all subjects at + 30 min, and it reached a peak at +120 min (median 61 mg/litre; range 46–104 mg/litre).

This study demonstrated that, despite rapid and substantial absorption of salicylate, there is negligible absorption of bismuth from standard oral doses of bismuth subsalicylate. Hence the bismuth is cleaved from the salicylate acid, but the bismuth is not absorbed.

Absorption of Bismuth from an Oral Dose of Bismuth Subnitrate (Roter Tablets) [25]

Plasma bismuth concentrations were measured before and after a single oral dose of bismuth subnitrate (two Roter tablets dissolved in 50 ml warm water) in ten fasting healthy subjects. Repeated blood samples were taken for 8 h post-dosing, but there appeared to be negligible absorption of bismuth – the median plasma bismuth concentration ranged between 1.5 and 3.0 ng/ml, with the highest observed plasma concentration of 11 ng/ml.

Discussion

The results of the experiments performed at the Royal Free Hospital show that bismuth is absorbed after oral dosing with De-Noltabs, but there is essentially no absorption of bismuth after oral dosing with either Pepto-Bismol liquid or Roter tablets (Fig. 5). The availability of bismuth for absorption must relate to the nature of

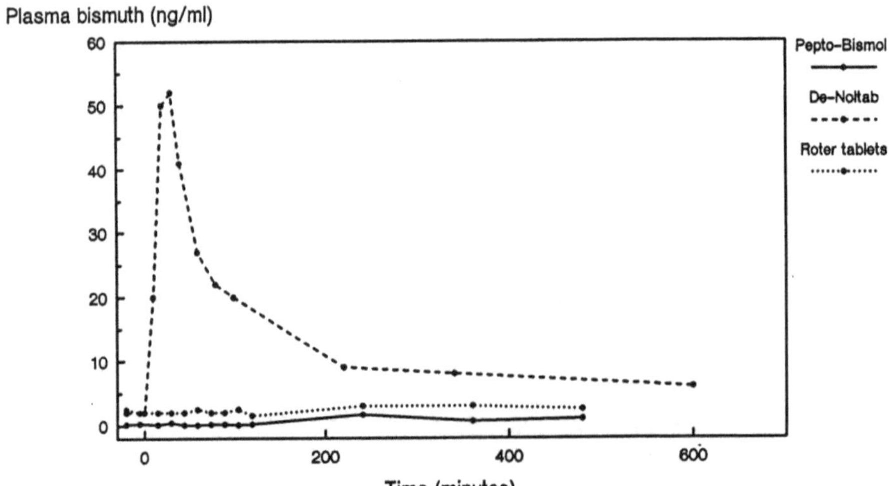

Fig. 5. Median plasma bismuth concentration in fasting healthy subjects after receiving tripotassium dicitrato bismuthate (2 De-Noltabs, $n = 16$), bismuth subsalicylate (Pepto-Bismol liquid 3 × 30 ml; $n = 10$), or bismuth subnitrate (2 Roter tablets; $n = 10$). Dosing started at 0 min

the bismuth salt present in each preparation as all three preparations contain substantial amounts of bismuth metal: Roter 2 tablets = 456 mg bismuth; Pepto-Bismol 90 ml = 897 mg bismuth; De-Noltab 2 = 214 mg bismuth. The site and mechanisms of bismuth absorption in man is unclear [26].

As the bioavailability of bismuth from the three compounds differs so much, it is now clearly important to define exactly which bismuth salt is used in any clinical study. Does bismuth act as a luminal agent, or is systemic absorption necessary for either short-term or long-term benefit? Is systemic absorption of bismuth a benefit, or a hazard? Prospective studies are necessary to compare the relative efficacy of the different bismuth-containing salts that are available for the management of gastritis and peptic ulceration.

References

1. Brinton W (1855) Royal Free Hospital: ulcer of the stomach treated successfully. Assoc Med J: 1125–1126
2. Lee SP, Lim TH, Pybus J, Clarke AC (1970) The tissue distribution of orally administered bismuth in the rat. Clin Exp Pharmacol Physiol 7:319–324
3. Brodgen RN, Pinder RM, Sawyer PR, Speight TM, Avery GS (1976) Tripotassium dicitrato bismuthate: a report of its pharmacological properties and therapeutic efficacy in peptic ulcer. Drugs 12:410–411
4. Tytgat GNJ (1987) Colloidal bismuth subcitrate in peptic ulcer – a review. Digestion 37 [suppl 2]: 31–41
5. Martin DF, Hollander D, May SJ, Ravenscroft MM, Tweedle DEF, Miller JP (1981) Difference in relapse rates of duodenal ulcer after healing with cimetidine or tripotassium dicitrato bismuthate. Lancet 7–10
6. Vantrappen G, Schuurmans P, Rutgeerts P, Janssens J (1982) A comparative study of colloidal bismuth subcitrate and cimetidine on the healing and recurrence of duodenal ulcer. Scand J Gastroenterol [Suppl 80]:23–30
7. Shreeve DR, Klass HJ, Jones PE (1983) Comparison of cimetidine and tripotassium dicitrato bismuthate in healing and relapse of duodenal ulcers. Digestion 28:96–101
8. Bianchi Porro G, Lazzroni M, Petrillo M, De Nicola C (1984) Relapse rates in duodenal ulcer patients formerly treated with bismuth subcitrate or maintained with cimetidine. Lancet II:698
9. Lee FI, Samloff IM, Hardman M (1985) Comparison of tripotassium dicitrato bismuthate tablets with ranitidine in healing and relapse of duodenal ulcers. Lancet I:1299–1302
10. Lane MR, Lee SR (1988) Recurrence of duodenal ulcer after medical treatment. Lancet I:1147–1149
11. Hamilton I, O'Connor HJ, Wood NC, Bradbury I, Axon ATR (1986) Healing and recurrence of duodenal ulcer after treatment with tripotassium dicitrato bismuthate tablets or cimetidine. Gut 27:106–110
12. Marshall BJ, Warren JR (1984) Unidentified curved bacilli in the stomach of patients with gastritis and peptic ulceration. Lancet I:1311–1315
13. Dooley CP, Cohen H (1988) The clinical significance of *Campylobacter pylori*. Ann Intern Med 108:70–79
14. Bartlett JE (1988) *Campylobacter pylori:* fact or fancy? Gastroenterology 94:229–238
15. Marshall BJ, Warren JR, Blincow ED, et al. (1988) Prospective double-blind trial of duodenal ulcer relapse after eradication of *Campylobacter pylori.* Lancet II:1437–1442
16. Lee SP (1981) Studies on the absorption and excretion of tripotassium dicitrato bismuthate in man. Res Commun Chem Pathol Pharmacol 34:359–364
17. Hamilton J, Axon ATR (1981) Controlled trial comparing De-Nol tablets with De-Nol liquid in the treatment of duodenal ulcer. Br Med J 282–362
18. Pounder RE (1984) Duodenal ulcers that will not heal. Gut 25:697–702

19. Gavey CJ, Szeto M-L, Nwokolo CU, Sercombe J, Pounder RE (1989) Bismuth accumulates in the body during treatment with tripotassium dicitrato bismuthate. Aliment Pharmacol Ther 3:21–28
20. Nwokolo CU, Gavey CJ, Smith JTL, Pounder RE (1989) The absorption of bismuth from oral doses of tripotassium dicitrato bismuthate. Aliment Pharmacol Ther 3:29–39
21. Bader J-P (1987) The safety profile of De-Nol. Digestion 37 [suppl 2]:59–53
22. Winship KA (1983) Toxicity of bismuth salts. Adv Drug React Ac Pois Rev 2:103–121
23. Nwokolo CU, Mistry P, Pounder RE (1990) The absorption of bismuth and salicylate from oral doses of Pepto-Bismol (bismuth salicylate). Aliment Pharmacol Ther 4:163–169
24. Trinder P (1954) Rapid determination of salicylate in biological fluids. Biochem J 57:301–303
25. Nwokolo CU, Prewett EJ, Sawyerr AM, Pounder RE (in press). Lack of bismuth absorption from bismuth subnitrate (Roter) Tablets. Hepatol Eur J Gastroenterol
26. Coghill SB, Hopwood D, McPherson S, Hislop S (1983) The ultrastructural localisation of De-Nol (colloidal tripotassium dicitrato bismuthate -TDB) in the upper gastrointestinal tract of man and rodents following oral and instrumental administration. J Pathol 139:105–114

The Absorption of Bismuth from Orally Administered Tripotassium Dicitrato Bismuthate and Bismuth Subsalicylate

H. MENGE, M. GREGOR, J. BLESSING, B. BROSIUS, R. HOPERT, and A. LANG

Introduction

Bismuth has a long history of use in medicine [1]. Its systemic administration as an antiinfective agent against syphilis and parasitic diseases was accompanied by a high incidence of toxicity. Orally administered medicinal preparations were used in gastro-intestinal complaints. Most of them contained water-insoluble salts of bismuth and hence were regarded – with some rare exceptions – as compounds of low toxicity. Since 1974, however, concern has been expressed, especially in Australia [2] and France [3], about the occurrence of encephalopathy associated with the use of these insoluble bismuth salts. Most of the patients had consumed large amounts of bismuth for long periods and exhibited high bismuth plasma levels at the time of clinical illness. Pharmacological studies revealed that neurotoxicity occurred only when the daily intake of bismuth exceeded 1,5 g and the bismuth blood concentrations were greater than 100 μg/l. Bismuth plasma concentrations below 50 μg/l were found to be without risk for encephalopathy [3]. In 1989 Nwokolo et al. [4] quantified the plasma bismuth concentrations during a course of treatment with tripotassium dicitrato bismuthate (colloidal bismuth subcitrate). The authors were able to demonstrate that bismuth is absorbed avidly from this compound. In some individuals peak plasma bismuth concentrations exceeded 100 μg/l, i. e., they were in the range hitherto considered to be associated with bismuth neurotoxicity. In the present study we have investigated whether the same is true for bismuth subsalicylate which is widely used in the treatment of travellers' diarrhea and *Helicobacter pylori*-associated diseases.

Subjects and Methods

The project was approved by the Ethics Committee of the Klinikum Steglitz of the Free University of Berlin. All volunteers gave written consent prior to its beginning. A total of 12 healthy students and clinical staff members were recruited for this study. All of them studied or worked at the Medical Department of the Academic Hospital Remscheid. They had never been treated with any bismuth-containing compounds, and none of them had been treated with antibiotics during the last 3 months. The volunteers were studied on two successive days. On day 1 six subjects were given bismuth subsalicylate (BSS), and on day 2 the other six subjects were given colloidal bismuth subcitrate (CBS). The study design is shown in Figure 1. The plasma concentrations of bismuth were analysed using atomic absorption spectrophotometry.

H. Menge et al. (Eds.)
Helicobacter pylori 1990

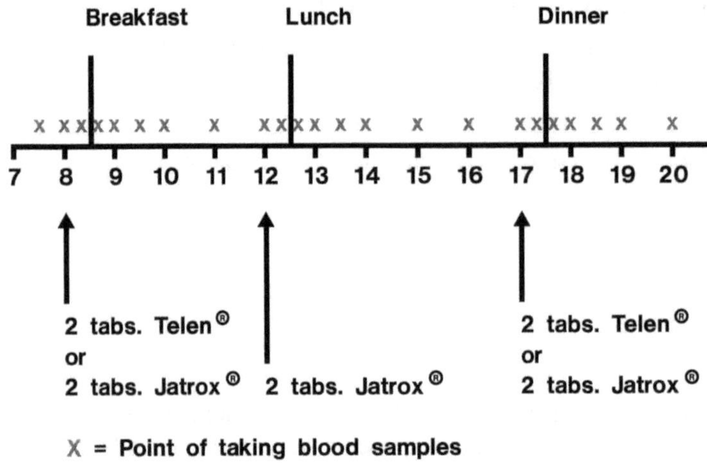

Fig. 1. Design of the present study. The 12 healthy subjects fasted from 20.00 hours on the evening before the study; meals were standardized; blood samples were taken at those moments indicated by an asterisk; each tablet of Telen contained 312 mg CBS and each tablet of Jatrox contained 300 mg BSS

Results

Before starting the study none of the volunteers had any detectable plasma bismuth.

Figure 2 and Figure 3 show the individual plasma bismuth concentrations of the six healthy subjects who were given BSS. From 8.00 hours, i. e., the time of the first dose of BSS, to 12.40 hours none of the volunteers had any bismuth detectable in plasma. At 13.00 hours bismuth was detectable in the plasma of one subject, and the same was true for three further volunteers at 17.00 hours, 17.20 hours, and 17.40 hours. The peak plasma concentration was 5.4 µg/l (measured in one volunteer at 13.30 hours).

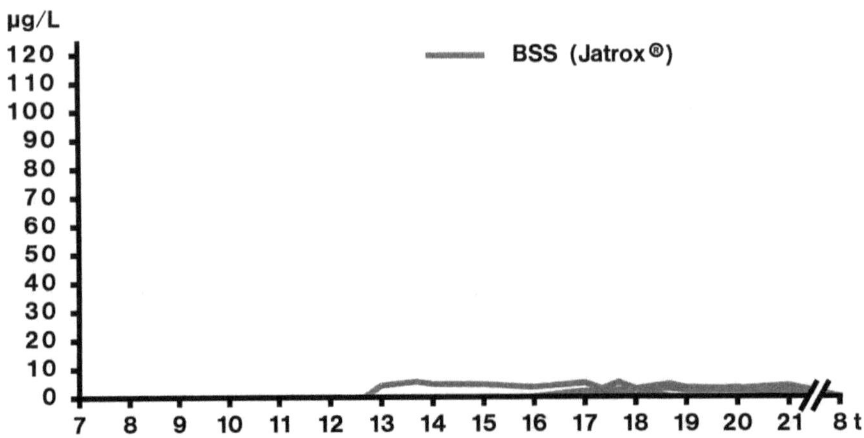

Fig. 2. Twenty-four-hour plasma bismuth concentrations in six healthy subjects receiving BSS

All plasma levels were transient. In two subjects, no bismuth was detectable in plasma during the study period of 24 h.

Figure 4 shows the 24-h plasma bismuth profiles of the six individuals who were given CBS. In contrast to the preceeding data, all volunteers exhibited detectable

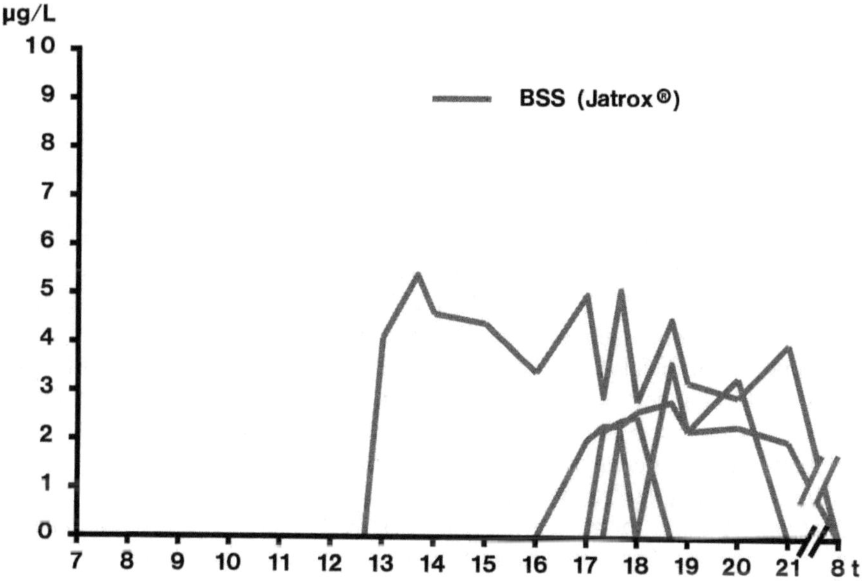

Fig. 3. Twenty-four-hour plasma bismuth concentrations in six healthy subjects receiving BSS (note the altered scale on the ordinate compared to Fig. 2)

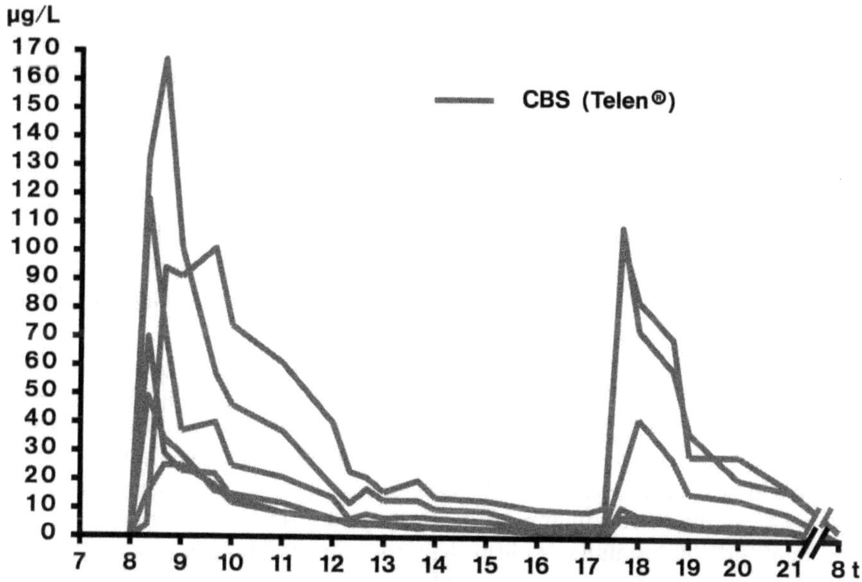

Fig. 4. Twenty-four-hour plasma bismuth concentrations in six healthy subjects receiving CBS

plasma bismuth levels with peak plasma concentrations being reached 20–40 min after the morning dose. These peak plasma concentrations showed great interindividual differences, ranging from 25 to 167 μg/l. They were transient and fell afterwards to steady state values, as is normally observed in bismuth-monitoring studies. A second transient but less pronounced increase in bismuth plasma concentrations was observed after the early evening dose of the drug.

Discussion

The present study demonstrates that the absorption of bismuth from BSS or CBS shows marked differences. After oral ingestion of BSS the highest plasma bismuth concentration is 5.4 μg/l, whereas the oral administration of CBS results in a peak plasma concentration of 167 μg/l. Additionally, the avidity of bismuth absorption is clearly dependent from the bismuth compound ingested. Traces of bismuth can be found in plasma only 5.0 h after the first BSS dose. By contrast, bismuth is found in plasma as early as 20 min after the first oral dose of CBS. The avidity of bismuth absorption from CBS is further documented by the fact that bismuth absorption was found in all volunteers taking CBS but only in four out of six volunteers taking BSS. The results concerning the bismuth plasma concentrations after administration of CBS are in good agreement with those obtained by Nwokolo et al. [4].

These observations indicate that bismuth is absorbed more effectively from CBS than from BSS, i.e., bismuth is absorbed from CBS more readily, more constantly, and to a larger amount. This difference in the behaviour of the two bismuth salts may result at least in part from their chemical nature [5, 6]. BSS is an ordinary inorganic salt of bismuth that is poorly soluble in water. Thus, this compound can hardly act as an important source of "bismuth ions" in an aqueous solution. By contrast, CBS represents an organic complex of bismuth in which bismuth is present in a complexed trivalent form, and therefore it can act as a source of bismuth ions. For this reason one may assume that CBS offers a larger amount of bismuth ions to the gastrointestinal mucosa than BSS does, which in turn could result in greater bismuth absorption and in higher bismuth plasma concentrations.

The early absorption of bismuth from CBS and the delayed absorption of the heavy metal from BSS points to different absorption sites for bismuth ions derived from these compounds. As yet, the transport mechanisms and the absorption sites for bismuth in the intestine remain uncertain. The early detection of bismuth in plasma after the first dose of CBS indicates that bismuth uptake from this compound takes place in the duodenum and proximal jejunum, since it is unlikely that any bismuth is absorbed by the gastric mucosa. This suggestion is supported by the findings of Coghill et al. [7] who demonstrated small particles of bismuth complex being endocytosed by the enterocytes of the duodenum and proximal jejunum after a single oral dose of De-Nol liquid. This early absorption implies that bismuth is readily liberated from CBS after its ingestion. Measurable bismuth plasma concentrations are found only 5 h after the first dosage of BSS. This time lag indicates that bismuth is absorbed from BSS in the distal jejunum or ileum or even in the large intestine. The water insolubility of this bismuth salt will probably not change during its passage to the distal intestine so that other factors will have to act to liberate the bismuth ions from BSS.

The most likely candidate for disintegrating the BSS molecule in the lower intestinal tract is the abundant bacterial flora of the ileum and large intestine. This idea is supported by the fact that the intestinal bacteria can break down another bismuth salt to form a nitrite, which in turn may cause methemoglobulinemia [8, 9].

After each CBS dose, the bismuth concentration in the plasma reaches a transient peak level. In some individuals this exceeds the arbitrarely set 50 μg/l and 100 μg/l, which represent the so called "safety" and "alert" zones of bismuth plasma concentration with regard to bismuth toxicity, according to French experience [3]. In the present study these high peaks were only of short duration and fell rapidly to low steady-state values, whereas in the cases of bismuth intoxication in France "high through values" were registered. The two situations thus cannot be compared and so far-reaching clinical conclusions in this regard should not be drawn from the data gained during this pharmacokinetic study.

References

1. Menge H (1988) Was ist gesichert in der Behandlung der Campylobacter-pylori-induzierten Gastritis und des Campylobacter-pylori-assoziierten peptischen Ulkus? Internist 29:745–754
2. Morgan FP, Billings JJ (1974) Is this subgallate poisoning? Med J Aust 2: 662–663
3. Lechat P, Kisch R (1986) Les encéphalopathies bismuthiques: réévaluation du risque. Gastroenterol Clin Biol 10:562–569
4. Nwokolo CU, Gavey CJ, Smith JTL, Pounder RE (1989) The absorption of bismuth from oral doses of tripotassium dicitrato bismuthate. Aliment Pharmacol Therap 3:29–39
5. Serfontein WJ, Mekel R (1979) Bismuth toxicity in man – II. Res Com Chem Pathol Pharmacol 2:391–411
6. Winship KA (1983) Toxicity of bismuth salts. Adv Drug React Ac Pois Rev 2:103–121
7. Coghill SB, Hopwood D, McPherson S, Hislop S (1983) The ultrastructural localisation of De-Nol (colloidal tripotassium dicitrato bismuthate TDB) in the upper gastrointestinal tract of man and rodents following oral and instrumental administration. J Path 139:105–114
8. Chaleil D, Allain P (1979) Influence de l'administration orale de nitrate basique de bismuth sur l'élimination et la distribution du radiobismuth administré par voie intrapéritonéale chez le rat. Ann pharmacol franc 37:285–290
9. Jacobsen JB, Huttel MS (1982) Methemoglobinemia after excessive intake of a subnitrate containing antacid. Ugeskr Laeger 144:2349–2350

Pharmacokinetics of Bismuth Compounds in Patients with Gastritis and Ulcer Disease During Standard Treatment

R. Raedsch, I. Walter-Sack, E. Weber, and J. Blessing

Introduction

Since *Helicobacter pylori* was identified as an important factor in the pathogenesis of gastritis and ulcer disease, bismuth compounds have been widely used in the treatment of these diseases. The bismuth compounds at present on the market comprise subcitrate, subsalicylate, nitrate, gallate, and aluminate salts. After oral ingestion of these preparations, bismuth is partly absorbed from the intestine. Encephalopathy has been reported as one of several side effects of bismuth therapy in patients using large doses of bismuth preparations. In these patients, bismuth concentrations exceeding 100 μg/l have been measured. From these findings, the recommendations were derived that bismuth treatment should be stopped if bismuth levels rise above 100 μg/l [1]. Recently, peak bismuth concentrations in plasma exceeding 100 μg/l have been reported in patients and healthy subjects after oral ingestion of standard doses of tripotassium dicitratobismuthate [2,3]. In the present study, we investigated the pharmacokinetics of the widely used compound bismuth subsalicylate and compared it with bismuth subcitrate.

Patients and Methods

Bismuth plasma concentrations were measured in ten patients during courses of standard treatment with bismuth compounds for gastritis and ulcer disease. Eight of the patients were treated with liquid bismuth subsalicylate 30 ml t.i.d. Two patients were on a standard therapy with bismuth subcitrate two tablets b.i.d. The course of treatment lasted for four weeks in each patient. The bismuth preparations were administered before breakfast and dinner (subcitrate), and before lunch and dinner, and at bedtime (subsalicylate).

On the 1st day of treatment, blood samples were collected at 10-min intervals both after administration of the first and the second doses of the bismuth compounds for 2-h periods. Furthermore, daily blood samples were taken in the morning before administration during the 1st week, and subsequently twice weekly during the 4 weeks treatment course. The plasma bismuth concentrations were measured by atomic absorption spectrometry using a graphite tube and ZEEMAN compensation. By this method, concentrations as low as 0.1 μg/l may be detected.

H. Menge et al. (Eds.)
Helicobacter pylori 1990

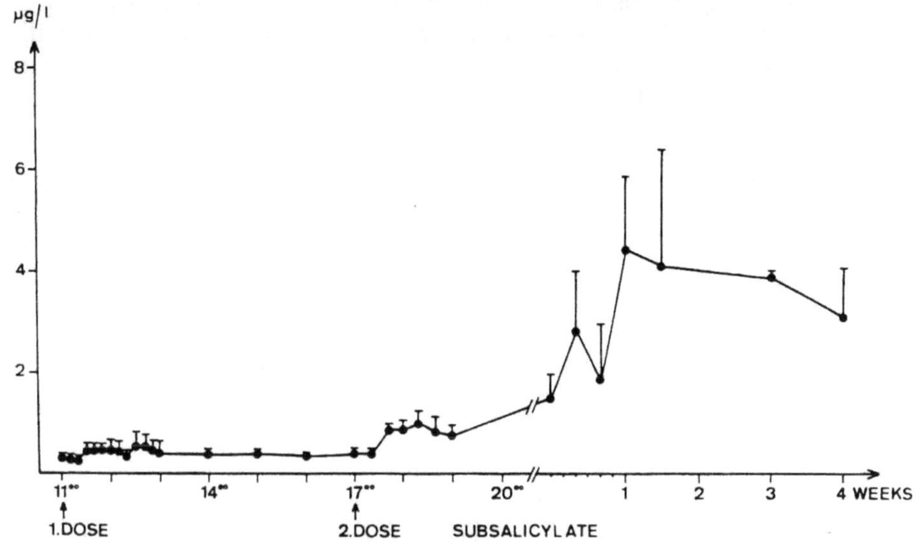

Fig. 1. Plasma bismuth concentrations in eight patients during 4 week courses of treatment with liquid bismuth subsalicylate. On the 1st day of treatment, an hourly scale is given from 1100 to 2000 hours. In contrast to bismuth subcitrate, no peak levels are measured after administration of bismuth subsalicylate. Plasma bismuth concentrations remain well below toxic levels throughout the treatment period

Results

In the two patients treated with bismuth subcitrate, bismuth peak levels in plasma of 100–120 µg/l were measured for 30–40 min after administration of each dose. Plateau levels measured in the morning before dosing did not exceed 15 µg/l during the 4-week treatment period. In the eight patients treated with bismuth subsalicylate, only minor concentrations of bismuth could be measured in plasma (Fig. 1.). No peak concentrations rose after dosing. During the 4 weeks of treatment with bismuth subsalicylate, plateau levels reached a mean of 3–4.5 µg/l (range 1–18 µg/l) and were found to be well below the toxic range of bismuth.

Summary and Conclusion

After oral ingestion of bismuth subcitrate tablets at standard doses, bismuth peak concentrations rise to levels in the range found in patients with bismuth-induced encephalopathy. The clinical significance of these peak levels is unknown. During treatment with liquid bismuth subsalicylate in standard doses, only minor bismuth concentrations were found in plasma and these were well below possible toxic levels. During a treatment course of 4 weeks with bismuth subsalicylate, no accumulation of bismuth in plasma was detected.

These results suggest that bismuth preparations differ greatly in the amount of bismuth absorbed out of them in the gut. Factors influencing bismuth absorption from various compounds must be defined. Pharmacokinetic studies of other bismuth compounds on the market should be initiated to ensure drug safety.

References

1. Bader JP (1987) The safety profile of De-Nol. Digestion 37 [Suppl 2]: 53–59
2. Gavey CJ, Szeto ML, Nwokolo CU, Sercombe J, Pounder RE (1989) Bismuth accumulates in the body during treatment with tripotassium dicitrato bismuthate. Aliment Pharmacol Therap 3: 21–28
3. Nwokolo CU, Gavey CJ, Smith JTL, Pounder RE (1989) The absorption of bismuth from oral doses of tripotassium dicitrato bismuthate. Aliment Pharmacol Therap 3: 29–39

Discussion

Classen: My question to the speakers is whether blood levels really are suitable parameters of bio-availability. What we should know are the mucosa levels of the various bismuth compounds. Blood levels may be a good parameter of absorption and perhaps toxicity but not of clinical efficacy for gastritis, ulcers, and so on. I do not have these data.

Nwokolo: I have not spoken about toxicity here. What we feel is that perhaps the absorption of bismuth may in fact be a good thing. As I said, I think that only when we have made direct clinical comparisons with the other bismuth containing agents can we have the answer to this question. We just have the feeling that the absorption of bismuth from De-Nol makes it different, and that to achieve this prolonged effect, a depot of bismuth may be needed which continues to leak out, so to speak, to reach the gastroduodenal endothelium in some way and which continues to improve the quality of the regenerating gastroduodenal epithelium. So, apart from the toxicity aspect, we feel that the absorption of small amounts of bismuth may be a positive factor.

Menge: I disagree with Dr. Nwokolo somewhat. Professor Tytgat and Dr. Rauws from Amsterdam have clearly demonstrated that the effect of bismuth on *H. pylori* is a local one. It is toxic to the bacterium. So, it is unimportant for this therapeutical problem whether bismuth is absorbed or not. As to Professor Classen's question: I agree with you. For the efficacy of the drug it is necessary to have high drug concentrations on or in the mucosa, but it is difficult to get data on these mucosal concentrations. Up to now, we have been doing the measurements only in the plasma and it is difficult to transform this method to biopsies. But it should be done.

Demling: My question is quite similar to Dr. Classen's question: We have heard that the different bismuth compounds are absorbed in different amounts, but I think the clinical effect of both preparations is quite similar, and the question arises whether a higher plasma concentration is really necessary to treat gastritis or ulcer. So, it could be that the preparation from subsalicylate is more tolerable for the patient and has the same effect, but the question is whether the eradication of *Helicobacter pylori* depends on a depot in the body and whether there is a depot which is better preserved by another preparation, maybe subcitrate.

Menge: In my opinion, and according to the data from Amsterdam, bismuth exerts a local, toxic effect on the bacterium and that's all.

Demling: So, you don't need a plasma level?

Menge: No. In my opinion these elevated plasma concentrations are only relevant for the toxicity of the drug. Dr. Nwokolo has found bismuth excretion over a period of 3 months. There must be a depot in the body which is not necessary for therapy but interesting for toxicity.

Graham: I think that we have some interesting data here, but part of the problem is that all of the data we are seeing on De-Nol is on a swallowable tablet and not necessarily on bismuth subcitrate. The pharmacology once a bismuth salt in the stomach is very, very similar and so we may well be seeing something that is only unique to that formulation of De-Nol and not to subcitrate. I take strong exception to your presentation, Dr. Menge, as to where things are happening. If you want to know where things are happening you have to measure where things are happening, you cannot make it up. And you made it up. You may be right, but I suspect you are wrong. We are seeing that the swallowable tablet empties in the stomach very rapidly.The further events are poorly understood. Does liquid De-Nol, which is standard use, have the same pharmacology as the swallowable tablet, or does a chewable tablet have a different pharmacology, where is it that these things happen, and where is the absorption site for bismuth? I think we need these experiments.

Menge: You want me to do too much. We only started these experiments after the paper of Dr. Nwokolo had been published, that means 5 months ago, you know.

Tytgat: Dr. Menge, is it known what percentage of bismuth is excreted in the urine after bismuth subsalicylate? For De-Nol there are estimates that 0.2% of the bismuth is absorbed and excreted in the urine. What is the percentage after bismuth subsalicylate.

Menge: We do not yet have these data.

Tytgat: So, the total amount of bismuth which is absorbed is presumably the same.

Menge: It can't be, according to our data. It is probable that less bismuth is absorbed from bismuth subsalicylate.

Tytgat: I would not be surprised if it is like that. The very early peaks depend greatly on the pharmacon used. The swallowable tablet is very different from the chewable tablet, which does not give a peak, and from the liquid. The most important point, however, is the following: the best fit for the pharmacology is a three-compartmental model. The half life of the rapid peak is about 4 h, but what is most important is that this fast peak is only responsible for, at most, 5% of the total area under the curve, which is therefore irrelevant. We should not spend too much time on that early peaking because it is, from the pharmacological point of view and from the toxicity point of view presumably irrelevant.

Marshall: We now have your reply, Dr. Nwokolo.

Nwokolo: I want to comment on the site of absorption. There is a paper from 1983 by Coghill et al. in the Journal of Pathology. He gave patients oral De-Nol liquid and took biopsies about 1 h later. He took biopsies from the oesophagus, stomach, and duodenum. He found endocytosis of bismuth particles in the duodenum, and not in the stomach. The gastric mucus prevented the bismuth particles from getting through to the mucosa. He also noticed a few particles of bismuth within some lipid vacuoles in oesophageal epithelial cells. I just thought that that might cast some light on the site of absorption.

Hazell: Dr. Nwokolo, correct me if I am wrong, the idea I got from your talk, was that you were suggesting that De-Nol had a residual effect because of this absorption and that this might account for the difference between H_2-antagonists and De-Nol, particularly in terms of ulcer relapse. McLean and associates some years ago reviewed the data on De-Nol in particular in comparison with H_2-antagonists and they came up with figures based on a number of published reports that the ulcer relapse rate following H_2-antagonist treatment was about 17% per month, whereas with bismuth they came up with about 7% per month. I took these figures and did some calculations. If we assume that approximately 20% of people treated with De-Nol have *H. pylori* effectively eradicated and then you take the residual population and look at the relapse rate, that residual population has a relapse rate that approximates the 17% following treatment with H_2-antagonists. So, the difference we are seeing could actually be a combination of effective therapy in a small group and ineffective therapy in the residual population.

Marshall: I would agree with that and this is a direct reply again to Dr. Nwokolo regarding our double-blind study. Only patients who took bismuth and had a eradication of *H. pylori* had a low relapse rate. In fact, the relapse rate in the 30% or so patients rendered *H. pylori* negative was the same, whether they were treated with antibiotics or not. This was less than 20%. The remaining patients who took the same dose of bismuth, but who still had *H. pylori* after therapy, did worse than the patients on H_2-blockers. Thus, there is no evidence whatsoever of an accumulated effect of bismuth, except if this could have helped to eradicate *H. pylori*. The correlation is not with bismuth or with any other drug but with *H. pylori*.

Nwokolo: I admit that *H. pylori* is a major determinant for relapse, but I am certain that it is not the only one. To answer this question I will refer to two studies. If you look at Lane's series from Auckland in New Zealand, he had a large series of about 468 duodenal ulcer patients followed prospectively over a period of 4 years and treated with a variety of agents. It is not that the patients whose ulcers were healed with tripotassium bismuthate did not relapse. They did so over a longer time. At the end of a period of 2 years, they approximated the relapse rates found with cimetidine. And I think that this suggests that, whatever the advantage TDB has, it is one that depreciates over time. This would support the theory of the depot becoming depleted in the months after healing. And secondly, I have also played with figures. I have applied Martin's percentages, probably because he was one of the early workers who provided us with the results showing the difference between the blockers and TDB. What I did, was to take 90 patients whose ulcers had been healed with TDB. I assumed that 30 (33%) of those patients would have had their *H. pylori* eradicated. The remaining 60 patients whose *H. pylori* was not eradicated would tend to behave as if their ulcers had been healed with cimetidine. If I sum that up and look at the theoretical curve that I obtain over a period of 18 months, the theoretical relapse rate is consistently higher than what is actually observed. I have done that for one or two of the studies and I have found this discrepancy. I have a transparency but have no time to show it. But there is a little shaded space on top which represents the discrepancy. I feel that there is something else apart from the antibacterial effect on *H. pylori*.

Marshall: One reason could be that those studies were not totally double blind because the patients were endoscoped while they were on the bismuth and so the black tongue was visible to the endoscopist.

Graham: A more reasonable explanation for the difference is, if the treatment does not eradicate but only suppresses, the natural history is still altered, and it takes the bacteria a while to regrow. I think that is what all of the rest of the data show. I disagree with you entirely, Guido that the early peak is irrelevant. If you assume that to get into the brain is bad, and I don't know this but I would assume that the high blood concentrations would increase the opportunity for bismuth getting into the brain, and if I can get the same therapeutic effect without that happening I would avoid it. If I were going to use De-Nol, I would use the chewable tablets or the liquid and avoid the swallowable tablets.

Tytgat: The only thing I said was that it was less than 5% of the total area under the curve. And it is the total area under the curve which is presumably important with respect to bioavailability and toxicity.

Graham: Do you know the bismuth concentration in the brain?

Tytgat: No, I don't know the brain concentration. There is no evidence in many people that these peaks are relevant. All the previous studies looked at plasma levels in the morning after the last dose the night before. These trough levels have nothing to do with the early peaking, and the whole story about safety levels are related to trough levels in the morning after dosing the day before. Many people have been treated with these compounds without adverse effects, so far, noticeable at least. Can I come back to Professor Menge with gastric absorption? I have looked at gastric material electronmicroscopically and I have never seen bismuth in the gastric mucosa, although plenty of bismuth is demonstrable electronmicroscopically in the small intestine in biopsies from the bulb or further down. So, I really wonder where gastric absorption is possible. On the other hand, if you take a tablet with water on an empty stomach, depending upon the size of the tablet it is very possible that the tablet is rapidly flushed through, because in an empty stomach the pylorus is presumably incompetent. Rapid release into the small intestine may cause this early peaking. So, I am not convinced that it is for certain true absorption in the stomach.

Menge: I agree with you. It will hardly be possible that bismuth absorption takes place in the stomach. It is most likely that the absorption starts in the duodenum or proximal jejunum.

Tytgat: What I am more interested in is finding out whether the peak depends upon the level of inflammation in the stomach, because other investigators studying healthy volunteers found much lower peaks. So my question is: could inflammation with disturbed permeability of the gastric lining be relevant for early absorption?

Menge: I can't answer this question, since the bismuth plasma concentrations were measured in young volunteers, 20–30 years of age.

Tytgat: Did you look at them histologically?

Menge: I could not persuade them to swallow the endoscope.

Nwokolo: We studied six patients, and six healthy volunteers. The healthy volunteers had higher peaks, although this was not significant statistically. You could see that on the graphs presented.

Pharmacology and Safety of Bismuth Compounds

A. SLIKKERVEER and F. A. DE WOLFF

Introduction

The increasing tendency to administer colloidal bismuth subcitrate (CBS) in the treatment of *Helicobacter pylori* infections has renewed interest in the therapeutic use of bismuth compounds. Because of the still unexplained, epidemic-like outbreak of poisoning caused by inorganic bismuth compounds in France between 1972 and 1978, interest in its possible toxicity was also revived.

In order to evaluate the possible risks of using medication containing bismuth, a short overview of the properties of the metal will be given. A full review has recently been published (Slikkerveer and de Wolff 1989).

Chemistry

In the periodic system of the elements, bismuth is located in group V, below nitrogen, phosphorus, arsenic, and antimony. It is a heavy metal with an atomic number of 83 and an atomic weight of 208.9. The only stable valence is 3^+. The metal has been used as a drug both as organic salts, such as thioglycollamate, and as inorganic salts, such as subnitrate and subcarbonate. The composition of bismuth salts is complex and often variable – the subnitrate is most often encountered as $(Bi_2O_3)_6(N_2O_5)_6(H_2O)_9$. The solubility of the inorganic salts in water is very low and can be influenced by acidity and by the addition of compounds containing sulfhydryl or hydroxy groups.

Analysis

At present, the method of choice for the measurement of bismuth is atomic absorption spectrophotometry (AAS). The hydride and electrothermal systems can both be used to detect bismuth in blood, plasma, serum, and urine. Significant differences in analytical approach in the described methods necessitate critical evaluation of the results. This also imposes the obligation to compare two methods thoroughly before any results can be compared or combined.

H. Menge et al. (Eds.)
Helicobacter pylori 1990

Pharmacokinetics

Absorption

The absorption of bismuth compounds from the gastrointestinal tract is very low. Excretion of bismuth in urine, measured after oral administration of CBS has been discontinued, suggests a bioavailability of only 0.2% (Gavey et al. 1989). In vivo experiments in rats demonstrated that the absorption of the subnitrate and the subsalicylate can be enhanced by the presence of sulfhydryl-containing compounds such as cysteine in the gastrointestinal tract (Chaleil et al. 1981). This effect was absent when cysteine was administered in the form of a cysteine-rich diet (D'Souza and Francis 1987).

Oral intake of bismuth compounds leads to a significant rise in bismuth concentrations in blood and plasma. After oral administration of bismuth subnitrate, silicate, or phosphate in healthy volunteers, blood bismuth concentrations varied from 17 ± 11 to 38 ± 8 μg/l. It should be noted that 15 ± 12 μg/l bismuth was measured in the blood of persons not receiving bismuth therapy (Conso et al. 1975). Recently, an early peak in blood or plasma bismuth concentration was demonstrated in patients and healthy volunteers after oral intake of CBS (Table 1). In 9 of 16 volunteers, peak concentrations above 100 μg/l were reached for 10–145 min (Nwokolo et al. 1989).

Table 1. Peak concentrations of bismuth after oral intake of colloidal bismuth subcitrate in several studies

Tablets (No)	Blood/ plasma	Bi (ng/ml)	Time of peak (min)	Author
?	p	25 ± 6	43 ± 5	McLean et al. 1988
1	b	4.7 - 21	15 - 60	Hespe et al. 1988
2	p	25 - 300	15 - 105	Nwokolo et al. 1989

In multiple dosing studies with CBS, an apparent steady state was reached in approximately 4 weeks with median plasma concentrations varying from 5 to 40 μ/gl (Gavey et al. 1989; Lee 1981).

The mechanism and the site of absorption are still unknown. The presence of early peaks in blood bismuth concentration after administration of CBS suggests either absorption from the stomach or from the proximal small bowel. Electron microscopy demonstrated the presence of CBS particles in the epithelial cells of the duodenum and proximal small bowel after oral intake of CBS in patients and experimental animals (Coghill et al. 1983). In rats, after short oral challenge with CBS, the uptake of bismuth in the mucosa, as studied by mucosal scrapings, was significantly higher in the proximal jejunum, ileum, and duodenum than in the stomach (Stiel et al. 1985).

Although the intestinal absorption of bismuth still needs to be investigated extensively, it seems that a very large variation in absorption within and between individuals is present.

Distribution

The circulating form of bismuth in blood is still unknown as are the compounds, most probably proteins, to which bismuth may be bound in vivo. Gel filtration of human blood incubated with bismuth subgallate demonstrated association of bismuth with high molecular weight proteins ($\geq$ 200.000 daltons) (Thomas et al. 1983).

Despite the large variation in compounds tested, the data on the distribution of bismuth over the organs are in remarkably close agreement and largely independent of the compound administered or the route of administration (Slikkerveer and de Wolff 1989). The highest concentration and the longest retention were always found in the kidney. An exemplary distribution was seen in rats after oral administration of CBS for 14 months (Lee et al. 1980): Kidney (13.9 μg/g) >> lung > spleen > liver > brain > heart > muscle (0.13 μg/g wet weight).

Metabolic Aspects

After exposure of patients to bismuth compounds for the treatment of syphilis, inclusion bodies were found in the proximal tubulus of the kidney in 86% of the patients (Beaver and Burr 1963). These inclusion bodies are sharply defined, round structures with a diameter of 5 μm. They are located in the nucleus and cytoplasm of the cells and contain bismuth, protein, carbohydrates, sulfur, and lipids (Ghadially 1979). In rats after exposure to subcutaneously injected $BiCl_3$, the binding of bismuth in the kidneys changed from high molecular weight proteins to a low molecular weight protein. This protein has been identified as a methallothioneine-like metal binding protein. The synthesis of this protein is induced de novo by the presence of bismuth and the process can be inhibited by selenium. As far as is known, this synthesis mainly takes place in the kidney. (Szymańska et al. 1978; Szymańska and Piotrowski 1980). The function of these proteins in the body is as yet unknown.

Elimination

Bismuth is eliminated from the body by urinary and fecal routes. The elimination in feces is thought to occur partly via the bile and partly via intestinal secretion (Gregus and Klaassen 1986). The contribution of both routes is still subject to discussion. Elimination from blood demonstrates multicompartment pharmacokinetics in humans and in rodents. Data on half-life times are still inconsistent. The only half-life times measured in humans are 3.5 min, and 15 min, and 3.2 h (de Bray et al. 1977). A compartment with a much longer half-life time, 17–22 years, may also exist in some or all patients (Buijs et al. 1985).

Toxic Effects

In the past, the use of bismuth compounds led to a variety of adverse effects. Clinically, the most important of these were nephrotoxicity and bismuth encephalo-

Table 2. Signs and symptoms of bismuth encephalopathy in 698 patients. (From Reinicke 1982)

Neurological symptoms	%	Psychic manifestations	%
Myoclonic jerks	80	Confusional syndrome	79
Trembling	59	Concentration incapacity	60
Memory disturbances	56	Deceleration of thought	58
Writing disturbances	53	Mental disturbance	36
Dysarthria	52	Excitation	35
Inability to walk	38	Depression	32
Rolling gait	36	Anxiety	27
Insomnia	35	Hallucinations	17
Sphincter troubles	30	Delirium	16
Convulsive crises	28	Other symptoms	%
Somnolence	25		
Cephalgia	25	Shoulder stiffness	8
Motor deficit	20	Renal impairment	5
Gait disturbances	20		
Abnormal movements	19	Osteonecrosis of the humeral head	3
Coma	13	Bismuth line on gums	0.4
Isolated Babinski	8		
Pyramidal signs	8		
Diplopia	5		

pathy. An epidemic-like outbreak of poisoning occurred in France between 1972 and 1978 and was caused by the intake of inorganic bismuth compounds. The signs and symptoms of bismuth encephalopathy are listed in Table 2. The exact etiology of these intoxications has never been clarified. It was suspected that another factor was responsible besides the intake of bismuth (Martin Bouyer et al. 1980, 1981).

Nephrotoxicity was seen in the form of acute reversible renal failure after use of bismuth tri- or thioglycollamate and diallylacetate (Urizar and Vernier 1966). Delayed reversible renal failure was noted after autointoxication with 100 tablets of De-Nol® (CBS) (Hudson and Mowat 1989). In the gastrointestinal tract, a bismuth line on the gums, gingivitis, stomatitis, and colitis have been described. Hepatitis has been mentioned as a side effect, but evidence is insufficient to prove a causal relationship. Osteoarthropathy has been described after treatment for syphilis and as a complication during bismuth encephalopathy.

It should be noted that adverse effects were always associated with one bismuth compound or a certain group of compounds.

Safety Evaluation

Although knowledge of bismuth is limited, some comments can be made on the safety of bismuth compounds in man. Generally, a standardized procedure is used for the evaluation of safety margins. This procedure starts with the evaluation of exposure, taking into account the nature of the compound studied, its occurrence and the quantities present. The route of exposure is investigated and an attempt is made to quantify the size of exposure. At present, interest in bismuth is limited to medicine, where the administered dose can be calculated from the amount per tablet and the number of tablets. What fraction really enters the body is still unknown. It may be assumed that this fraction is very low. For the moment, the concentration of bismuth in blood will have to be taken as the most accurate estimate of exposure. The next step in the evaluation of safety is to gather information on the pharmacokinetics of the compound and on the adverse effects in relation to dose or blood concentration. The relation between dose and adverse effects of bismuth is still obscure. The last step in safety evaluation is the comparison of the exposure to the existing safety limits or the formulation of new safety limits if none exist.

The only tentative safety limits for bismuth were proposed by Hillemand et al. (1977): a bismuth concentration in blood below 50 μg/l can be considered safe, between 50 μg/l and 100 μg/l the patient should be checked regularly, and above 100 μg/l treatment should be stopped immediately.

Before testing bismuth levels against these criteria, it is necessary to evaluate the safety limits themselves. These levels were based on a comparison of two groups of patients. The first group – nonintoxicated patients – was undergoing oral bismuth subnitrate therapy, in doses between 10 and 20 g/day, according to the Bensaude rule (20 days of treatment followed by 10 days of rest). Blood samples were taken at random during therapy, so they could have been taken during the rest period too. The other group consisted of patients suffering from bismuth encephalopathy, whose data were taken from the literature. There are three main points of criticism of the Hillemand paper:

1. The data from both intoxicated and nonintoxicated groups of patients were not sufficiently standardized to be combined.
2. Comparison of data of two groups from two separate sources is only acceptable for drawing preliminary conclusions and not for far-reaching conclusions concerning international safety levels.
3. The analytical techniques, with which the data for the calculations were obtained, differed greatly, and the data should not have been compared.

However disputable, these safety margins are the only ones available in the literature. If we really wish to use them in evaluating the current data on bismuth levels, at least two kinetic criteria should be distinguished: the trough values and the peak values. At the moment no conclusions can be drawn, as the safety levels of bismuth will need to be (re)assessed in a controlled experiment with validated analytical and epidemiological methods.

References

Beaver DL, Burr RE (1963) Bismuth inclusions in the human kidney. Archives of Pathology 76:89–94

Buijs WC, Corstens FH, Beentjes LB (1985) Long-term retention of ^{207}Bi in the body after injection of ^{206}Bi. Health Phys 49:1267–1269

Chaleil D, Lefevre F, Allain P, Martin GJ (1981) Enhanced bismuth digestive absorption in rats by some sulfhydryl compounds: nmr study of complexes formed. J Inorg Biochem 15:213–221

Coghill SB, Hopwood D, McPherson S, Hislop S (1983) The ultrastructural localisation of De-Nol® (colloidal tripotassium dicitrato-bismuthate-TDB) in the upper gastrointestinal tract of man and rodents following oral and instrumental administration. J Pathol 139:105–114

Conso F, Bourdon R, Gaultier M (1975) Bismuth sanguin et urinaire après traitement bref par différents sels "insolubles" de bismuth. Eur J Toxicol 8:137–141

De Bray J-M, Emile J, Moreau R, Daver A, Cheguillaume J, Allain P (1977) Pathogénie des encéphalopathies bismuthiques. Étude préliminaire à l'aide du bismuth 206 chez l'homme. Nou Presse Med 6:1394

D'Souza RW, Francis WR (1987) Bioavailability and pharmacokinetics of bismuth in the rat. Pharm Res 4 [Suppl]:115

Gavey CJ, Szeto M-L, Nwokolo CU, Sercombe J, Pounder RE (1989) Bismuth accumulates in the body during treatment with tripotassium dicitrato bismuthate. Aliment Pharmacol Ther 3:21–28

Ghadially FN (1979) Ultrastructural localization and in situ analysis of iron, bismuth and gold inclusions. CRC Crit Rev Toxicol 6:303–350

Gregus Z, Klaassen CD (1986) Disposition of metals in rats: a comparative study of fecal, urinary and biliary excretion and tissue distribution of eighteen metals. Toxicol Appl Pharmacol 85:24–38

Hespe W, Staal HJM, Hall DWR (1988) Bismuth absorption form the colloidal subcitrate. Lancet II:1258

Hillemand P, Pallière M, Laquais B, Bouvet P (1977) Traitement bismuthique et bismuthémie. Semaine des Hôpiteaux de Paris 53:1663–1669

Hudson M, Mowat NAG (1989) CBS (De-Nol®) self-poisoning – reversible toxicity. Br Med J 299:159

Lee SP (1981) Studies on the absorption and excretion of tripotassium dicitrato-bismuthate in man. Res Commun Chem Pathol Pharmacol 43:359–364

Lee SP, Lim TH, Pybus J, Clarke AC (1980) Tissue distribution of orally administered bismuth in the rat. Clin Exp Pharmacol Physiol 7:319–324

Martin-Bouyer G, Foulon B, Guerbois H, Barin C (1980) Aspects épidémiologiques des encéphalopathies après administration de bismuth par voie orale. Therapie 35:307–313

Martin-Bouyer G, Foulon G, Guerbois H, Barin C (1981) Epidemiological study of encephalopathies following bismuth administration per os. Characteristics of intoxicated subjects: comparison with a control group. Clin Toxicol 18:1277–1283

McLean AJ, Froomes P, McNeill JJ, Wan AT, Harrison PM (1988) Bismuth subcitrate handling in man; abstract. Clin Pharmacol Ther 186

Nwokolo CU, Gavey CJ, Smith JTL, Pounder RE (1989) The absorption of bismuth from oral doses of tripotassium dicitrato bismuthate. Aliment Pharmacol Ther 3:29–39

Reinicke C (1982) Bismuth. In: Dukes MNG (ed) Dukes side effects of drugs (annual 6), Excerpta Medica, Amsterdam, pp 217–221

Slikkerveer A, de Wolff FA (1989) Pharmacokinetics and toxicity of bismuth compounds. Med Toxicol Adverse Drug Exp 4:303–322

Stiel D, Murray DJ, Peters TJ (1985) Uptake and subcellular localisation of bismuth in the gastrointestinal mucosa of rats after short term administration of CBS. Gut 26:364–368

Szymańska JA, Piotrowski JK (1980) Studies to identify the low molecular weight bismuthbinding proteins in rat kidney. Biochem Pharmacol 29:2913–2918

Szymańska JA, Zychowicz M, Zelazowski AJ, Piotrowski JK (1978) Effect of selenium on the organ distribution and binding of bismuth in rat tissues. Arch Toxicol 40:131–141

Thomas DW, Sobecki S, Hartley TF, Coyle P, Alp MH (1983) Variable absorption and excretion of bismuth and its potential for toxicity. In: Brown SS, Savory J (eds) Chemical toxicology and clinical chemistry of metals. Academic, London, pp 391–394

Urizar R, Vernier RL (1966) Bismuth nephropathy. JAMA 198:207–209

Discussion

Demling: You showed us a list of side effects, but we learned that those side effects don't only depend on the area under the curve of observed material, but also on the form of the curve. If there is a peak, you may be getting into the region of toxicity; on the other hand, if there is a flat but long curve, you may get into a region of no effect, so the effect of a drug depends on the form of the curve.

Slikkerveer: I do not think I said that, because I do not agree. We do not know whether the height of the peak, i. e., the form of the curve is important for the toxicity. Most toxic effects are long-term effects, and the peak is an acute phenomenon.

Demling: Yes, but an acute peak can mean toxicity, as we know from antibiotics.

Slikkerveer: But we do not see this toxicity. Toxicity is only seen after long-term exposure and there are no real acute effects of bismuth.These are all long-term effects but perhaps you are right. Perhaps when the peak goes up too high something changes in the body. But I honestly do not know. I think it's more the case that all the effects are the long-term; the central nervous system effects are an accumulative type of effect.

Demling: You repeat this peak every day?

Slikkerveer: You may know, but I do not whether the peak is the same every day.

Graham: The patient that took 100 tablets certainly did not experience a long-term side effect.

Slikkerveer: No, he experienced kidney disturbances but no central nervous system disturbances.

Demling: But I mean if you take some bismuth tablets every day and thus have a peak every day I think you can get into the range of toxicity.

Slikkerveer: If what you say is true. If you have every day a high peak, if you are one of those "high absorbers" if they exist, then you will probably enter the toxic range. But I do not know whether there are people who have peaks every day, every time they take the bismuth or whether they are as high every day.

Demling: I mean subcitrate for example.

Slikkerveer: Yes, they are the ones with the peaks, but I still do not know whether there are high peaks every day.

Volkheimer: What is the diameter of the particles?

Slikkerveer: They were 5 μm.

Menge: Professor Tytgat, you want to contribute to this discussion.

Tytgat: Yes. The colloidal particles are small, but bismuth is not absorbed as an entire particle. It is absorbed as bismuth, and that is a small molecule which is taken up by the small intestine. It is bound to metallo-protein and then, when this is saturated, it may enter the systemic circulation, where it is in all probability bound to proteins. I fully agree with Dr. Slikkerveer that the very short duration of that early peaking is presumably irrelevant, because virtually everything is protein bound. The total amount of bismuth absorbed after a full course of therapy is 0.2%, which is a very small amount, and this is fully excreted in the urine. It takes some time to excrete from the third compartment, which is presumably the kidney.

Graham: Was your statement about irrelevancy opinion or fact?

Tytgat: You promised me that you would do the studies with four quadrant serial biopsies every day in your patients for about 1 year, so we anxiously await your data, Dr. Graham.

Blessing: You have mentioned that one must be critical about the methods of determining of bismuth. I have a question to Dr. Nwokolo. In one of your figures you have shown a maximal concentration of 530 μg/L; is this a correct result or may it be a contamination effect because in similar studies we performed recently, we only found concentrations up to 170 μg bismuth per litre plasma?

Nwokolo: These results were measured by an analytical chemist in the UK and we accepted the results *at face value*. It is possible to argue that levels were excessive – we were not expecting to see such levels anyway – we were quite surprised when those results came back, so we were not in a position to say it is impossible to have bismuth levels above 500 ng/ml. This was new ground, completely new ground. It is possible that 530 ng/ml is an outlyer and perhaps we should ignore it, but I think the message of that particular study is that there is an early peak.

Tytgat: Were all the samples obtained through an in-dwelling catheter? Or did you use separate punctures? I'm asking that because I'm still not sure that bismuth cannot stick to plastic.

Slikkeveer: It will react later.

Nwokolo: In the methodology, we used in-dwelling catheters. We couldn't puncture the subjects every 10 min, so we had an in-dwelling intravenous catheter. We used 40 units of heparin to maintain its patency.

Slikkerveer: I would like to react to the analytical problems first. It is not logical that there is contamination in bismuth analysis. It is when something happens that you lose the bismuth, so you should probably believe the higher rather than the lower numbers. It is in the low numbers that you run into problems. That is the first point, and the second is that as far as we know, we have developed a suitable method for analyzing bismuth. There is no problem with plastic, nor is there a problem with glass. As far as we know up to now, bismuth is not lost.

Veldhuyzen van Zanten: Based on your review, is there a method you recommend strongly, for measuring bismuth in blood samples?

Slikkerveer: I could say my own, but that would not be honest.

Menge: And what method do you use?

Slikkerveer: I do use a method with electrothermal atomic absorption spectrophotometry, but it is difficult to give a definitive answer as to which is the true method, because to decide this quality control is necessary and there are too few people doing the bismuth measurements to make a quality control system possible. When we know how many people are measuring bismuth, we perhaps can start such a system. There is a center in the United Kingdom which does all the metal quality control systems, and we would like to place our system there. There are some other methods but it is difficult to say which is best, because in the literature the analytical specifications are not specific enough to judge the method. You have to be careful and you should remember to check the method. That is the most important message.

Menge: Okay, we have got the point.

Wadström: What method can be used for tissue concentrations. You emphasise that this is much more difficult.

Slikkerveer: It is much more difficult, because there are more interfering factors. I think there is at the moment no method published which I could recommend. I think you should be careful in what you are doing. This is the only thing I can say at the moment, because there are all kinds of techniques – you need acid digestion or a microwave to digest the sample, and then you need to do the measurement itself. I cannot give an answer.

Menge: You mentioned that some measurements were done in blood samples and others in plasma samples. Do you know whether there are differences in bismuth concentrations using blood or plasma samples?

Slikkerveer: It seems – these are preliminary data – that when people take bismuth for a longer time, the ratio between blood and plasma changes. And that could mean that bismuth enters the red blood cells or other blood cells, but that is why I warn you about it. I think at the moment you should take both to be sure.

Nwokolo: Just a comment on toxicity – something I've tried desperately to get away from. In France, there was massive ingestion of bismuth containing salts. I think it was an average of about 15–20 g a day or was it milligrams?

Slikkerveer: No, grams. You are right, yes.

Nwokolo: And the observation was that it was surprising that only perhaps 80 people died and 980 cases of intoxication have been reported. Considering the tonnage of the stuff that was ingested this seems to suggest that there may be a small group within the population that is more susceptible than others, perhaps a small percentage. I think that our work demonstrates that there is marked interindividual variation in the amount of bismuth absorbed following oral dosing.

Menge: In France the toxic agent was mainly bismuth subnitrate, and in Australia it was mainly subgallate. Do you think intoxication will be possible with all other bismuth compounds as well?

Slikkerveer: I think that is a question which basically cannot be answered. But the subgallates which were responsible for intoxication in Australia, were also responsible in France for some of the cases. So, this cannot be answered. But there were a large number of preparations involved.

Graham: I would like to at least put this into perspective. We are discussing bismuth toxicity with question marks. I mean, does it occur with the doses we are giving and if it occurs, is it important, because everyone agrees it is totally reversible. You stop the drug and the patients recover. At the same time we are giving our patients potent antibiotics and every time we do that we know that they may cause side effects. But what percentage of our patients are going to have a major side effect, and is it reversible? So we are really talking about a drug that is incredibly safe compared with drugs that we feel much more comfortable with, but which are inherently much more dangerous. I think we should not lose sight of that.

Ober: I think the answer is out on which bismuth salts caused toxicity and encephalopathy in France. All those that were used, all those that were available caused at least one case of bismuth toxicity. There was only a slight shift in the proportion in favor of nitrates. If the consumption of the salts was divided by the number of intoxications, the highest quotient was obtained for nitrates.

Slikkerveer: Yes, you are right.

Section 4

Clinical Trials for *Helicobacter pylori* Treatment

Treatment Regimens to Eradicate *Helicobacter pylori*

G. BÖRSCH

Introduction

It is the aim of this contribution to give a brief review of present-day modalities to eradicate *Helicobacter* (formerly *Campylobacter*) *pylori* from its gastroduodenal habitat. Treatment options, however, must be viewed against the background of the natural history and the pathophysiological relevance of *H. pylori* colonization in humans. Careful note should therefore be taken of the work published by Langenberg et al. [15, 16] and many others that *H. pylori* infection leads to a chronic and stable colonization of gastric antral epithelium. These bacteria then act as a direct cause of chronic active type B gastritis [28] and likewise take part in the composite causes of idiopathic or gastritis-associated ulcer disease [12], which may be termed GAUD [3].

It has to be stressed that *H. pylori* colonization is indeed a stable condition; hence spontaneous clearance – if at all possible – represents a rare phenomenon. Thus active treatment of some kind will presently provide the only reasonable approach to achieve bacterial clearance, in the event that this should appear to be desirable in individual patients from a clinical point of view.

When treating *H. pylori* one should definitely aim at bacterial eradication rather than mere temporary suppression of the bacterial density, since only then – in theory and in practice – can the true potential of *H. pylori* therapy be fully exploited, e.g., the profound modification of the natural history of chronic gastritis and of gastritis-associated ulcer disease, at least gastritis-associated duodenal ulcer disease.

Attempts at eradication are not fruitless endeavors from the bacteriological point of view, since – as has been shown among others in Amsterdam by Rauws et al. [25], in Virginia by Marshall et al. [18], in Australia by Borody et al. [8, 9], and by our own group in the Federal Republic of Germany [7] – reinfection is a rare phenomenon in the event that true eradication has indeed been achieved, which should not be assessed prior to 3 or even 4 weeks after cessation of the index therapy [6, 25].

Clearly, the initial clinical results so far published, especially the dramatic reduction of the frequency of duodenal ulcer relapses after *H. pylori* eradication [8, 9, 10, 17] in addition to the infrequent bacterial reinfections from outside sources, now render top clinical priority to research aimed at identifying suitable treatment regimens to eradicate *H. pylori*. How then can eradication of *H. pylori* be achieved, but in a safe, effective, and reasonably inexpensive manner?

H. Menge et al. (Eds.)
Helicobacter pylori 1990

Antibiotic Monotherapy

The following discussions will be confined to bacteriological, not clinical results. They will address studies that have assessed the posttherapeutic *H. pylori* state of treated patients not before 3–4 weeks after cessation of the index therapy, unless the inefficiency of the treatment regimen under study has been sufficiently documented by demonstrating posttherapeutic persistence of *H. pylori* colonization immediately after therapy. With very few exceptions, all antibiotics are highly active in vitro against *H. pylori*. All of these are highly ineffective in vivo in the natural gastric environment, and the reasons why that might be so may reside in the very complex interrelations of topical and systemic actions of these drugs and their pharmacokinetic properties in the wide pH range which is so characteristic of the thin epithelial mucus layer [20]. A list of antibiotics, the efficacy of which as monotherapy against *H. pylori* has so far been assessed, is given in Table 1. Detailed references are summarized elsewhere [4, 5, 13].

Table 1. List of antibiotics so far applied and proven ineffective as monotherapy against *H. pylori*. Detailed references are given elsewhere [4, 5, 13]

Ciprofloxacin	Oral penicillin
Ofloxacin	Bacampicillin
Norfloxacin	Pivmecillinam
Nitrofurantoin	Doxycycline
Furazolidone	Erythromycin
Fusidic acid	Josamycin
Nifuroxazide	Spiramycin
Paromomycin	Rifampicin
Tinidazole	Amoxycillin
Metronidazole	

All these drugs have so far been proved ineffective with eradication rates generally well below 30%, at least at the doses and treatment durations so far applied. In addition, there are oral or personal communications that oral cephalosporins and clindamycin are likewise ineffective drugs.

Of considerable interest are, however, initial Swedish data that describe a beneficial effect of a profound pH modification on the efficacy of antibiotic monotherapy, communicated by Unge et al. [29]. In the hands of these investigators, amoxycillin 1.5 g/day for 14 days as monotherapy led to bacterial eradication in a meagre 14% of patients treated. However, in stomachs rendered anacidic by omeprazole, there was a surprising eradication rate of five out of eight carriers (63%) by amoxycillin alone. There have been speculations on the antibacterial action of omeprazole itself, possibly eradicating *H. pylori* by allowing a wide array of gut bacteria to colonize an anacidic and thus rather defenseless stomach, making the stomach a bowel-like environment from a bacteriological point of view. Gut bacteria are then said to compete with *H. pylori* for space or rather mucus, finally eradicating these spirals by depriving them of their ecological niche. However, Unge et al. [29] clearly suggest that this is not so, by describing an eradication rate for omeprazole after 2 weeks of treatment of none in eight [29]. Nevertheless, these initial observations open the path to a reinvestigation of the whole range of antibiotics which had previously been proved to be ineffective, but which may behave differently and effectively after profound pH modifications of the natural gastric environment.

Bismuth Monotherapy

While bismuth salts may effectively suppress *H. pylori,* they rarely eradicate. The best results of bismuth monotherapy with an eradication rate of 43% have been published by the O'Morain group from Dublin, Ireland [24]. Most other authors reported eradication rates after bismuth monotherapy between 10% and 30% [4, 13]. Note should also be taken of Lambert's recent work that colloidal bismuth subcitrate (CBS) given as 2 × 2 tablets is apparently less effective (15% eradication) than CBS in a dose of 4 × 1 tablets (yielding 30% eradication) [14].

Oral Triple-Drug Therapy

Antibiotic monotherapy and the bismuth work left *H. pylori* enthusiasts with a bacterium, with intelligent and elegant pathogenetic models to describe its potential role in gastroduodenal disease, but – unfortunately – without any effective therapy. It was in this state of therapeutic despair that investigators like Borody from Australia [8, 9] focused their attention on what has long been standard for Koch's *Mycobacterium tuberculosis:* oral triple therapy. Amazingly, the Borody modification with bismuth and tetracycline for 4 weeks plus metronidazole for 2 weeks (Table 2) yielded an eradication rate of 94% in a large population of duodenal ulcer and nonulcer

Table 2. Eradication of *H. pylori* by oral triple-drug therapy

Author	Drug	Dosage	Duration (days)	*n*	Indication	Study type	Eradication after 4 weeks
O'Riordan et al. 1989 [24]	CBS Amoxycillin Metronidazole	4×120 mg 3×500 mg 3×400 mg	28 7 7	20	DU	Controlled	17/20=85%
Börsch et al. 1989 [6, 7]	BSS Metronidazole Amoxycillin	3×600 mg 3×500 mg 3×500 mg	7–14 7–14 7–14	96	Ulcer and/or NUD	Controlled	77/96=80%
Borody et al. 1988 [8]	CBS Tetracycline Metronidazole	4×120 mg 4×500 mg 4×200 mg	28 28 14	100	DU NUD	Pilot	94/100=94%
McNulty et al. 1989 [21]	CBS Achromomycine Metronidazole	4×120 mg[a] 4×250 mg 4×200 mg	28 28 14	30	NUD	Pilot	17/30=65%

BSS, bismuth subsalicylate tablets; CBS, colloidal bismuth subcitrate; NUD, nonulcer dyspepsia
[a] Swallow tablets

dyspepsia patients, thus giving unequivocal proof that *H. pylori* colonization of the upper gastrointestinal tract is a condition which can be treated with predictable and high success rates. McNulty et al. [21] were unable completely to confirm Borody's high Australian success rates, finding eradication by a British adaption of the Borody triple therapy in only 65% (Table 2). However, as we know from the work of Glupczynski et al. [11], full drug compliance is exceptionally rare in such patients. Also, swallow tablets as used by McNulty et al. [21] might yield results different from those of other CBS galenic preparations.

The work of our own group using bismuth subsalicylate (BSS), metronidazole, and amoxycillin 3 × 500 mg for as short as 1 week showed eradication in approximately 80% of patients finishing treatment [5, 6, 7]. This has recently been confirmed by O'Riordan et al. [24] for a similar therapeutic regimen.

Therefore, oral triple therapy in various modifications is effective against *H. pylori,* with eradication rates ranging from 80% to 94%, disregarding McNulty's 65% results [21]. However, the safety of oral triple therapy has not been proven in large controlled clinical trials, and at present such therapy is not commendable for routine clinical work.

Double-Drug Therapy

But is it indeed oral triple therapy which is really being needed? In a systematic manner, the Irish O'Morain group [24] has added 1 week of treatment with amoxycillin 3 × 500 mg, metronidazole 3 × 200 or 3 × 400 mg, or metronidazole plus amoxycillin to a 4-week course of CBS. CBS plus metronidazole 3 × 400 mg gave an equivalent eradication rate (85%) to triple-drug therapy with CBS plus metronidazole plus amoxycillin. The latter thus might be superfluous in most patients.

Therefore, it might be double-drug therapy which may represent the treatment of choice to eradicate *H. pylori,* if such treatment should appear desirable from a clinical point of view in an individual patient. Bismuth plus amoxycillin [25] or bismuth plus ofloxacin [1] are not particularly effective combinations. The best results so far have been achieved by bismuth plus metronidazole. Three doses of 400 mg is superior (85%) to 3 × 200 mg (57%) [24]. Giving the drug three times daily may also be advantageous, since Marshall et al. [17] obtained slightly lower eradication rates of 70% by giving tinidazole, which is comparable to metronidazole, twice daily 500 mg for 10 days in addition to CBS for 56 days. Prior in vitro identification of the 20% metronidazole resisters could likewise help to improve results even further [19].

Apparently, bismuth does not play an essential part in double therapeutic regimens. Our own initial data suggest that metronidazole plus amoxycillin for 1 week yields eradication rates of 78% [5], while Oderda et al. [23] in children even obtained eradication in 94%, albeit by 6 weeks drug treatment of this double combination.

Experimental Approaches

Up to now there have not been any convincing clinical results concerning interesting experimental approaches such as mucus modifiers or urease inhibitors. Of course, active *H. pylori* vaccination, if ever possible, could very well prove virtually to eradicate chronic active gastritis and duodenal ulcer disease and also to modify the prevalence of gastric cancer disease. However, at issue is mucosal – not systemic – immunity, the induction of which could represent an extremely difficult, if at all feasible, endeavor.

More practically oriented experimental approaches to treat *H. pylori* presently center around the reinvestigation of antibiotic efficacy after prior induction of profound pH changes in the gastric environment, for example via omeprazole-induced anacidity [29].

Conclusion

The main question to be addressed in this contribution – how can eradication of *H. pylori* be achieved – is much more easily answered in 1989 than it had been possible during the 1987 First International Symposium on *Helicobacter pylori* in Kronberg [22]. The main answers are that for achieving eradication, antibiotic monotherapy is ineffective (< 30%). Bismuth monotherapy is not superior (< 30%). Oral triple therapy may be 80%–94% effective, but since it is of yet unproven safety it is presently not commendable for routine clinical application. Double therapy with bismuth/metronidazole or amoxycillin/metronidazole as the most suitable candidates presently appears more appealing especially in the light of initial data from Ireland [24] and Australia [17] that it may yield results similar to those of oral triple therapy with eradication rates of 85% or higher. One can also infer from what is known about the safety of metronidazole therapy from its extremely broad application for female genital tract colonizations by *Trichomonas vaginalis* or gram-negative bacteria that single short-term therapeutic courses of this nitroimidazole will not be hampered by safety considerations [2, 26, 27].

A new and highly interesting experimental approach presently makes use of profound alterations of gastric pH to improve the in vivo efficacy of antibiotic monotherapy, but only very limited data are available in this important research field so far.

In summary, it may therefore be concluded that effective and reasonably safe regimens to eradicate *H. pylori* now exist, and that they should suffice to give further clear experimental proof of the *H. pylori* hypothesis by eradicating these organisms safely and predictably in a large number of ulcer and dyspepsia patients, preferentially entered in large and well-conducted randomized controlled therapeutic trials.

References

1. Bayerdörffer E, Simon T, Bästlein C, Ottenjann R (1987) Bismuth/ofloxacin combination for duodenal ulcer. Lancet II:1467–1468
2. Beard CM, Noller KL, O'Fallon WMO, Kurland LT, Dahlin DC (1988) Cancer after exposure to metronidazole. Mayo Clin Proc 63:147–153
3. Börsch G (1987) *Campylobacter pylori:* new and renewed insights into gastritis-associated ulcer disease (GAUD). Hepatogastroenterology 34:191–193
4. Börsch G (1988) Therapie der *Campylobacter pylori*-Infektion. Leber Magen Darm 18:40–45

5. Börsch G (1990) Antibiotische Eradikations-Therapie bei *Campylobacter pylori*-Besiedlung. In: Ottenjann R, Schmitt W (eds) 2. Münchener *Campylobacter pylori*-Symposium. Thieme, Stuttgart (in press)
6. Börsch G, Wegener M, Mai U, Opferkuch W (1989) Efficiency of oral triple therapy to eradicate *C. pylori*. In: Mégraud F, Lamouliatte H (eds) Gastroduodenal pathology and *Campylobacter pylori*. Elsevier, Amsterdam, pp 595–598
7. Börsch G, Wegener M, Reitemeyer E, Mai U, Opferkuch W (1989) Clinical results and medium term follow-up studies after eradication of *Campylobacter pylori*. In: Mégraud F, Lamouliatte H (eds) Gastroduodenal pathology and *Campylobacter pylori*. Elsevier, Amsterdam, pp 599–603
8. Borody T, Cole P, Noonan S, Morgan A, Ossip G, Maysey J, Brandl S (1988) Long-term *Campylobacter pylori* recurrence post-eradication. Gastroenterology 94:A43
9. Borody T, Noonan S, Cole P, Hyland L, Morgan A, Lenne J, Moore-Jones D, Brandl S (1989) Duodenal ulcer recurrence in patients remaining *C. pylori* (CP) negative long term post-eradication. Gastroenterology 96:A52
10. Coghlan JG, Gilligan D, Humphries H, McKenna D, Dooley C, Sweeney E, Keane C, O'Morain C (1987) *Campylobacter pylori* and recurrence of duodenal ulcers – a 12-month follow-up study. Lancet II:1109–1111
11. Glupczynski Y, Nyst JF, Burette A, Vanderlinden MP, Deltenre M (1989) Lack of antibiotic compliance in patients treated for *Campylobacter pylori*-associated gastritis. The Vth international workshop on *Campylobacter* infections, Puerto Vallarta, Mexico
12. Graham DY (1989) *Campylobacter pylori* and peptic ulcer disease. Gastroenterology 96:615–625
13. Hirschl AM, Pletschette M (1989) Antibiotic treatment of *Campylobacter pylori* infection. In: Rathbone BJ, Heatley RV (eds) *Campylobacter pylori* and gastroduodenal disease. Blackwell, Oxford, pp 217–224
14. Lambert JR, Borromeo M, Eaves ER, Hansky J, Korman M (1988) Efficacy of different dosage regimens of bismuth in eradicating *Campylobacter pylori*. Gastroenterology 94:A248
15. Langenberg W, Rauws EAJ, Houthoff HJ, Oudbier JH, van Bohemen CG, Tytgat GNJ, Rietra PJGM (1988) Follow-up study of individuals with untreated *Campylobacter pylori*-associated gastritis and of noninfected persons with non-ulcer dyspepsia. J Infect Dis 157:1245–1249
16. Langenberg W, Rauws EAJ, Widjojokusumo A, Tytgat GNJ, Zanen HC (1986) Identification of *Campylobacter pyloridis* isolates by restriction endonuclease DNA analysis. J Clin Microbiol 24:414–417
17. Marshall BJ, Goodwin CS, Warren JR, Murray R, Blincow ED, Blackbourn SJ, Phillips M, Waters TE, Sanderson CR (1988) Prospective double-blind trial of duodenal ulcer relapse after eradication of *Campylobacter pylori*. Lancet II:1437–1441
18. Marshall BJ, Caldwell SH, Hoffman SR, Frierson HF, Guerrant RL, McCallum RW (1989) Can *C. pylori* be eradicated? Long-term follow-up on 28 successfully treated patients. Gastroenterology 96:A321
19. Marshall BJ, Barret LJ, McCallum RW, Guerrant RL (1989) *C. pylori* therapy: is in vitro disc testing with metronidazole worthwhile? The Vth international workshop on *Campylobacter* infections, Puerto Vallarta, Mexico
20. McNulty CAM (1989) Bacteriological and pharmacological basis for the treatment of *Campylobacter pylori* infection. Gastroenterol Clin Biol 13:96B–100B
21. McNulty CAM, Eyre-Brook IA, Uff JS, Dent JC, Wilkinson SP (1989) Triple therapy is not always 95% effective. The Vth international workshop on *Campylobacter* infections, Puerto Vallarta, Mexico
22. Menge H, Gregor M, Tytgat GNJ, Marshall BJ (eds) (1988) *Campylobacter pylori*. Springer, Berlin Heidelberg New York
23. Oderda G, Vaira D, Hoton J, Ainley C, Altare F, Ansaldi N (1989) Amoxycillin plus tinidazole for *Campylobacter pylori* gastritis in children: assessment by serum IgG antibody, pepsinogen I, and gastrin levels. Lancet I:690–692
24. O'Riordan T, Tobin A, Beattie S, Sweeney E, Keane C, O'Morain C (1989) Adjuvant antibiotic treatment improves eradication of *Campylobacter pylori* in duodenal ulcer. Gastroenterology 96:A378
25. Rauws EAJ, Langenberg W, Houthoff HJ, Zanen HC, Tytgat GN (1988) *Campylobacter pyloridis*-associated chronic active antral gastritis. A prospective study of its prevalence and the effect of antibacterial and antiulcer treatment. Gastroenterology 94:33–40

26. Rosenblatt JE, Edson RS (1989) Metronidazole. Mayo Clin Proc 62:1013–1027
27. Scully BE (1988) Metronidazole. Med Clin North Am 72:613–621
28. Tytgat GNJ, Rauws A (1989) The role of *Campylobacter pylori* in gastroduodenal disease. A "believer"'s point of view. Gastroenterol Clin Biol 13:118B–121B
29. Unge P, Olsson J, Gad A, Gnarpe H (1989) Does omeprazole 40 mg o. m. improve antimicrobial therapy directed towards gastric *Campylobacter* in patients with antral gastritis? A pilot study. In: Mégraud F, Lamouliatte H (eds) Gastroduodenal pathology and *Campylobacter pylori*. Elsevier, Amsterdam, pp 641–645

Discussion

Classen: You mentioned in your talk that double-drug therapy is effective and you recommended bismuth and metronidazole. At the same time you said a combination of antibiotics and acid depressing drugs is interesting. Now, how do you proceed particularly in those patients who have first treatment with bismuth and metronidazole without eradicating *H. pylori.*

Börsch: We are just starting these investigations all together. I do not know of any group with experience in sequence therapy, such as trying one antibiotic combination first and trying another one in the patients with persisting colonization. We do not have experience with that, I don't know whether the Dutch group has. I start in my clinical practice with patients who want treatment with the bismuth plus metronidazole combination. If this does not eradicate the bacteria, I change back to conventional treatment with H_2-blockers. I have not tried other drug regimens in these patients.

Rauws: We have treated resistant patients who remained *Helicobacter*-positive after colloidal bismuth subcitrate monotherapy, amoxicillin monotherapy, or therapy with a combination of these two drugs. Only these patients were offered triple therapy, and in this negatively selected group of patients, eradication of about 85%–88% was observed.

Veldhuyzen van Zanten: I would like to ask what you think is the minimum requirement to assess eradication. I personally feel it should include a breath test. We have several patients where the breath test was positive and initial histology negative. When the histology was reviewed, *H. pylori* organisms were now found, but in low numbers. Can you comment on that?

Börsch: Yes, we stick to the Dutch data, and we have defined eradication by negative test results of urease test plus a very good culture 4 weeks after cessation of therapy. Patients who have been negative in these tests 4 weeks after therapy have in my own clinical work a very low rate of recurrence of *H. pylori* infection, below 10%. This is clinical proof for the fact that the 4-week interval after therapy is enough for really assessing eradication.

Veldhuyzen van Zanten: So, you don't think a breath test is necessary?

Börsch: I do not think so and it is clinically not available for most of us. I think, a good culture and urease test are enough to define eradication, but you have to do it 4 weeks after cessation of therapy.

Vaira: I really enjoyed your talk. I would like just to ask you a very simple question: don't you think we should perform a double-blind trial with bismuth plus tinidazole versus amoxicillin plus tinidazole, before saying that the bismuth plus tinidazole is the best treatment?

Börsch: We could do double-blind trials but it is much work for many doctors and many patients and the facts that we can derive from literature are very clear. A double combination of bismuth plus amoxicillin yields eradication at the most in 50% and many other studies have yielded results below that, 30% or even 25%. The results on metronidazole plus bismuth are almost uniform and in the high range of about 80%, and so are the amoxicillin/metronidazole combinations. I am not sure whether we should do a controlled trial to compare the efficacy of these two regimens. We should be more concerned about performing randomized trials to evaluate clinical end points.

Vaira: Very simple, very quickly. You may forget that unfortunately bismuth is not licensed, neither in the UK nor in Italy. I don't know about Germany. The children have therefore no chance of being treated differently. So, I think, we must consider this as well, don't you think so?

Börsch: The way to solve this problem would be to use amoxicillin plus metronidazole in such countries.

Tytgat: If you use that combination what is the frequency of resistance and what is the incidence of side-effects with amoxicillin plus metronidazole?

Börsch: My own experience is with bismuth-containing triple therapy, and getting the treatment duration down to 1 week, I have not seen serious side effects. There were quite a few minor effects such as burning of the throat or sensations of glossitis. I do not know about the Oderda's data in the children. I have no data of my own on resistance with metronidazole plus amoxicillin.

Vaira: Of course, they were not my patients. All the patients were in the pediatrics department in Turin. What Dr. Oderda told me was that we had a very low compliance rate. There were just three children; two got a little bit of nausea, and one had diarrhea for 1 or 2 days, but none of them had to stop therapy. I would like to remind you that they took the therapy for 6 weeks.

Effect of Eradication of *Helicobacter pylori* on Nonulcer Dyspepsia Syndrome and Chronic Gastritis

E. A. J. Rauws

Introduction

"Dyspepsia" is a syndrome with symptoms of postprandial epigastric pain, early satiety, nausea, vomiting, belching, and bloating. It is very common. The prevalence of nonulcer dyspepsia syndrome ranges from 20% to 30% [1, 2], and the annual incidence is over 1% [3]. Nonulcer dyspepsia is not only very common, but also costly, because it often results in empirical treatment intended to heal nonexisting peptic ulcer, resulting in expensive diagnostic tests and time lost from work [4].

Despite extensive investigation, only about 20% of patients have distinct mucosal lesions [5]. If there is no focal lesion or systemic disease, the patient is considered to have the "nonulcer dyspepsia" syndrome [6].

Different authors, however, define nonulcer dyspepsia differently, and often even their definitions for the main symptoms of this syndrome differ [6–10]. In practice, doctors use the term dyspepsia for a combination of symptoms attributed to the upper gastrointestinal tract, which are episodic, recurring, or chronic and persistent.

There is no generally accepted method of scoring dyspepsia. A positive placebo effect in about 30% makes interpretation of any therapeutic result even more difficult.

One of the best ways to score and monitor dyspeptic symptoms is probably to assess the symptoms on a duration-intensity-behavioral scale (DIBS) that contains at least seven steps [11, 12]. The symptom scoring should be started at least 1 or 2 weeks before even placebo treatment is given, to eliminate any influence of attention given to the patient's complaints on the symptoms. Treatment should then be started in a double-blind placebo-controlled study, while self-scoring of symptoms continues, four times a day (morning, lunchtime, dinnertime, and bedtime).

Progress in treatment has been hampered by the heterogeneity and our lack of knowledge of the pathophysiology of nonulcer dyspepsia. The role of acid or pepsin in its etiology is speculative. In practice, patients with apparently acid-related dyspeptic symptoms are treated with H_2-receptor antagonists, mucosal protective agents, or antacids. Dysmotility-like symptoms are usually treated with prokinetic drugs. Psychoactive drugs are tried when psychogenic factors are prominent.

In general, the treatment of nonulcer dyspepsia syndrome is rather diasppointing.

Use of antacids or H_2-receptor blockers in dyspeptic patients is usually no more effective than placebo [13, 14]. The effect of antacids or H_2-receptor antagonists can be partly explained by acid neutralization in patients with unrecognized gastroesophageal reflux [13]. Evidence of any beneficial effect of tranquilizers is lacking.

H. Menge et al. (Eds.)
Helicobacter pylori 1990

In some selected cases prokinetic drugs [15–17] and H_2-receptor blockers [18, 19] have been shown to improve symptoms.

The relation of *Helicobacter pylori*-associated gastritis to symptoms is controversial. The high prevalence of *H. pylori* colonization in nonulcer dyspepsia patients, compared for instance with that in age-matched blood donors, supports, however, the role of this microorganism in the etiology of active chronic gastritis and the dyspeptic symptoms.

However, active chronic gastritis is also common in an asymptomatic population [20–23] increasing with age [24] to affect more than half of those over 50 years of age. The link between *H. pylori* and gastritis, and the association between gastritis and dyspepsia led to therapeutic attempts to eradicate the microorganisms, with the aim of reducing gastric inflammation, thereby ameliorating dyspeptic symptoms.

If *H. pylori*-associated gastritis is a cause of nonulcer dyspepsia syndrome, then eradication of these microorganisms and normalization of the gastric mucosa would be expected to result in an improvement or even complete disappearance of the dyspeptic symptoms. This statement, however, is not that easy to prove or disprove.

Literature survey

McNulty et al. [25], in an investigator-blind study, compared bismuth subsalicylate, erythromycin ethylsuccinate, and placebo in the treatment of *H. pylori*-associated gastritis. They performed endoscopy and biopsy for culture and histological examination before and immediately after treatment, and asked patients about the presence and severity of nausea, vomiting, heartburn, belching, and indigestion. Usually within 48 h after treatment, patients were asked if their symptoms were the same, better, or worse.

Eleven of 12 patients with dyspeptic symptoms (92%) who were cleared of *H. pylori* reported improvement in symptoms compared with 21 of 32 patients with symptoms (66%) in the group with persistent infection. The difference did not reach statistical significance. These authors found no association between the severity of gastritis and symptoms before treatment or between the resolution of gastritis and improvement of symptoms after treatment.

Lambert et al. [26] in a double-blind randomized controlled trial treated 33 *H. pylori*-positive nonulcer dyspepsia patients with placebo or colloidal bismuth subcitrate (CBS) for 4 weeks.

Endoscopy with biopsy was repeated 1 week after cessation of therapy. A 5-day symptom score was completed before and after treatment. Clearance of *H. pylori* occurred in 11 of 15 (73%) of CBS-treated patients and in 1 of 18 (6%) placebo-treated patients. CBS therapy significantly relieved pain, day and night ($P < 0.01$). There was no significant improvement in the severity of heartburn, feeling of fullness, nausea, vomiting, or flatulence. More important, however, in subjects cleared (that is not "eradicated"!) of *H. pylori* there was a significant improvement in nausea, vomiting, and day and night pain ($P < 0.001$) in parallel with significant improvement in acute and chronic inflammatory changes of the mucosa ($P < 0.01$).

Borody et al. [27] related symptoms to *H. pylori* and histological gastritis in a double-blind trial of 4 weeks of CBS or placebo. Abdominal pain, heartburn, nausea, abdominal distension, and food intolerance were scored for 7 days on diary cards. Gastric mucosal biopsies were taken before and 2 weeks after stopping treatment. Placebo and CBS-treated patients were then all treated for another 4 weeks with CBS and restudied. In the CBS-treated, but not in the placebo-treated patients, there was significant improvement in abdominal pain ($P < 0.001$), abdominal distension ($P < 0.01$), and nausea ($P < 0.002$). Patients receiving CBS after initial placebo treatment also experienced significant improvement in abdominal pain and burning ($P < 0.01$). After active therapy there was a significant correlation between clearance of *H. pylori* and improvement in chronic gastritis. Unfortunately, there were no data on the relationship between symptoms and the *H. pylori* status.

Borody et al. [28] in another uncontrolled study scored for symptoms before and 2 weeks after treatment with CBS (4 weeks) plus tinidazole (10 days), with or without amoxicillin, erythromycin, or tetracycline. In 31 of 40 nonulcer dyspepsia patients *H. pylori* was no longer present on Warthin-Starry stain and/or urease test.

Epigastric pain or burning disappeared in 22 of 27 and improved by 50% in 4 of 27 patients with this symptom. Postprandial abdominal distension disappeared in 4 of 17 and improved in 11 of 17 patients. Nausea disappeared in four of nine and improved by 50% also in four of nine nonulcer dyspepsia patients. In patients who became *H. pylori* negative after treatment, gastritis disappeared in 9 of the 31 patients, and in 20 of the 31 patients there was a 50% improvement in the severity of active and/or active chronic gastritis.

Kang et al. [29] studied the effect of CBS on symptoms and gastric histology in patients with nonulcer dyspepsia syndrome. Patients were randomized to receive CBS or placebo one tablet qid for 8 weeks. Fifty-one patients completed the trial: 28 patients in the CBS group and 23 patients in the placebo group. Overall there was no difference between the two groups in terms of symptom relief, reduction of gastritis, or eradication of *H. pylori.* Among patients with histological gastritis, those ($n = 23$) who took CBS used significantly less antacids during the first 6 weeks of therapy ($P < 0.02$), they were more likely to become asymptomatic ($P < 0.05$), their gastritis was more likely to resolve ($P < 0.03$), and *H. pylori* was more likely to be cleared ($P < 0.001$), when composed with patients taking placebo. In contrast, nonulcer dyspepsia patients without gastritis in their index biopsies ($n = 28$) fared similarly whether they received CBS or placebo and used antacids in equal amounts. These authors concluded that administration of CBS benefited nonulcer dyspepsia patients with gastritis, but had no effect on those patients without gastritis. They suggested that histological gastritis is one of the several causes of nonulcer dyspepsia.

Morgan et al. [30 performed a double-blind, placebo-controlled randomized treatment study in adults with *H. pylori*-associated gastritis. Patients received furazolidone ($n = 14$), nitrofurantoin ($n = 24$), or a placebo ($n = 31$) for 14 days, and kept a daily diary of the severity of their symptoms of dyspepsia (belching, nausea, vomiting, heartburn, anorexia, indigestion, and abdominal pain). All symptoms were rated on the following scale: 0 = absent; 1 = mild; 2 = moderate; 3 = severe.

Follow-up data were gathered 2 and 6 weeks after treatment had ended. Endoscopy was carried out at baseline, 1 day after cessation of therapy, and 6 weeks after the end of treatment to verify colonization by *H. pylori* and to determine the severity of gastric inflammation. A total of 106 adult outpatients with *H. pylori*-associated gastritis and nonulcer dyspepsia were randomly assigned to the various therapeutic regimens.

Thirty-seven patients (35%) were excluded from the analysis for various reasons. In 12 patients (11 of 46 on nitrofurantoin and 1 of 45 on placebo) treatment had to be stopped because of adverse reactions. Exclusions during the posttreatment period (11 additional patients) were due to voluntary withdrawal.

Analysis of the symptom data revealed no significant differences between the three treatment groups in the length of time to relief of any of the seven symptoms assessed. The high rates of adverse reactions (nausea, headache) associated with treatment with nitrofurantoin and the low numbers of patients ($n = 15$) treated with furazolidone obscured any changes in symptoms that might have resulted from improvement of the underlying inflammation.

In a double-blind randomized study, Rokkas et al. [31] tested the efficacy of colloidal bismuth subcitrate in the clearance of *H. pylori* and symptoms. Sixty-six patients with dyspeptic symptoms (epigastric pain, nausea, vomiting, heartburn, halitosis, flatulence, postprandial bloating) with normal abdominal and upper gastrointestinal endoscopy were randomly allocated to 8 weeks of placebo two tablets bid, or CBS two tablets bid therapy. In addition all patients were given a supply of antacid tablets (Gelusil) for symptomatic relief and a diary on which to record daily the presence or absence of epigastric pain, its duration, and the number of antacid tablets taken.

The patient's overall well-being was quantified using a scale from 0 (= no symptoms) to 100, representing severe, unbearable symptoms. Antral biopsies and symptoms were assessed using a questionnaire, before and after treatment. Of the 52 patients completing the trial, 25 (12 *H. pylori*-positive) were on CBS and 27 (8 *H. pylori*-positive) on placebo.

Colloidal bismuth subcitrate cleared *H. pylori* from 10 of 12, and placebo cleared 0 of 8 *H. pylori*-positive patients. In the *H. pylori*-positive subgroup treated with CBS, the symptom score improved significantly over the pretreatment score. There were no improvements in symptom scores in the *H. pylori*-negative subgroup treated with CBS, or in the placebo (*H. pylori*-positive and -negative) group.

In the whole group of 66 patients there was a significant correlation between *H. pylori* and postprandial bloating ($P < 0.05$). In the subgroup of *H. pylori*-positive patients CBS abolished postprandial bloating in eight of ten patients with this symptom ($P = 0.002$), whereas placebo did not.

Remarkably, these authors found seven *H. pylori*-negative patients receiving placebo to be positive at the end of treatment. Five of these seven patients initially had gastritis, and it was suggested that they may have been colonized by *H. pylori* which was for some reason undetected. Another explanation suggested was that these patients were infected by *H. pylori*-contaminated fiberoptic endoscopes. The change from *H. pylori*-negative to -positive was associated with significant deterioration in symptoms, supporting the latter explanation.

Lambert et al. [32] studied 82 nonulcer dyspepsia patients in a prospective randomized placebo-controlled study to assess the efficacy of CBS in improving symptoms. All 82 nonulcer dyspepsia patients (50 patients were *H. pylori* positive) were randomized to receive either placebo or CBS (108 mg qid) for 4 weeks. Endoscopy with mucosal biopsies for histological and bacteriological examination was performed before and 1 week after therapy. Symptoms of day pain, night pain, heartburn, bloating, flatulence, and nausea/vomiting were scored from 0 (none) to 4 (severe) before and after cessation of therapy during 5 days by self-recording on symptom score cards.

The total symptom score before treatment was significantly higher in *H. pylori*-positive individuals compared with *H. pylori*-negative patients ($P < 0.05$).

Forty-eight of the 50 *H. pylori*-positive patients completed the study. Clearance of *H. pylori* occurred in 13 of 22 (59%) CBS-treated patients compared with only 1 of 26 placebo-treated patients. There was a significant improvement ($P < 0.05$) in the total symptom score in patients who cleared *H. pylori* after treatment. The improvement in symptoms occurred with all symptoms, but was most marked with abdominal pain.

Thirty of the 32 *H. pylori*-negative subjects completed the study. In these patients a nonsignificant change in both placebo and CBS-treated group was observed.

The authors concluded that eradication of *H. pylori* significantly improves symptoms and histological gastritis in nonulcer dyspepsia patients. In *H. pylori*-negative patients a small nonsignificant improvement in both placebo and CBS-treated patients was observed, demonstrating a certain placebo response rate in *H. pylori*-negative nonulcer dyspepsia patients.

The Amsterdam Study

In an open study nonulcer dyspepsia patients entered a 4-week trial with CBS, amoxicillin or CBS and amoxicillin combination, or CBS-amoxicillin-metronidazole combination therapy. Biopsies were taken, and symptoms of epigastric pain, nausea, vomiting, heartburn, and abdominal distension were recorded for severity and graded from 0 to 3 (absent = 0, mild = 1, moderate = 2, severe = 3). All *H. pylori*-positive nonulcer dyspepsia patients were included, irrespective of their symptom score.

The symptoms were evaluated by direct questioning before treatment (day 0), immediately after treatment (day 28–30), and 1 month after stopping treatment. The total "symptom score" was the sum of these individual assessments and varied from 0 (no symptoms) to a maximum of 15 (maximal symptom score).

Results

In this retrospective analysis, 117 nonulcer dyspepsia patients at the start of therapy, all *H. pylori*-positive, were evaluated. The results on the symptom score, regardless of therapeutic regimen, which aimed at eradicating *H. pylori*, are summarized in Table 1. We compared the symptom scores of these patients who remained *H. pylori*-positive after treatment (group A; n = 77 patients) with those who became and

Table 1. Symptom scores (mean) for nonulcer dyspepsia, in *H. pylori*-positive patients before treatment, immediately after treatment, and 1 month after stopping treatment, in relation to *H. pylori* status

	Before treatment	After treatment	One month after treatment
Group A (n = 77)	5.3	3.6	3.7
Group B (n = 40)	4.9	2.5	2.3

remained *H. pylori*-negative for at least 1 month after stopping treatment (group B; $n = 40$ patients).

In both groups A and B, symptom scores immediately after treatment were significantly lower than the pretreatment scores (Wilcoxon's matched-pairs signed rank test; $P < 0.001$). Symptom scores 1 month after stopping treatment did not differ significantly from those immediately after treatment in either group A (still *H. pylori*-positive) or group B (*H. pylori*-eradicated) ($P > 0.40$ in both groups).

When the two groups were compared with regard to symptom reduction (before treatment versus 1 month after treatment) there was a trend toward more improvement in the group in whom *H. pylori* was eradicated ($P = 0.10$).

Discussion

Histological evidence of gastritis in association with *H. pylori* is found in about 50%–90% of dyspeptic patients referred for upper gastrointestinal endoscopy. The higher prevalence of *H. pylori* in nonulcer dyspepsia patients than in asymptomatic persons, and the close association of *H. pylori* with active chronic gastritis, suggests that these organisms may be causally related to nonulcer dyspepsia.

Ingestion of *H. pylori,* as in two volunteer studies [33, 34], may result in acute dyspeptic symptoms, which resolved spontancously in both volunteers. In one study, the microorganism and the concomitant gastritis disappeared spontaneously [33] but in the other *H. pylori* and the subsequent gastritis persisted [34].

The histological improvement in the gastric mucosa after successful eradication of *H. pylori* [25, 35–37], especially after amoxicillin monotherapy [36, 37], is additional evidence for the causative role of *H. pylori* in active chronic gastritis. Our study [36] shows that successful eradication of *H. pylori* may lead to full histological normality of the gastric mucosa during prolonged follow-up.

The association between the resolution of gastritis following treatment and improvement of symptoms remains less clear.

Bismuth-containing drugs have been used as popular, over-the-counter medication for the relief of dyspepsia for many decades.

In the studies in which CBS was compared with placebo, there was usually a significantly better improvement in symptoms of nonulcer dyspepsia in the CBS-treated group, in parallel with improvement in gastritis severity and *H. pylori* clearance [26, 27, 31]. In none of these studies, however, was the follow-up period after treatment more than 2 weeks, so no study could demonstrate whether real eradication of *H. pylori* leads to an improvement in dyspeptic symptoms.

We were the first to study the relationship between symptom improvement and true eradication. In our retrospective analysis there was a trend toward better symptom improvement 1 month after stopping therapy in patients in whom *H. pylori* had been eradicated than in those in whom the bacterium persisted. Prospective studies, designed to eliminate effects due to placebo response, and that take into account the possible induction of dyspeptic symptoms by antibiotics, are needed to prove or disprove that the trend we reported indeed reflects that *H. pylori* is the cause of part of the spectrum of nonulcer dyspepsia. Double-blind-placebo-controlled therapeutic studies, using generally accepted scoring systems [11, 12], should then be carried out to evaluate the long-term effects on symptoms of *H. pylori* eradication.

References

1. Krag E (1982) Non-ulcer dyspepsia introduction: epidemiological data. Scand J Gastroenterol 79 [Suppl]:6–8
2. Thomson WG, Heaton KW (1980) Functional bowel disorders in apparently healthy people. Gastroenterology 79:283–288
3. Bonnevie O (1982). Outcome of non-ulcer dyspepsia. Scand J Gastroenterol 79 [Suppl]:135–138
4. Nyrén O, Adami HO, Gustavsson S, Lööf L (1986) Excess sick-listing in social and economic non-ulcer dyspepsia. J Clin Gastroenterol 8:339–345
5. Health and Public Policy Committee, American College of Physicians (1985) Endoscopy in the evaluation of dyspepsia. Ann Intern Med 102:266–269
6. Anonymous (1988) Management of dyspepsia: report of a working party. Lancet I:576–579
7. Dombal de FT (1981) Analysis of foregut symptoms. In: Baron JH, Moody FG (eds) International Medical Review I. Foregut. Butterworths, London, pp 49–66
8. Heatley RV, Rathbone BJ (1987) Dyspepsia: a dilemma for doctors? Lancet II:779–781
9. Lagarde SP, Spiro HM (1984) Non ulcer dyspepsia. In: Peptic ulcer disease. Saunders, London, pp 437–446 (Clinics in gastroenterology, vol 13, no 2)
10. Lennard-Jones JE (1983) Functional gastrointestinal disorders. N Engl J Med 308:431–435
11. Nyrén O, Adami HO, Bates S et al. (1986) Absence of therapeutic benefit from antacids or cimetidine in non-ulcer dyspepsia. N Engl J Med 314:339–343
12. Sjödén PO, Bates S, Nyrén O (1983) Continuous self-recording of epigastric pain with two rating scales: compliance, authenticity, reliability, and sensitivity. J Behav Assess 5:327–344
13. Graham DY, Smith JL, Patterson DJ (1983) Why do apparently healthy people use antacid tablets? Am J Gastroenterol 78:257–260
14. Weberg R, Berstad A (1988) Low-dose antacids and pirenzepine in the treatment of patients with non-ulcer dyspepsia and erosive prepyloric changes. (A randomized, double blind, placebo-controlled trial). Scand J Gastroenterol 23:237–243
15. Albibi R, McCallum RW (1983) Metoclopramide: pharmacology and clinical application. Ann Intern Med 98:86–95
16. Brogden RN, Carmine AA, Heel RC et al. (1982) Domperidone: a review of its pharmacological activity, pharmacokinetics and therapeutic efficacy in the symptomatic treatment of chronic dyspepsia and as an antiemetic. Drugs 24:360–400
17. Rösch W (1987) Cisapride in non-ulcer dyspepsia. Results of a placebo-controlled trial. Scand J Gastroenterol 22:161–164
18. Delattre M, Malesky M, Prinzie A (1985) Symptomatic treatment of non-ulcer dyspepsia with cimetidine. Curr Ther Res 37:980–991
19. Talley NJ, McNeil D, Hayden A, Piper DW (1986) Randomised, double-blind, placebo-controlled cross-over trial of cimetidine and pirenzepine in non-ulcer dyspepsia. Gastroenterology 91:149–156
20. Kreuning J, Bosman FT, Kuiper G et al. (1978) Gastric and duodenal mucosa in "healthy" individuals. An endoscopic and histopathological study of 50 volunteers. J Clin Pathol 31:69–77
21. Langenberg ML, Tytgat GNJ, Schipper MEI, Rietra PJGM, Zanen HC (1984) *Campylobacter*-like organisms in the stomach of patients and healthy individuals. Lancet I:1348
22. Myren J, Serck-Hanssen A (1975) Gastroscopic observations related to bioptic histology in healthy medical students. Scand J Gastroenterol 10:353–355
23. Villako K, Ihamäki T, Tamm A et al. (1984) Upper abdominal complaints and gastritis. Ann Clin Res 16:192–194
24. Graham DY, Klein PD, Opekun AR, Boutton TW (1988) Effect of age on the frequency of active *Campylobacter pylori* infection diagnosed by the [13C] urea breath test in normal subjects and patients with peptic ulcer disease. J Infect Dis 157:777–780

25. McNulty CAM, Gearty JC, Grump B et al. (1986) *Campylobacter pyloridis* and associated gastritis: investigator blind, placebo controlled trial of bismuth salicylate and erythromycin ethylsuccinate. Br Med J 293:645–649
26. Lambert JR, Borromeo M, Korman MG, Hansky J (1987) Role of *Campylobacter pyloridis* in non-ulcer dyspepsia. A randomised controlled trial (abstract) Gastroenterology 92:1488
27. Borody T, Hennessy W, Daskalopoulos G et al. (1987) Double-blind trial of De-Nol in non-ulcer dyspepsia associated with *Campylobacter pylori* gastritis. Gastroenterology 92:1324
28. Borody T, Daskalopoulos G, Brandl S et al. (1987) Dyspeptic symptoms improve following eradication of gastric *Campylobacter pyloridis* (abstract) Gastroenterology 92:1324
29. Kang JY, Tay HH, Wee A et al. (1988) The effect of colloidal bismuth subcitrate on symptoms and gastric histology in non-ulcer dyspepsia – a double-blind placebo – controlled study. Gut 10:A1440
30. Morgan D, Kraft W, Bender M, Pearson A (1988) Nitrofurans in the treatment of gastritis associated with *Campylobacter pylori.* Gastroenterology 95:1178–1184
31. Rokkas T, Pursey C, Uzoechina E et al. (1988) Non-ulcer dyspepsia and short term De-Nol therapy: a placebo controlled trial with particular reference to the role of *Campylobacter pylori.* Gut 29:1386–1391
32. Lambert JR, Dunn K, Borromeo M et al. (1989) *Campylobacter pylori* – a role in non-ulcer dyspepsia? Scand J Gastroenterol 24 [Suppl 160] 7–13
33. Marshall BJ, Armstrong JA, McGechie DB, Glancy RJ (1985) Attempt to fulfil Koch's postulates for pyloric campylobacter. Med J Aust 142:436–439
34. Morris A, Nicholson G (1987) Ingestion of *Campylobacter pyloridis* causes gastritis and raised fasting gastric pH. Am J Gastroenterol 82:192–199
35. Marshall BJ, Hislop I, Glancy R, Armstrong J (1984) Histological improvement of active chronic gastritis in patients treated with De-Nol. Aust NZ J Med 14 [Suppl 4]:907
36. Rauws EAJ, Langenberg W, Houthoff HJ, Zanen HC, Tytgat GNJ (1988) *Campylobacter pyloridis*-associated chronic antral gastritis. Gastroenterology 94:33–40
37. Glupczynski Y, Burette A, Labbe M, Deprez C, De Reuck M, Deltenre M (1988) *Campylobacter pylori*-associated gastritis: a double-blind placebo-controlled trial with amoxycillin. Am J Gastroenterol 83:365–372

Discussion

Talley: I am wondering how you define nonulcer dyspepsia. I noticed, for example, that you included heartburn as one of the symptoms. I wonder if patients with heartburn really have gastroesophageal reflux disease and whether that is a very different group from other nonulcer dyspeptic patients. I have one other question and that is: Is *H. pylori* truly increased in nonulcer dyspepsia? We know that the prevalence of *H. pylori* in the general population of say 50 year olds is about 50%, and in most studies on nonulcer dyspeptics the mean age is typically around 50 years and *H. pylori* is found in about 50% (at least that is what several groups have reported). Therefore, is the prevalence of *H. pylori* truly increased in nonulcer dyspepsia?

Rauws: Well, to start with your last question, I think by using breath tests or serological tests it has been shown now in many countries that the incidence of *H. pylori* is higher in dyspeptic patients than in blood donors or whatever your control group is. We agree that there is a big difference when you compare groups of different ages. In our asymptomatic group of 34 individuals, the mean age was only 38 years and in the dyspeptic group this was 58 years. There is a difference of 20 years. I think we should also be very careful while including and comparing individuals with different ethnical background, and I think we should very carefully define our study group. Another problem is defining symptoms. I think when you ask a patient if he complains of nausea and then ask him immediately after that question, “what do you mean by nausea?”, he does not have an answer to that question. I think that, especially for a symptom such as heart burn, it is very difficult to say what you mean for the patient but also for the doctor asking that question.

Graham: But the question was if you have evaluated the patient by symptoms and if you would have made a diagnosis of gastroesophageal reflux, would you have this patient in for a nonulcer dyspepsia trial, and would he be included in your retrospective evaluation?

Rauws: If a patient has signs of reflux esophagitis he is excluded from our study on nonulcer dyspepsia patients. But we did not do any 24-h pH measuring.

Graham: I think we all accept that the clinical reasons are good enough.

Börsch: Dr. Rauws, you have given average results of improvement. It is my opinion that a small fraction of the patients improves rather dramatically while the other fraction of the patients rather stays the same. So we should also ask about the proportion of patients who really improved. In my opinion, this is about one-third. Can you give an estimate from your data?

Rauws: I fully agree. We have a few excellent results, patients complaining for more than 20 years and after triple therapy or whatever therapy they do not have any more complaints after successful *H. pylori* eradication. I think, in about a quarter or one-third patients will remain asymptomatic or improve by at least 50% in symptoms after real eradication of the micro-organism. But we should find a way to clearly select or define those patients who benefit from this type of therapy. If there are still patients with IBS included in the nonulcer dyspepsia patient group, you cannot expect any benefit from this type of therapy for the whole group. We should very carefully define what kind of patients we are studying.

Colin-Jones: Can I follow that up by asking whether, from your study, you observed any particular symptoms which seem to show a better response when *H. pylori* was cleared, compared with others?

Rauws: Well, we have many more data and we stopped analyzing when we found out that the way of scoring symptoms, as we did, is not a proper way to do it. We stopped analyzing and we stopped to find out if one or two symptoms improved better than the whole group of symptoms. We took the whole bunch of symptoms and then came to these results. It might be that, if we have a good scoring system, one or two symptoms will improve more than the whole group of five or six symptoms.

Petersen: Everyone having had to do with nonulcer dyspepsia must agree that this is a difficult condition containing a heterogeneous group of patients. It is very hard to believe that one type of treatment, such as bismuth, can help the majority of these patients. So, if it is true that bismuth and *H. pylori* eradication really helps in nonulcer dyspepsia and you are able to show that in the conventional study this may mean that there is a relatively small group of patients having a really great benefit, I find it very unlikely that all of them should improve a little.

Rauws: I think it is very difficult to give an answer. Most studies are published as abstracts. When you give double-blind placebo versus a bismuth preparation it is never double-blind, because of the stool discoloration. It might be that if this occurs the patient suspects that he has not taken placebo but an active agent and it may be that this is the only placebo effect you are measuring with this type of study. I should say you should try to compare colloidal bismuth versus colloidal bismuth with metronidazole. Because colloidal bismuth in our hands eradicates *H. pylori* in about 10% and colloidal bismuth in combination with metronidazole in a range of 80%, you can do a study double blind, the patient knows and the doctor knows that the stools will be black or gray and everyone is more blinded than they are when comparing colloidal bismuth versus placebo.

Graham: Professor Tytgat, did you have a question?

Tytgat: Yes, it is more of a kind of a philosophical comment. I think we all agree that it is extremely difficult to do these studies and we all agree that the studies performed so far all have major flaws and we all agree that these studies have to be repeated hopefully in many centres with a sufficient number of patients, followed up for a long enough time and monitoring eradication carefully throughout these studies. On the other hand, it is obvious from what has been presented, that there is a trend in these studies. All studies available so far point in the same direction that patients who are *H. pylori* positive tend to improve in their dyspeptic symptoms. I think this is sufficient to now allow large scale studies. Hopefully this afternoon the experts will tell us how to do these studies. These studies will be difficult and they have to be prolonged for at least about a year because the follow-up of the histology told us that it takes almost about a year before the histology truly comes back to normal. If you are successful in eradicating *H. pylori,* the polymorphs disappear very rapidly, but the mononuclear inflammatory infiltrate takes a long time to disappear, and I am rather enthusiastic about *H. pylori* – related dyspepsia. From a purely clinical point of view, and this is indeed casuistic information, I have been impressed by some patients with long-standing, truly severely disabling dyspepsia who tell you spontaneously that they are reborn with complete clearing of all their symptoms. I think this is really very stimulating and should encourage us to continue these studies in the future.

Section 5

Optimal Design of Clinical Trials

Histological Definition and Scoring of Gastritis

J. I. Wyatt and M. F. Dixon

Introduction

The presence of inflammation in the gastric mucosa is recognized morphologically by changes in cellularity, vascularity, and epithelial integrity. Acute purulent gastritis, which is rarely encountered by the histopathologist, is characterized by a neutrophil infiltrate and surface purulent exudate; such an effect has been attributed to the acute stage of *Helicobacter pylori* infection [1].

Chronic gastritis is very common, being familiar to all histopathologists. Inflammatory cells are sparse in the normal gastric mucosa (Fig. 1) and an increase in their number is the defining characteristic of chronic gastritis. As with all subjective changes in histology, there is inevitably some degree of interobserver variation in the diagnosis of chronic gastritis. This, together with variability between different systems of classification and grading of chronic gastritis, has led to some lack of comparability within the literature on chronic gastritis.

Pathogenetic Classification of Gastritis

The presence of *H. pylori* in histological sections can now be used to distinguish *Helicobacter*-associated gastritis histologically, and this appears to define a pattern of inflammatory response which differs from cases of *Helicobacter*-negative gastritis. The latter group includes a heterogeneous collection of conditions, some of which are associated with specific pathogenetic mechanisms (Table 1) [2]. In this chapter, most discussion will concern *Helicobacter*-associated gastritis, and its scoring with respect to the design of clinical trials. However, the patterns of the *Helicobacter*-negative gastritis will first be briefly described in order to define *Helicobacter*-associated gastritis within a broader context of gastric inflammation.

Table 1. Pathogenetic classification of chronic gastritis

	Pathogenesis	Aetiology
Type A	Autoimmunity	?
Type B	Bacterial infection	*Helicobacter pylori*
Type C	Chemical injury	Enterogastric reflux, NSAIDs, alcohol
Lymphocytic	? abnormal response to mucosal antigen	? role of *H. pylori*
Eosinophilic	allergic response	
Granulomatous	idiopathic	

H. Menge et al. (Eds.)
Helicobacter pylori 1990

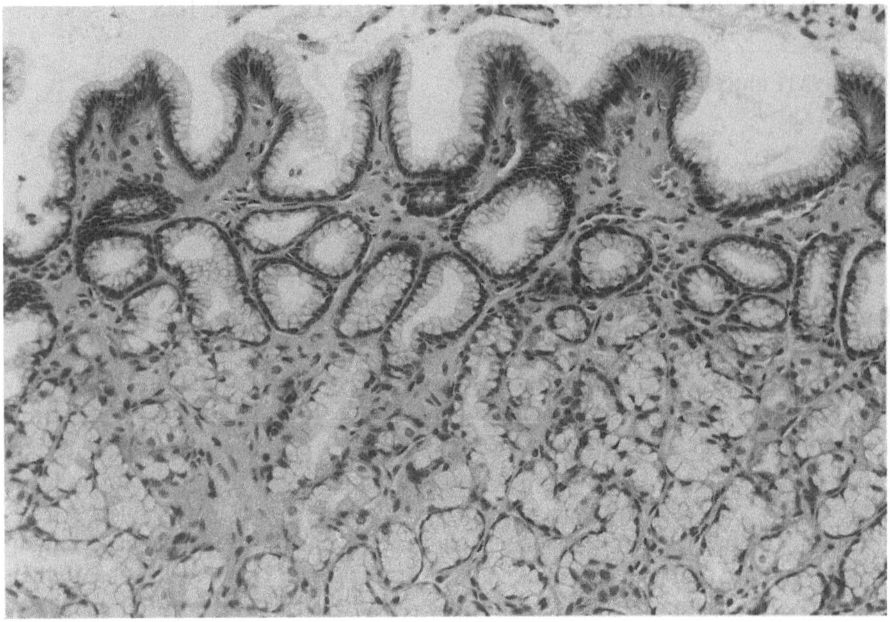

a

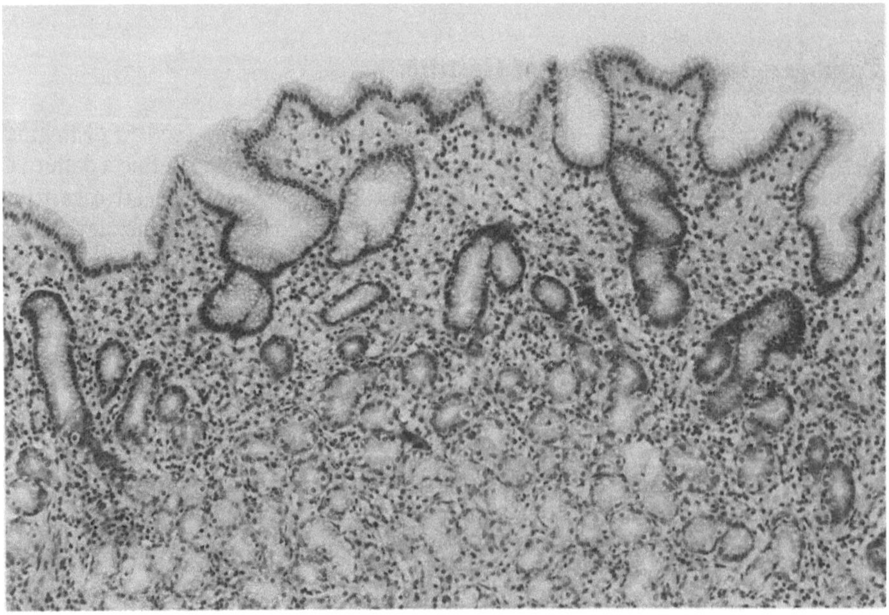

b

Fig. 1a, b. a Normal antral mucosa to show sparsity of inflammatory cells in the lamina propria. **b** *Helicobacter*-associated gastritis; a mild increase in mononuclear cells (grade 1) for comparison with **a**

In autoimmune chronic gastritis, the inflammation and destruction of gastric glands is largely restricted to body type mucosa, with little or no antral gastritis, leading to atrophy of the body mucosa with extensive intestinal metaplasia [3, 4]. Functionally, this results in achlorhydria and pernicious anaemia. This inflammation is accompanied by organ-specific circulating autoantibodies, and *H. pylori* is absent in the great majority of affected patients [5, 6].

"Reflux gastritis" is a pattern of mucosal injury seen most markedly in patients who have had a partial gastrectomy or gastroenterostomy. It is characterized by the predominance of the non-cellular components of the inflammatory response, namely oedema, vascular congestion and epithelial hyperplasia, resulting in elongation and serration of the gastric pits [7, 8]. Inflammatory cells are present in normal numbers or only mildly increased. A similar but milder pattern of mucosal injury is seen without previous surgery in a proportion of *Helicobacter*-negative patients with non-ulcer dyspepsia, some of whom consume alcohol or non-steroidal anti-inflammatory agents (NSAIDS). This suggests that this pattern is a reflection of chemical injury to the gastric mucosa, by agents which include bile and ingested irritants [2].

About 2% of patients with chronic gastritis have a very characteristic pattern with large numbers of intraepithelial lymphocytes, and varying degrees of lamina propria cellularity. This "lymphocytic" gastritis is sometimes associated with endoscopically distinctive raised eroded lesions in the body mucosa [9]. *H. pylori* is not usually seen histologically, although there is a serological response to *H. pylori* antigens in some affected patients [10].

In our experience, most cases of granulomatous gastritis are not associated with *H. pylori*. This category represents a group of aetiologically distinct conditions including Crohn's disease and sarcoidosis [11], and the absence of *H. pylori* in such patients may serve to alert the pathologist to look out for an unusual cause for inflammation.

Eosinophilic gastritis and Menetriere's disease [12] are the rarest of these rare lesions. Both appear to be associated rarely with *H. pylori* although numbers are too small to comment on its significance. These observations serve to emphasize that chronic gastritis can be divided into a number of separate entities on pathogenetic and morphological grounds. However, the majority of patients with gastritis – between 60% and 90% – have the *Helicobacter*-associated gastritis which forms the subject of the rest of this chapter.

Helicobacter-Associated Chronic Gastritis

Histologically patients with *H. pylori* infection have diffuse antral inflammation which typically has both a mononuclear cell and a neutrophil polymorph component. Additionally the body mucosa is nearly always colonized by *H. pylori*, and in most but by no means all patients there is also inflammation in the body mucosa [13, 14]. There are commonly changes in the surface epithelial cells, with irregularity, mucin depletion, and crypt hyperplasia, but these changes are less uniform than the inflammatory cell changes within and between biopsies from the same patient. Lymphoid follicles appear to be a specific feature of *Helicobacter*-associated gastritis, and are present in about 30% of affected biopsies [15], but their dependence on sampling error makes them an unreliable feature for grading inflammation. In our experience, *H. pylori* may be associated with any degree of glandular atrophy, and is present irrespective of the presence or absence of intestinal metaplasia in the stomach (as long as there is sufficient gastric type, nonmetaplastic epithelium in the biopsy for *H. pylori* to be detected).

The sensitivity of histology as a means of detecting *H. pylori* is comparable to that of other biopsy methods (culture, gram smear, biopsy urease test [16]). The reliability of any of these techniques assumes diffuse distribution of the organism in the gastric mucosa, and although "patchiness" of colonization has been cited as the cause of false-negative results [17], this in practice is a relatively rare problem in the antrum. We agree with Bayerdörffer [18] that two antral biopsies are sufficient for practical purposes to establish *H. pylori* status. Morris has recently demonstrated [16] that the biopsy techniques are equally valid in post-treatment biopsies. It is our experience that the untreated patients in whom bacteria are seen in a minority of biopsies [19] are those in whom the bacterial density in the positive biopsies is very low. Whether these patients with low bacterial load are a clinically distinct group is currently unclear.

Grading of Chronic Gastritis

Systems used for grading chronic gastritis centre on either its distribution and the degree of glandular atrophy and presence of intestinal metaplasia [4, 20, 21] or on the character and density of the inflammatory cell infiltrate [22–29]. These two systems give different information about the gastritis. On one hand, assessments of glandular loss and intestinal metaplasia give information about the natural progression and duration of chronic gastritis, and have formed the basis for population-based studies of the dynamics of atrophic gastritis [30]. Such grading systems are not appropriate to the assessment of short-term response to treatment, and have not been applied in treatment trials. Alternatively, assessment of the density of inflammatory cells in the mucosa reflects the intensity of the inflammatory process at any one time, and grading systems based on this have clearly shown that improvement in gastric inflammation follows eradication of *H. pylori* [22, 26–29].

A commonly used classification of chronic gastritis is into chronic superficial and chronic atrophic gastritis, depending on the location of the inflammatory cell infiltrate (i.e. limited to the thickness of the foveolar zone in superficial gastritis, extending more deeply in atrophic gastritis) [20]. This is best seen in body-type mucosa, where deep inflammation is associated with atrophy of specialized glandular tissue. However, it is rarely appropriate in the antrum in that here inflammatory cells frequently encroach on the glandular layer. "Chronic atrophic" gastritis is used by many histopathologists to describe deep infiltration by inflammatory cells whether or not there is discernible glandular atrophy. As explained by Kekki et al. [21], only glandular atrophy carries appreciable functional consequences; these authors advocate restriction of "atrophic" gastritis to those cases where loss of glands is visible. Diffuse inflammation without appreciable glandular loss is typically present in the antrum of duodenal ulcer patients; Correa [4] describes this as diffuse antral gastritis which he distinguishes from the multifocal "environmental" gastritis with intestinal metaplasia seen in populations with high prevalence of gastric ulcer and gastric carcinoma.

Warren's original report [31] noted the association of *H. pylori* specifically with activity of the gastritis, defined by the presence of intraepithelial polymorphs. This is a very characteristic feature of chronic gastritis and is absent from most biopsies showing *H. pylori*-negative gastritis. The frequency of *H. pylori* in active and inactive gastritis quoted by several workers has been recently tabulated by Dixon [32], who emphasizes the almost universal finding of *H. pylori* in active gastritis whether this is categorized as superficial or atrophic. Bayerdörffer [18] has shown that if sufficient material is examined the gastritis in patients with *H. pylori* is always active somewhere.

Scoring of Gastritis for Treatment Trials

The acute, neutrophil polymorph component of the gastritis quickly subsides after treatment of *Helicobacter*-associated gastritis, whether by antibiotics or by bismuth compounds [27]. The mononuclear infiltrate persists in the lamina propria, but apparently is eventually reduced to normal levels if *H. pylori* has genuinely been eradicated. Most grading systems in published studies assess the infiltration by mononuclear and polymorphonuclear cells separately as mild, moderate, or severe [24–27] (see Table 2 for a comparison of grading systems in published treatment trials). This simple system is adequate to show the significant differences between patients cleared and not cleared after treatment in trials with relatively small numbers of subjects. Additional parameters have been included in several studies, for example, the degree of mucin depletion [26, 28], epithelial and lamina propria polymorphs scored separately [27], and surface erosions [27].

These assessments are subjective, and will therefore not be totally reproducible. Variation is reduced where the same pathologist grades all material in the study, and may be further reduced if two separate observers grade the biopsies and the results are combined. In practice, the changes following treatment are sufficiently marked that significant alterations have been demonstrated in all the trials to date by simple, subjective methods performed by a pathologist "blinded" with respect to the treatment group of the patient.

Table 2. Some systems used to grade the severity of *Helicobacter*-associated gastritis

Reference	Polymorphs	Mononuclear cells	Mucin depletion	Erosions
Coghlan et al. 1987 [22]	0–3		–	–
Malfertheiner et al. 1987 [23]	0–3		–	–
Hui et al. 1987 [24]	0–3	0–3	–	–
Carrick et al. 1989 [25]	0–3	0–3	–	–
Marshall et al. 1987 [26]	0–3	0–3	0–3	–
Rauws et al. 1988 [27]	0–3 l. p. 0–3 i. e.	0–2	–	0–2
McNulty et al. 1986 [28]	0–4	0–4	–	–
Morgan et al. 1988 [29]	0–4	–	0–4	–

l. p., lamina propria neutrophils; i. e., intraepithelial polymorphs

Quantitation of cell types by morphometric techniques has been applied to gastritis [33, 34], and goes some way to avoiding the difficulties of reproducibility and subjectivity. However, such techniques are extremely demanding to perform and appear to be unnecessarily burdensome for current treatment trials. For example, the counting of cell types in gastritis recently reported by Collins et al. [33] required 2.5 h to assess each patient.

Work by McNulty et al. [35] introduces a new aspect into histological grading in treatment studies. Patients initially with more severe mucin depletion and polymorph infiltration appeared to be more likely to achieve eradication of *H. pylori* following a triple-therapy regimen. If efficacy of treatment is affected by the severity of gastritis, then stratification of treatment arms according to the histological grade may need to be incorporated into the optimal study design for clinical trials. This is an area which urgently needs further study. Similarly, there are differences in the severity [33] and pattern of distribution [22, 36] of inflammation in gastric patients with and without duodenal ulcer, and it must therefore be determined whether the efficacy of treatment is similar in different clinical groups.

References

1. Salmeron M, Desplaces N, Lavergne A, Houdert R (1986) *Campylobacter*-like organisms and acute purulent gastritis. Lancet II:975–976
2. Wyatt JI, Dixon MF (1988) Chronic gastritis – a pathogenetic approach. J Pathol 154:113–124
3. Strickland RG, Mackay IR (1973) A reappraisal of the nature and significance of chronic atrophic gastritis. Dig Dis Sci 18:426–440
4. Correa P (1988) Chronic gastritis: a clinico-pathological classification. Am J Gastroenterol 83:504–509
5. O'Connor HJ, Axon ATR, Dixon MF (1984) *Campylobacter*-like organisms unusual in type A (pernicious anaemia) gastritis. Lancet II:1091
6. Flejou PF, Bahame P, Smith A et al. (1989) Pernicious anaemia and campylobacter-like organisms: is the gastric antrum resistant to colonisation: Gut 30:60–64
7. Dixon MF, O'Connor HJ, Axon ATR, King RFJG, Johnston D (1986) Reflux gastritis; distinct histopathological entity? J Clin Pathol 39:524–530
8. O'Connor HJ, Wyatt JI, Dixon MF, Axon ATR (1986) *Campylobacter*-like organisms and reflux gastritis. J Clin Pathol 39:531–534
9. Haot J, Delos M, Wallez L et al. (1986) Intraepithelial lymphocytes in inflammatory gastric pathology. Acta Endoscop 16:61–67
10. Dixon MF, Wyatt JI, Burke DA, Rathbone BJ (1988) Lymphocytic gastritis – relationship to *Campylobacter pylori* infections. J Pathol 154:125–132
11. Fisher C, Price AB (1989) Granulomatous gastritis. J Pathol 158:351
12. Ormand JE, Talley NJ, Shorter RG et al. (1989) *Campylobacter pylori* prevalence in specific forms of gastritis: further evidence supporting a pathogenic role for *C. pylori* in chronic antral gastritis. Gastroenterology 96:378
13. Wyatt JI, Rathbone BJ, Heatley RV (1986) Local immune response to gastric *Campylobacter* in non-ulcer dyspepsia. J Clin Pathol 39:863–870
14. Hazell SL, Hennessy WB, Borody TF et al. (1987) *Campylobacter pyloridis* gastritis II: distribution of bacteria and associated inflammation in the gastroduodenal environment. Am J Gastroenterol 82:297–301
15. Wyatt JI, Rathbone BJ (1988) Immune response of the gastric mucosa to *Campylobacter pylori.* Scand J Gastroenterol 23 [Suppl 142]:44–49
16. Morris A, Ali MR, Brown P, Lane M, Patton K (1989) *Campylobacter pylori* infection in biopsy specimens of gastric antrum: laboratory diagnosis and estimation of sampling error. J Clin Pathol 42:727–732

17. Goodwin CS, Armstrong JA, Marshall BJ (1986) *Campylobacter pyloridis,* gastritis, and peptic ulceration. J Clin Pathol 39:353–365
18. Bayerdörffer E, Oertel H, Lehn N et al. (1989) Topographic association between active gastritis and *Campylobacter pylori* colonisation. J Clin Pathol 42:834–839
19. Wyatt JI, Primrose J, Dixon MF (1988) Distribution of *Campylobacter pylori* in gastric biopsies. J Pathol 155:350
20. Whitehead R (1985) Mucosal biopsy of the gastrointestinal tract. 3rd edn Saunders, Philadelphia
21. Kekki M, Siurala M, Varis K et al. (1987) Classification principes and genetics of chronic gastritis. Scand J Gastroenterol 22 [Suppl 141]:1–28
22. Coghlan JG, Humphries GH, Dooley C et al. (1987) *Campylobacter pylori* and recurrence of duodenal ulcers – a 12 month follow-up study. Lancet II:1109–1111
23. Malfertheiner P, Stanescu A, Baczako K, Bode G, Ditschuneit H (1988) Chronic erosive gastritis – a therapeutic approach with bismuth. Scand J Gastroenterol 23 [Suppl 142]:87–92
24. Hui W-M, Lam S-K, Chau P-Y et al. (1987) Persistence of *Campylobacter pyloridis* despite healing of duodenal ulcer and improvement of accompanying duodenitis and gastritis. Dig Dis Sci 32:1255–1260
25. Carrick J, Lee A, Hazell S, Ralston M, Daskalopoulos G (1989) *Campylobacter pylori* duodenal ulcer and gastric metaplasia: possible role of functional heterotopic tissue in ulcerogenesis. Gut 30:790–797
26. Marshall BJ, Armstrong JA, Francis GJ, Nokes NT, Wee SH (1987) Antimicrobial action of bismuth in relation to *Campylobacter pyloridis* colonisation and gastritis. Digestion 37 [Suppl 2]:16–30
27. Rauws EAJ, Langenberg W, Houthorr HJ, Zanen HC, Tytgat GN (1988) *Campylobacter pyloridis*-associated chronic active antral gastritis: a prospective study of its prevalence and the effects of antibacterial and antiulcer treatment. Gastroenterology 94:33–40
28. McNulty CAM, Gearty JC, Crump B et al. (1986) *Campylobacter pyloridis* and associated gastritis: investigator blind, placebo controlled trial of bismuth salicylate and erythromycin ethyl succinate. Br Med J 293:645–649
29. Morgan D, Kraft W, Bender M, Pearson A (1988) Nitrofurans in the treatment of gastritis associated with *Campylobacter pylori.* Gastroenterology 95:1178–1184
30. Ihamaki T, Kekki M, Sipponen P, Siurala M (1985) The sequelae and course of chronic gastritis during a 30–34 year follow up study. Scand J Gastroenterol 20:485–491
31. Warren JR (1983) Unidentified curved bacilli on gastric epithelium in active chronic gastritis. Lancet I:1273
32. Dixon MF (1989) *Campylobacter pylori* and chronic gastritis. In: Rathbone BJ, Heatley RV (eds) *Campylobacter pylori* and gastroduodenal disease. Blackwell, Oxford
33. Collins JA, Hamilton PW, Watt PCH, Sloan JM, Love AHG (1989) Superficial gastritis and *Campylobacter pylori* in dyspeptic patients – a quantitative study using computer-linked image analysis. J Pathol 158:303–310
34. Toukan AV, Kamal MF, Amr SS, Arnout MA, Abu-Romiyeh AS (1985) Gastroduodenal inflammation in patients with non-ulcer dyspepsia. A controlled endoscopic and morphometric study. Dig Dis Sci 30:313–320
35. McNulty CAM, Eyre-Brook IA, Uff JS, Dent JC, Witkinson SP (1989) Triple therapy is not always 95% effective. In: Ruig-Palacios GM (ed) Campylobacter V: Proceedings of the fifth international workshop on Campylobacter infections. Mexico 1989
36. Schrager J, Spink R, Mitra S (1967) The antrum in patients with duodenal and gastric ulcers. Gut 8:497–508

Discussion

Hazell: I have raised objections to the argument that two antral biopsies are sufficient on previous occasions. In a series we did a few years ago and those just recently completed by Bayerdörffer et al. (Journal of Clinical Pathology) it was shown that you do get body-only gastritis due to *Helicobacter pylori*. If you take only antral biopsies in a few cases you are going to miss *Helicobacter pylori*, probably in 5% of cases.

Wyatt: Yes I agree, although in the series of patients I looked at with multiple biopsies, I myself did not find any with bacteria only in the body mucosa. In some *Helicobacter pylori* and gastritis were confined to the antrum. However, I accept your findings and those of Bayerdörffer.

I think the important point here is that the patchiness of the bacteria is a reflection of their density, that is, that false negative biopsies due to patchy colonization are found in patients in whom the overall bacterial density is low. Most patients with *H. pylori*, however, will have large numbers of bacteria in all, or nearly all, of their biopsies, and in these, sampling error, by any biopsy technique, should not be a problem.

We do not know if the density of colonization by *H. pylori* is important in determining the patients' response to treatment, and this question should be addressed in the design of treatment trials.

Another overlooked point in the question of sensitivity of histology is the size of the biopsy taken. Clearly, the bigger the biopsy forceps, the less the risk of a false negative result.

Demling: It is generally accepted that immunological gastritis goes into atrophy. How is it with *Helicobacter pylori* B gastritis? Do you think there is also an endstage atrophy and, therefore, a premalignant condition?

Wyatt: Yes, I am sure there is. There is a sizable body of literature on the progression of chronic gastritis, written before the recognition of *H. pylori*. We can now combine this with our knowledge of *H. pylori* and its associated pattern of gastritis to deduce that atrophic and premalignant changes probably develop on a background of *Helicobacter*-associated gastritis.

Demling: So, you can avoid atrophic gastritis by using this kind of treatment?

Wyatt: This will be the other very interesting aspect of treatment studies. It should be possible to discover whether the development of intestinal metaplasia, and dysplasia, is prevented by treating *Helicobacter*-associated gastritis at its early, superficial stage. A further question will be whether intestinal metaplasia persists after treatment has led to the resolution of the inflammatory cell component of atropic gastritis.

Varkonyi: What is your experience, how frequently does the intestinal metaplasia in *Helicobacter*-induced chronic gastritis occur and is it the small intestinal or colonic type?

Wyatt: Intestinal metaplasia is not uncommon in patients with *H. pylori*. Its frequency increases with the patient's age. Of course, *H. pylori* does not colonize intestinal metaplasia, and so our ability to diagnose *Helicobacter*-associated gastritis depends on having sufficient gastric type surface epithelium also in the biopsy.

Having said that, the frequency of finding intestinal metaplasia in gastric biopsies increases in patients with gastritis with increasing age; in my experience, nearly half the patients aged over 70 years with gastritis will have intestinal metaplasia in their biopsies. The metaplasia may be either "complete" (small intestinal, type I) or less commonly "incomplete" (large intestinal, sulphomucin-positive, type II) type.

Tytgat: Should it not be scored in the scoring system?

Wyatt: Intestinal metaplasia is one of the features which is very dependent on sampling error. While inflammation is diffuse, and its severity relatively uniform in the antrum, the sensitivity for diagnosing intestinal metaplasia will depend on the number of biopsies examined. Multiple biopsies from many patients with intestinal metaplasia will need to be examined after *H. pylori* eradication to study the effect of treatment.

Tytgat: Correct, but it is the only way to know whether it is reversible, otherwise we will never know.

Wyatt: Yes, I agree.

Stadelmann: The hypersecretory type of gastritis you mentioned is of course a typical *H. pylori* gastritis. But in my opinion the term hypersecretory gastritis is not justified because you have in this type of gastritis mostly no hypersecretion. There are patients with duodenal ulcer who have in a greater part a hypersecretion. There are patients with gastric ulcer and there are patients in this group with *H. pylori* gastritis without ulcers; most of them don't have hypersecretion. Therefore, the term "hypersecretory type" is not justified.

Wyatt: Correa himself now uses the term "diffuse antral gastritis" to describe this condition in preference to "hypersecretory gastritis."

Graham: Although pathologists like categorizing 1, 2, 3, it is possible that if these are really ordered categories, they should not be called 1, 2, and 3 but should rather be handled nonparametrically. I think if we ever find out how they are to be analyzed and whether they are ordered categories, you should call them A, B, C, D, which prevents anybody from coming out with a new plus or minus C-type of inappropriate analysis.

Sipponen: One comment. The nomenclature used in the classification of chronic gastritis is confusing at present. In the early beginning, Stricland and MacKay indicated with the B gastritis an entity in which there is severe, at least moderate, atrophic gastritis in the antrum in connection with the presence of normal mucosa in the gastric body. So, it does not follow these original principles if we use the term B gastritis to indicate any gastritis lesions in the antrum.

McNulty: If we consider that the severity and extent of the gastritis is important should we be taking body specimens from all patients pretreatment?

Wyatt: The site and number of biopsies taken before and after treatment will be determined by the questions addressed by the study.

If the question is simply "can we eradicate *H. pylori* and does the gastritis improve?" then the outline I have given is as appropriate as any. However, if the question then becomes "does the success of a particular treatment depend on the pattern and the characteristics of the gastritis?" then clearly we have got to design the histology protocol in a rather different way.

The efficacy of treatment varies considerably between different trials so far performed, and one factor in this may be heterogeneity in the pattern of severity of gastritis. Biopsies should be collected prospectively from defined sites to explore this point.

Ober: A question unrelated to the classification. In the presence of *Helicobacter pylori,* how often do you not see acute inflammatory PMN's?

Wyatt: About 80% of our individual biopsies with *H. pylori* have intraepithelial polymorphs, that is, show active gastritis. However in the very good paper by Bayerdörffer, the conclusion was that if you take enough biopsies from somebody with *Helicobacter* then there will always be active gastritis somewhere, if you look hard enough for it.

Tytgat: Does it matter where in the antrum the biopsies are taken?

Wyatt: I have not found the site in the antrum to affect the detection of *H. pylori* in any consistent way, and I do not know of any literature which suggests it may.

Tytgat: Is there a difference in the bacterial load between the first and the second biopsy? Do you transfer organisms after you contaminate your biopsy forceps.

Wyatt: I have found no consistent difference in the density of bacteria between first and second biopsy. I would not expect bacteria possibly contaminating the biopsy surface from the forceps to mimic the close association with the epithelial cell surface seen with *H. pylori* genuinely present in the stomach.

Tytgat: If you see macroscopically visible abnormalities, should we aim for those abnormalities or should we stay away from these erosions?

Wyatt: Ideally we do both. You should send the pathologist a biopsy from the abnormal area (to exclude specific pathology – dysplasia, malignancy). But for the purposes of grading the severity of inflammation I think an additional biopsy away from a macroscopic abnormality would be better.

Tytgat: But are you sure that if you sample erosions the yield is the same as if you sample the normal non-erosive mucosa? I think it is the opposite. I think you should stay away from erosions.

Wyatt: Yes, I think that the bacterial load in a biopsy from the margin of an erosion may be lower than elsewhere in a macroscopically uninvolved area of mucosa.

Tytgat: Do you have data to support that?

Wyatt: No, nothing published, but this is my impression from my experience in looking at large numbers of biopsies.

Measuring Symptoms in *Helicobacter pylori*-Associated Gastritis and Non-Ulcer Dyspepsia

S. J. O. Veldhuyzen van Zanten

Introduction

Methodological issues in measuring symptoms of *Helicobacter pylori*-associated gastritis (HPAG) and non-ulcer dyspepsia (NUD) for use in clinical trials to date have not received sufficient attention. To avoid confusion both the term HPAG and NUD will be defined first. The term HPAG is reserved for patients who are symptomatic and in whom after upper gastrointestinal endoscopy a firm diagnosis of histologically proven *H. pylori* gastritis is established. NUD patients are those persons that have histological evidence neither of gastritis nor of *H. pylori*. It should be stressed that we are not talking about patients with active duodenal ulceration, although symptom relief in these patients is also an important outcome measurement in clinical trials.

Why is symptom measurement so important in HPAG and NUD patients? At the moment the true importance of harbouring *H. pylori* in the stomach is still unclear. Therefore what should one do when one has a patient with HPAG but no ulcer? Clinical trials are certainly necessary to study which treatments are efficacious in eradicating *H. pylori*, but more than looking at eradication is necessary.

Looking at Table 1 it should become clear that symptom measurement is crucial and that one should only treat patients with HPAG and NUD if it has been convincingly shown that treatment controls the symptoms of the patient. The fact that we at the moment are uncertain about long-term effective therapy for eradication of *H. pylori* is another strong argument that improvement in symptoms should be a primary outcome in clinical trials.

Reliability of Symptom Measurement

There is a lot of scepticism about whether it is possible to measure upper gastrointestinal symptoms *reliably* at all. Upper gastrointestinal symptoms are vague, they vary a

Table 1. Importance of symptom measurement in clinical trials of *Helicobacter pylori* and NUD

1. *Crucial:* Physician cannot make rational decision to treat without information on the effect of treatment on symptoms
2. *Important:* information on effect of symptoms likely to aid physician in making optimal treatment decision
3. *Secondary:* information on effect of symptoms may be of interest but will not likely affect treatment decision
4. *Irrelevant* or *not feasible*

H. Menge et al. (Eds.)
Helicobacter pylori 1990

great deal over time, and many physicians consider it therefore not worth the effort to spend much time on them. Knill-Jones and colleagues tried to predict the presence of duodenal or gastric ulcer based on symptoms and demographic factors and this was not very successful [1]. The fact that no study to date has linked the presence of *H. pylori* to certain symptoms may reinforce this belief.

However, the fact that symptoms do not predict a disease or discriminate among diseases does *not* rule out their usefulness to evaluate the effect of a treatment. This important distinction was first pointed out by Kirschner and Guyatt [2]. It is shown in Table 2.

Table 2. Purpose of symptom measurement

1. To *discriminate:* used to distinguish patients in different categories, e.g. HPAG versus NUD
2. To *predict:* used to classify patients based on symptoms in a certain category, e.g. DU or gastric ulcer
3. To *evaluate:* used to *measure change* of symptoms over time. This allows for *quantification of a treatment effect*

Having concluded that the aim of measuring symptoms is to evaluate whether treatment is effective and if possible to quantify the amount of improvement, the question then is "can symptoms in HPAG and NUD be measured reliably so that they can be used as outcome measurements in clinical trials?"

What does it mean when we say symptom measurement has to be reliable? Table 3 lists the three essential attributes that are necessary in order for symptom measurement to be reliable outcome measurements in clinical trials.

Validity in general terms means that symptoms measure what they are supposed to measure.

Reproducibility implies that symptom measurements are stable in patients who have not changed clinically. For the latter the term test-retest reliability is often used.

Responsiveness is also called sensitivity to change. It is the ability of symptom measurement to detect clinical change in a patient if indeed such a change took place.

Establishing the validity of the measurement of symptoms is difficult and probably the reason that many investigators have paid relative little attention to it. One can what is called "construct" validity by comparing the "soft" measurement of symptoms

Table 3. Essential prerequisites when symptoms are used as outcome measurements

Measurement should be:

1. *Valid*
   a) "Symptoms should measure what they are supposed to measure"
2. *Reproducible*
   a) Same result is obtained in stable subjects
   b) Test-retest stability
3. *Responsive*
   a) If a patient's symptoms change (improve or deteriorate) measurement must register a change

with other "hard" data. For example one can correlate the severity and extent of ulcerative colitis in a patient with symptoms such as fatigue, left lower abdominal pain and frequency of bowel movements [3]. For the case of *H. pylori*-associated gastritis one can try to correlate change in severity of histological inflammation with change in symptoms. An important consequence of what was just mentioned is that it often will be necessary to establish reproducibility, validity, and responsiveness in a separate study prior to its use in an actual trial.

Back to the measurement of symptoms in HPAG and NUD patients using the concepts of validity, reproducibility and responsiveness, how have symptoms been measured in clinical trials of HPAG and NUD to date? We did a fully recursive literature search going back to 1980 [4]. All published clinical trials of NUD and HPAG that were randomized and placebo controlled were retrieved. In total 15 trials were identified. When looking at how symptoms were measured, major shortcomings in most of the trials became evident. For example some measured symptoms retrospectively or only asked whether symptoms had changed. In only 1 of 15 trials was a validated way of measuring symptoms used. This was the NUD trial by Nyren et al. published in the New England Journal of Medicine in 1986 [5]. A possible limitation of this study was that it only measured epigastric pain. One other study by Talley et al. looked rather convincing because of its comprehensiveness, although the symptom measurement used was never validated in a separate study [6].

We have tried to study whether measurement of upper gastrointestinal symptoms can fulfil the criteria of validity, reproducibility and responsiveness. The main questions we wanted to answer were whether symptoms are stable when their measurement is repeated within a short period, whether treatment results in improvement of symptoms and finally whether an improvement in symptoms is valid.

Methods

Eight symptoms were measured prior to endoscopy ($T = 0$) in 55 patients who had symptoms of dyspepsia. All patients underwent endoscopy with gastric biopsies taken from the antrum for histology and culture. In addition a [^{14}C]urea breath test was also performed. Patients with duodenal ulcer, gastric ulcer, or reflux esophagitis were excluded. The presence of the irritable bowel syndrome assessed by using the Manning criteria was also an exclusion criterion [7]. This was carried out to avoid the possible confounding of irritable bowel syndrome symptoms with those of gastritis.

Table 4 indicates that symptoms were measured using a five-point Likert scale: 1 = no problem, 2 = mild problem, 3 = moderate problem, 4 = severe problem, 5 = very severe problem. The explanation for the severity that was given to the patient is also shown.

In all patients symptoms were remeasured 1 week later ($T = 1$). In 22 HPAG patients symptom measurement was repeated after 1 month of treatment with bismuth and ampicillin ($T = 4$). It was also repeated in 17 NUD patients who were either treated with an antacid or an H_2-receptor antagonist. In the HPAG patients after treatment endoscopy was repeated. Histological examination of biopsies after treatment was used to correlate change in symptoms with histological improvement. A four-point histology scale grading the severity of the gastritis was used: 1 = no

Table 4. Five-point Likert scale for measuring symptoms

1. *No problem*
2. *Mild problem,* can be ignored when I do not think about it
3. *Moderate problem,* cannot be ignored but does not influence daily activities
4. *Severe problem,* influences your concentration on daily activities
5. *Very severe problem,* markedly influences your daily activities, and/or requires rest

gastritis, 2 = only occasional inflammatory cells present, 3 = intermediate inflammatory cell infiltration and 4 = dense infiltration of inflammatory cells.

When Likert scales are used the distance between each scale cannot be considered equal and therefore one has to use non-parametric tests for statistical testing. We used the Wilcoxon signed rank test and the Mann-Whitney U test for analysis.

Results

Of the 55 enrolled patients, 30 turned out to be *H. pylori*-positive by histology, culture and [^{14}C]urea breath test. The other 25 patients were *H. pylori*-negative and labelled NUD. The results are summarized in Table 5.

The following points need to be made:

1. Symptoms were *reproducible*. There was no statistically significant difference between the initial measurement ($T = 0$) and the one of 1 week later ($T = 1$), with the sole exception of epigastric pain in the HPAG group. However, the mean scores were slightly lower after 1 week ($T = 1$) and these are shown in Table 5. The difference before and after treatment was a comparison of the after treatment score with $T = 1$.

Table 5. Results symptom measurement

	HPAG			NUD		
	$T = 0,1$		$T = 4$	$T = 0,1$		$T = 4$
	Mean	SE	Mean	Mean	SE	Mean
Epigastric pain	3.1	0.13	2.4*	2.5	0.17	2.0*
Burping/belching	2.8	0.16	2.1*	2.4	0.16	1.9*
Heartburn	2.7	0.14	2.1*	2.5	0.22	2.0*
Bloating	2.3	0.15	2.0	2.2	0.13	1.7*
Flatulence	2.2	0.15	1.8*	1.8	0.15	1.6
Sour tase	2.1	0.20	1.6*	2.3	0.18	2.0
Nausea	1.9	0.14	1.7	1.8	0.18	1.6
Halitosis	1.9	0.17	1.6	2.1	0.25	1.8

SE, standard error; *, statistically significant, $P < 0.05$

Symptoms were *reproducibel:* no significant difference between symptoms at $T = 0$ and $T = 1$, indicating that symptoms were stable, except for epigastric pain HPAG

Symptoms were *valid* and *responsive:* the improvement in symptoms in HPAG patients at $T = 4$ correlated with histological improvement in severity of gastritis on a four-point scale: 2.7 before, 1.9 after treatment

For further explanation see text

2. Symptoms were *responsive* and *valid*. They were responsive because they showed an improvement after treatment. As indicated in Table 5 in five symptoms in HPAG patients and in four in the NUD group, this difference was statistically significant. It was already mentioned that in this area it is difficult to establish validity. For HPAG we are fortunate in that we can use the histological severity of gastritis for construct validity. We predicted that if symptoms showed a response it would correlate with improvement in the histological severity of the gastritis. Before treatment the average histological severity of gastritis received a score of 2.7 and it improved to 1.9 after treatment. For NUD unfortunately this is not possible and one has to rely on the "face validity" of the symptom measurement.

Discussion

Most published randomized trials in HPAG and NUD have not used validated methods of symptom measurement. As pointed out the aim of measuring symptoms in *H. pylori*-associated gastritis and NUD is *evaluation* of treatment not prediction or discrimination among diseases. We have shown that using five-point Likert scales symptoms are stable when measured over a 1-week interval. Symptom measurement was also responsive. It was able to detect change in severity of symptoms in treated HPAG and NUD patients. An important advantage of these scales is that they make a quantification of the treatment effect possible. We used histological improvement of gastritis successfully to "construct"-validate responsiveness of symptoms.

It needs to be stressed that treatment was not randomized in this study. It does show that symptom measurement is reproducible and responsive but it does not say anything about the effectiveness of the treatment itself. It seems likely that in future trials of HPAG it will not be necessary to measure all eight symptoms. One could take for example the four most severe symptoms and/or combine the total scores of these. However, this will have to be established in a separate study since the data shown do not allow for this kind of a post hoc analysis.

Finally, using five-point Likert scales is one way of measuring symptoms reliably, but it seems likely that other methods may be feasible as well.

References

1. Knill-Jones RP (1985) A formal approach to symptoms in dyspepsia. Clin Gastroenterol 14:517–529
2. Kirshner B, Guyatt GH (1985) A methodological framework for assessing health indices. J Chronic Dis 14:27–36
3. Mitchell A, Guyatt GH, Singer J et al. (1988) Quality of life in patients with inflammatory bowel disease. J Clin Gastroenterol 10:306–310
4. Veldhuyzen van Zanten SJO, Tytgat KMAJ, Jalali S, Goodacre RL, Hunt RH (1989) Can gastritis symptoms be evaluated in clinical trials? A review of treatment of gastritis, non-ulcer dyspepsia and *Campylobacter pylori* associated gastritis. J Clin Gastroenterol 11:496–501
5. Nyren O, Adami HO, Bates S et al. (1986) Absence of therapeutic benefit from antacids or cimetidine in non-ulcer dyspepsia. N Engl J Med 314:339–343

6. Talley NJ, McNeil D, Hayden A, Piper DW. Randomized, double blind, placebo controlled crossover trial of cimetidine and pirenzepine in non-ulcer dyspepsia. Gastroenterology 91:149–156
7. Manning AP, Thompson WG, Heaton KW, Morris AF (1978) Towards positive diagnosis of the irritable bowel syndrome. Br Med J 2:653–654

Discussion

Graham: That was a very nice discussion, but there is one factor you meet in validity responsiveness reproducibility, that you did not mention but which is meaningful. The patients do not care if they have a score of 3 which falls to 2.4 and which is statistically significant. What counts to patients are things like pain-free days. So I think that while these scales are nice, and may give statistically valid results, they are irrelevant for the patients themselves. I would go further in that direction and say that we have to define what we are going to call a success, not a statistical success, but a clinical success.

Talley: Can I respond to Dr. Graham? David, I think that's garbage, basically.

Graham: I'm pleased that you believe that.

Talley: In one respect you're right. It's important to have a global responsive scale and actually look for abolition of symptoms. However, if you want to pick out different groups that perhaps are going to respond, and I suspect that there are various subgroups that will respond differently, then you need to utilize well-validated scales to study this property. You will want to see the individual symptoms improving as well as global improvement to conclude that a treatment is efficacious. In my opinion, just saying "good response" or "no response" is naive.

Petersen: We have had the same problems, the same aims, but have not been as successful as you are. We have had several problems. First of all, it is very hard to get a patient to grade more than one symptom. And then it is the reproducibility, which is poor because of the natural fluctuations in symptoms. At least, that is a very disturbing fact. In our experience this is a disturbing factor that depends a little on how you face the patient.

Veldhuyzen van Zanten: To Dr. Graham I would like to respond that it is my belief that most patients may not reach the stage of being pain-free. However, symptoms may still improve substantially and thus be worthwhile for the patient. The trial by Rokkas had several problems one of them being that many patients became *H. pylori* positive after the second endoscopy. A problem still is to determine what improvement is clinically significant. This was not addressed in my talk.

To Dr. Peterson I would like to say that I would not advocate measuring symptoms just before and then immediately after the endoscopy. We have shown that symptoms are reasonably stable within a 1-week interval.

Westblom: I would like to propose another scale to evaluate the symptoms. We have used a method where we asked the patients to put an *x* on a line which is 100 mm long and has the two extremes as its ends. If you ask about pain, for instance how often they have it, these extremes would be "never" and "all the time". They put the x on the line and then when they come back they are asked to put another x on a similar line. When we analyze these data we measure the difference in millimeters between the first and the second marking, and transfer that change into plus or minus the number of millimeters. Has anyone used a similar scale?

Veldhuyzen van Zanten: Those scales which are called visual analog scales are used quite a bit in the psychometric literature. Most investigators have commented on the fact that it is quite difficult to explain to patients and therefore I think there is a disadvantage to using those measurements, but other than that there is no problem in using them.

Westblom: We haven't seen any problems so far. The patients seem to be able to understand what it is all about.

Demling: Just a short question. How did you treat your nonulcer dyspepsia patients?

Veldhuyzen van Zanten: The *Helicobacter* patients were treated with a combination of bismuth and ampicillin. The nonulcer dyspepsia patients were treated with either an antiacid or an H_2-receptor antagonist.

Demling: Is there an unspecific effect on complaints coming from nonulcer dyspepsia?

Veldhuyzen van Zanten: I tried to make very clear that I do not think our data say anything about the effectiveness of treatment on symptoms. The data only say something about the way they were measured.

Logan: I would like to come back to Dr. Petersen's point about reproducibility. In the real world, not the ideal, patients' symptoms do change from week to week. If you are going to look at reproducibility, therefore, you ought to be looking at reproducibility from day to day.

Veldhuyzen van Zanten: I agree with you. Nyren and coworkers in their trial used the assumption of what they called temporal stability of symptoms. They compared each symptom to the score of the one of the next day. They showed that symptoms are reasonably stable over consecutive days. I think in practice if you are going to delay treatment and wait for biopsy results you bring patients back in about a week. Given our results you can assume symptoms will be reasonably stable.

Talley: I just wanted to make a comment about visual analog scales. My colleague tried to use visual analog scales in Sydney a few years ago, and we found that patients marked them rather erratically.

Tytgat: In addition there is some confusion. Some physicians allow the patient to see the initial or preceding mark. In principle, it is forbidden to let them see the previous marks. Do you have problems with the visual analog scale too, Dr. de Koster?

De Koster: This is a paper about the methodology of scoring symptoms, so I think you should also go into the methodology of statistics. One of the major flaws in what you showed was in fact your repetitive measurements. You had eight symptoms. For all of these you used a cut-off point of 5% and said it was statistically significant. You cannot do that and in fact one of the advantages of using visual analog scales is you have at that moment a continuous variable you can perform parametric tests with.

Veldhuyzen van Zanten: We used nonparametric testing. This is appropriate in this situation. The nonparametric tests are more consecutive than, for example, a repeated measures analysis of variance. I think you are trying to say there may be a problem of multiple outcomes.

De Koster: But it is repetitive, you used it many times. If you score 100 symptoms, you are going to have five symptoms which are significantly different. So you should use other tests.

Veldhuyzen van Zanten: Which test would you suggest?

De Koster: I would suggest for instance analysis of covariants.

Veldhuyzen van Zanten: I don't think that is appropriate in this situation. The nonparametric tests are more consecutive and do not require any assumptions like the analysis of variance does.

De Koster: Dr. Graham, bring us back to Earth.

Graham: It's a foreign language that you're talking up there. I agree with you entirely that you have to have a lead-in period in which you have to make sure the patients have stable symptoms. Patients like to help and if they know the doctor wants them to have symptoms, they have more symptoms than they do a week or two later. But, I am concerned about my duodenal ulcer patients, the ones Barry Marshall just talked about and in whom he called it a failure if they had a recurrence of symptoms. He demanded that they should not have symptoms to be considered a success. And yet in NUD, you and Dr. Talley and others would be happy to have them have only 20% or 30% or 60% of their previous symptoms and you would call that a success. I just cannot understand why we should treat them as symptomatically different from the ulcer patients. An ulcer patient does not care if he has a crater, he or she cares if it hurts.

Veldhuyzen van Zanten: Well, first of all NUD patients are definitely a different entity and symptom measurement has another purpose there. It is not the same as in peptic ulcer disease where the actual ulcer is an important outcome as well.

Graham: Not as far as the patients are concerned. I mean, a patient only comes to us because he has symptoms or a complication, and they do not care if we heal their ulcer or not as long as they feel well.

Veldhuyzen van Zanten: You are alluding to the question, of what is a clinically important difference and, for nonulcer dyspepsia, that is probably the toughest question of them all. What do we agree on is a clinically significant difference? The quality of life literature provides some answer to how you can do it, but in general terms I think that is something we all have to agree on. How should NUD trials be designed, what outcomes do we use and how do we determine what is a clinically significant difference.

Graham: Rokkas was able to show in his study that a large proportion of the patients became pain free, really had pain-free days, and it would seem to me that this would be meaningful. When he stopped that study the symptoms in many of those patients returned 2 or 3 months later. I think this is strong evidence that possibly he was doing some good. But pain-free days is what we use in our studies and I think that is the only thing that my patients care about.

Veldhuyzen: It would be nice if patients become completely symptom free. But I think in NUD patients this will be unlikely. And I believe it certainly may well be that patients improve in a way that is meaningful for them without being completely symptom free. I would not want to have a trial design that would fail to register this kind of an improvement.

Optimal Study Design for Therapeutic Trials in *Helicobacter pylori*-Associated Nonulcer Dyspepsia

N. J. Talley

Hunches and intuitive impressions are essential for getting the work started, but it is only through the quality of numbers at the end that the truth can be told.

Lewis Thomas: *Science 1977*

Introduction

Although more than 20 definitions have been proposed, dyspepsia is probably best considered to be chronic upper abdominal pain (or discomfort) that is intermittent or continuous and may be related to meals (Talley and Phillips 1988). It is a very common symptom; in the United States, the prevalence of recurrent upper abdominal pain in 30- to 64-year-olds has been estimated to be 16% (Talley et al. 1990). The majority of patients with dyspepsia who present for medical evaluation are eventually labeled as having nonulcer dyspepsia. Broadly defined, nonulcer dyspepsia represents a syndrome characterized by symptoms that are suggestive of peptic ulcer disease; however, no acute or chronic peptic ulceration is present on investigation (Talley and Phillips 1988).

Helicobacter pylori gastritis is found in approximately 50% of patients with nonulcer dyspepsia in industrialized nations (Marshall and Warren 1984; Rokkas et al. 1987; Rathbone et al. 1988; Andersen et al. 1988; Loffeld et al. 1988; Börsch et al. 1988; Sobala et al. 1989). However, the prevalence of *H. pylori* in apparently healthy persons in the community may approach a similar level (Dooley et al. 1989; Graham et al. 1988). Despite this, the concept of targeting antibacterial therapy for patients with nonulcer dyspepsia who are infected with *H. pylori* has emerged (Talley, 1988). Clearly, such an idea needs to be put through rigorous testing before it can be accepted, and indeed some randomized controlled trials have been published (McNulty et al. 1986; Glupczynski et al. 1988; Gastrointestinal Physiology Working Group 1988; Rokkas et al. 1988; Karg et al. 1990) (Tables 1, 2). While these studies have all made important contributions, each has suffered from potential biases that makes interpretation of the results difficult. This chapter will focus on the principle causes of bias in randomized controlled trials (Fig. 1), discuss some of the problems encountered in previous studies of patients with nonulcer dyspepsia associated with *H. pylori*, and offer possible solutions.

Study Population

The first major consideration in a randomized controlled trial is careful characterization of the study population, as this will determine who is enrolled; therefore, the definition used by the investigator is critical. Unfortunately, there is no universally accepted definition of nonulcer dyspepsia (Talley and Phillips 1988). Moreover, no symptom complex identifies patients with nonulcer dyspepsia who are *H. pylori*-

H. Menge et al. (Eds.)
Helicobacter pylori 1990

Table 1. Randomized placebo-controlled trials of bismuth in *H. pylori* (HP)-associated nonulcer dyspepsia

Author	*n*	Population studied	Active medication	Symptom Improvement on active therapy %	Placebo Response %	HP suppression on active therapy %
McNulty 1986[a]	50	HP +ve only	Bismuth subsalicylate	92	66	78
Borody 1987[b]	43	HP +ve only	Bismuth subcitrate	Symptom score improved*	?	?
Rokkas 1988[b]	52	HP +ve and HP −ve	Bismuth subcitrate	60 (92 HP +ve)	26 (25 HP +ve)*	83
Lambert 1989[b]	82	HP +ve and HP −ve	Bismuth subcitrate	Symptoms improved more in HP +ve*	Similar to active therapy overall	59
Kang 1990	51	HP +ve and HP −ve	Bismuth subcitrate	73 (in HP +ve)*	25 (in HP +ve)	89

[a] Investigator blind
[b] Double blind
* Statistically significant
? Not stated

Table 2. Randomized placebo-controlled trials of antibiotics in *H. pylori* (HP)-associated nonulcer dyspepsia

Author	*n*	Population studied	Active medication	Symptom improvement on active therapy %	HP suppression on active therapy %
McNulty 1986[a]	50	HP +ve only	Erythromycin	64 (67% on placebo)	7
Glupczynski 1988[b]	45	HP +ve only	Amoxycillin	No difference from placebo	91
Gastrointestinal Physiology Working Group 1988[b]	69	HP +ve only	Furazolidone or nitrofurantoin	No difference from placebo	86 and 58

[a] Investigator blind
[b] Double blind

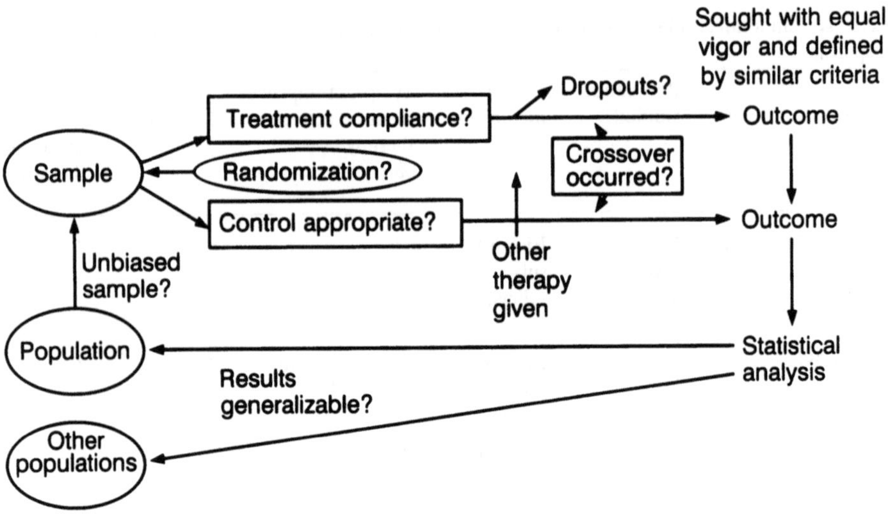

Fig. 1. Potential sites of bias in randomized controlled trials of patients with nonulcer dyspepsia (adapted from Fletcher RH, Fletcher SW, Wagner EH, Clinical Epidemiology: the essentials, 2nd ed Baltimore: Williams and Wilkins, 1988, with permission)

positive from those who are negative (Andersen et al. 1988; Loffeld et al. 1988; Börsch et al. 1988; Sobala et al. 1989). The studies to date have generally used very vague symptom definitions, usually just stating that the subjects had upper gastrointestinal symptoms (Gastrointestinal Physiology Working Group 1988; Glupczynski et al. 1988; Rokkas et al. 1988). Because of this, it is difficult to compare the available results.

Ideally, an "operational definition" to determine which patients will be included should be used; such an approach puts subjective variables in an observable framework (Klein 1988). For example, rather than just requiring the presence of abdominal discomfort without a peptic ulcer, it would be preferable to specify something like "3 months or more of pain in the epigastrium occurring at least three times per week that is severe enough to influence concentration on daily activities, where endoscopy shows no acute or chronic ulcer, esophagitis or malignancy."

The exclusion criteria applied are also critical. In recent years, it has been increasingly appreciated that the irritable bowel syndrome and gastroesophageal reflux can often be associated with ulcer-like dyspepsia (Talley and Piper 1985); in theory, such cases would be unlikely to respond to antibacterial therapy. Most of the trials have not addressed this important concern (McNulty et al. 1986; Gastrointestinal Physiology Working Group 1988; Glupczynski et al. 1988; Karg et al. 1990).

Randomization

Clearly, allocation of patients into the study groups must be performed without bias, and therefore randomization is the preferred method. However, a number of the studies have only randomized *H. pylori*-positive patients, which confounds their interpretation (McNulty et al. 1986; Borody et al. 1987a; Gastrointestinal Physiology Working Group 1988; Glupczynski et al. 1988).

It must also be remembered that randomization is no guarantee that by chance important differences between the groups are not present. This particularly applies to studies with small sample sizes (Rothman 1977). Investigators therefore usually try to determine if such a bias exists by comparing baseline demographic and disease-related variables in the pretreated study groups. It may then be possible to control for confounding by known or suspected risk factors in the analysis. The trials that have been published have evaluated their study groups for baseline differrnces (McNulty et al. 1986; Gastrointestinal Physiology Working Group 1988; Glupczynski 1988; Rokkas et al. 1988; Karg et al. 1990). While such baseline comparisons can be helpful, the absence of significant differences does not rule out important, unrecognized characteristics. For example, less than a decade ago, *H. pylori* status would not have been considered.

Placebo Control and Blinding

The placebo response in nonulcer dyspepsia, like the irritable bowel syndrome, is usually considerable, although it is variable. Placebo responses of between 20% and 60% have been found (Tallcy and Phillips 1988). If no placebo control is included, it is therefore impossible to be certain that even marked symptom improvement is related to therapy in nonulcer dyspepsia. For this reason, anecdotal reports of therapeutic success in *H. pylori*-associated nonulcer dyspepsia patients treated with antibacterial therapy should be considered very preliminary at best (Borody et al. 1987b; Rauws et al. 1988).

A major source of bias in placebo-controlled trials is that patients taking the active drug may experience side effects which effectively unblind the investigator. For example, bismuth, unlike placebo, typically causes black discoloration of the stools, teeth, and tongue; investigators who bccomc awarc of this may unconsciously score such a patient's symptoms differently to reflect their preconceived ideas. It is difficult to determine how important this bias might have been in the trials to date. Self-report questionnaires may help overcome this problem. In addition, if therapy itself is a confounder (for example, if the antibiotics in the active treatment arm cause major upper gastrointestinal distress), the results may be very difficult to interpret.

Symptom Rating Methods

Measurement of clinical efficacy using symptom-rating scales is critical in nonulcer dyspepsia trials as no objective markers exist. The measurements approaches undertaken to date, however, have been unsatisfactory (Talley et al. 1989). Investigators have usually asked patients at interview about their symptoms often without using standardized methodology (McNulty et al. 1986; Glupczynski et al. 1988; Rokkas et al. 1988; Karg et al. 1990).

Optimally, studies should measure the frequency, duration, and severity of relevant individual symptoms (e.g., epigastric pain, nausea) as well as global change

(Talley et al. 1986). The severity of symptoms can be obtained by using a visual analog scale or a Likert scale (e.g., a seven- to ten-point pain scale ranging from no pain to very severe pain) (Guyatt 1987). Nyrén et al. (1987) have shown that pain duration and intensity are independent measures; therefore, a pain index can be calculated by the product of duration and intensity. The global measure should integrate change in all major symptoms and weigh each according to its importance to the patient (Klein 1988). More convincing evidence that antibacterial therapy is effective would come if significant changes in both global measures and specific symptoms could be shown with active medication (Klein 1988). However, few published studies have included such an approach (Rokkas et al. 1988).

Another important outcome measure is antacid or other medication use during the trial, as such use is another gauge of symptom severity. On the other hand, certain medications may interfere with the interpretation of the results; even if instructed otherwise, patients may take medicines during a trial. It is essential that any such use be recorded and, if necessary, adjusted for in the analysis. Similarly measuring patient compliance needs to be carefully addressed.

Whatever clinical measures are used, they must be obtained reliably and measure what they are supposed to measure, i.e., they have to be valid (Guyatt 1987). We have recently developed a valid self-report scale to evaluate symptoms in patients with functional bowel disorders (Talley et al. 1989), and we are testing newer versions to determine their validity and responsiveness to change in randomized controlled trials. Eventually, we hope to have available a disease-specific standardized questionnaire for use in nonulcer dyspepsia trials (Talley, unpublished observations).

Trial Length

Like the irritable bowel syndrome (Klein 1988), nonulcer dyspepsia is a chronic, often relapsing and remitting disease (Talley et al. 1987). While suppression of *H. pylori* is easily achievable, eradication is more difficult (Rauws et al. 1988; Ormand and Talley 1989). Eradication is now defined as the absence of *H. pylori* 1 month or more after cessation of therapy (Rauws et al. 1988). For this reason, studies need to follow-up patients for a suitable period following cessation of antimicrobial therapy. The symptom scores over time can then be correlated with the gastritis scores. As it may take more than 6 months for chronic gastritis to resolve following eradication of *H. pylori* (Rauws et al. 1988), a follow-up of at least this amount of time would be ideal.

Statistical Considerations

The statistical analysis can be misleading. If too few patients are enrolled, it is possible to miss a clinically important difference between a treatment and placebo (a type II error) (Freiman et al. 1978). The power of the study therefore needs to be stated if no difference between treatments is detected. None of the negative published studies have included a statement about their power (McNulty et al. 1986; Gastrointestinal Physiology Working Group 1988; Glupczynski et al. 1988). On the other hand, if 20 symptoms are measured and analyzed, by chance alone one of the comparisons may be significant at the 5% level statistically (a type I error) (Tukey 1977). While significance testing can be very misleading, reporting confidence intervals is more useful as they represent a set of possible values given the degree of variability in the data (Rothman 1986).

It is also important that an analysis be performed on all patients who were randomized (an intention to treat analysis) as well as on those who actually complied with the treatment (Sackett and Gent 1979). An intention to treat analysis gives a conservative estimation of any treatment effect as some patients will not have taken their medications. On the other hand, analyzing only those who received treatment may be biased as the groups remaining can be quite dissimilar. Ideally, both types of analyses should be reported. A number of the published studies did not perform an intention to treat analysis (McNulty et al. 1986; Gastrointestinal Physiology Working Group 1988; Glupczynski et al. 1988; Rokkas et al. 1988).

Generalizability

The ability to generalize the results is a relevant consideration. The kinds of patients included determine the applicability of the findings. If only young patients are enrolled, the results may not apply in the elderly, while a study in Hispanics in Los Angeles may not apply to Caucasians in southern Minnesota. Moreover, the study populations in trials usually comprise a highly selected and often biased sample of all patients with the disease of interest, as many, if not most, patients refuse to participate or are excluded (Brazer et al. 1989). For this reason, it is essential to have information on all patients screened for entry into a trial to give an indication whether the results apply to patients not represented in the trial (Hampton 1981). The addition of a patient registry to carefully determine the number and characteristics of all eligible, ineligible, and excluded patients allows a trial's applicability to be judged and should be reported.

Table 3. Optimal study design for randomized controlled trials of *H. pylori*-associated nonulcer dyspepsia

Population
– Define the study population approached and who refused to participate
– Use a comprehensive operational definition of nonulcer dyspepsia
– Exclude patients with irritable bowel syndrome and symptomatic gastroesophageal reflux
Study Design
– Enroll an adequate sample size
– Randomize *H. pylori*-positive and -negative patients
– If necessary, use stratified randomization or control for potential confounders
– Always have a placebo arm, and ensure adequate blinding of both patients and investigators
Evaluation
– Use valid symptom and global rating scales
– Measure other medication use (e.g., antacids) and compliance
– Follow up patients for a suitable period following completion of the therapy
Analysis
– Report the study power
– Report confidence intervals rather than just significance tests

Recommendations for Future Studies

It is apparent that better studies can be designed in the future. A list of recommendations is given in Table 3. Use of a strict operational definition will determine the nature of the patients enrolled. The measures of improvement should then include each of the important elements in the definition. A patient registry should be kept so that generalizability of the results can be assessed. It is also very important to spell out whether the study will focus on nonulcer dyspepsia patients who have no evidence of the irritable bowel syndrome, gastroesophageal reflux, or disease elsewhere, or whether a heterogeneous population is to be entered. Studies of heterogeneous patients are less likely to yield a convincing result. An adequate sample size must also be enrolled; the results are more likely to be accepted as a true reflection of reality if a reasonable number have been studied. It is crucial that a valid, symptom-rating approach be used, and measures of both individual symptoms and global improvement (or deterioration) should be incorporated. In the statistical analysis, the reporting of confidence intervals and the power of the study adds useful information.

Such an approach will hopefully result in better trials; it should also allow the results of new studies to be objectively evaluated and make meta-analysis more feasible. Eventually, better management of patients with nonulcer dyspepsia should result.

References

Andersen LP, Elsborg L, Justesen T (1988) *Campylobacter pylori* in peptic ulcer disease III. Symptoms and paraclinical and epidemiologic findings. Scand J Gastroenterol 23:347–350

Borody T, Hennessy W, Carrick J, Daskalopoulas G, Hazell S (1987a) Double-blind trials of De-Nol in non-ulcer dyspepsia associated with *Campylobacter pyloridis* gastritis (abstract). Gastroenterology 92:1324

Borody TJ, Carrick J, Hazell SL (1987b) Symptoms improve after the eradication of gastric *Campylobacter pyloridis* (letter). Med J Aust 46:450–451

Börsch G, Schmidt G, Wegener M et al. (1988) *Campylobacter pylori:* prospective analysis of clinical and histological factors associated with colonization of the upper gastrointestinal tract. Eur J Clin Invest 18:133–138

Brazer SR, Tyor MP, Pancotto FS et al. (1989) Randomized, double-blind comparison of famotidine with ranitidine in treatment of acute, benign gastric ulcer disease. Community-based study coupled with a patient registry. Dig Dis Sci 34:1047–1052

Dooley CP, Cohen H, Fitzgibbons PL, Bauer M, Appleman MD, Perez-Perez GI, Blaser MJ (1989) Prevalence of *Campylobacter pylori* infection and histologic gastritis in asymptomatic persons. N Engl J Med 321:1562–66

Freiman JA, Chalmers TC, Smith H, Kuebler RR (1978) The importance of beta, the type II error and sample size in the design and interpretation of the randomized controlled trial: survey of 71 "negative" trials. N Engl J Med 299:690–694

Gastrointestinal Physiology Working Group of Cayetano Heredia and the John Hopkins Universities, Morgan D, Kraft W, Bender M, Pearson A (1988) Nitrofurans in the treatment of gastritis associated with *Campylobacter pylori.* Gastroenterology 95:1178–1184

Glupczynski Y, Burette A, Labbe M, Deprez C, De Reuck M, Deltenre M (1988) *Campylobacter pylori* associated gastritis: a double-blind placebo-controlled trial with amoxycillin. Am J Gastroenterol 83:365–372

Graham DY, Klein PD, Opekun AR, Boutton TW (1988) Effect of age on the frequency of active *Campylobacter pylori* infection diagnosed by the [C13] urea breath test in normal subjects and patients with peptic ulcer disease. J Infect Dis 157:777–780

Guyatt GH (1987) Measuring quality of life: a review of means of measurement in clinical trials of new medicines. Pharm Med 2:49–60

Hampton JR (1981) Presentation and analysis of the results of clinical trials in cardiovascular disease. Br Med J 282:1371–1373

Kang JY, Tay HH, Wee A, Guan R, Math MV, Yap I (1990) Effect of colloidal bismuth subcitrate on symptoms and gastric histology in non-ulcer dyspepsia – a double-blind placebo controlled study. Gut 31:476–480

Klein KB (1988) Controlled treatment trials in the irritable bowel syndrome: a critique. Gastroenterology 95:232–241

Lambert JR, Borromeo M, Korman MG, Hansky J (1989) *Campylobacter pylori* and non-ulcer dyspepsia – randomized controlled trial. Gastroenterology 96:A284

Loffeld RJLF, Potters HVPJ, Arends JW, Stobberingh E, Flendrig JA, Von Spreeuwel JP (1988) *Campylobacter* associated gastritis in patients with non-ulcer dyspepsia. J Clin Pathol 41:85–88

Marshall BJ, Warren JR (1984) Unidentified curved bacilli in the stomach of patients with gastritis and peptic ulceration. Lancet I:1311–1315

McNulty CAM, Gearty JC, Crump B et al. (1986) *Campylobacter pyloridis* and associated gastritis: investigator blind placebo-controlled trial of bismuth salicylate and erythromycin ethyl-succinate. Br Med J 293:645–649

Nyrén O, Adami HO, Bates S et al. (1987) Self-rating of pain in non-ulcer dyspepsia. J Clin Gastroenterol 9:408–414

Ormand JE, Talley NJ (1990) *Campylobacter pylori:* controversies and an approach to management. Mayo Clin Proc 65:414–426

Rathbone BJ, Wyatt J, Heatley RV (1988) Symptomatology in *C. pylori*-positive and negative non-ulcer dyspepsia. Gut 29:A1473

Rauws EAJ, Langenberg W, Houthoff HJ, Zanen HC, Tytgat GNJ (1988) *Campylobacter pyloridis*-associated chronic antral gastritis. Gastroenterology 94:33–40

Rokkas T, Pursey C, Uzocchina E et al. (1987) *Campylobacter pylori* and non-ulcer dyspepsia. Am J Gastroenterol 82:1149–1152

Rokkas T, Pursey C, Uzeochina E, et al. (1988) Non-ulcer dyspepsia and short-term De-Nol therapy: a placebo controlled trial with particular reference to the role of *Campylobacter pylori.* Gut 29:1386–1391

Rothman KJ (1977) Epidemiologic methods in clinical trials. Cancer 39:1771–1775

Rothman KJ (1986) Modern epidemiology. Little, Brown, Boston, pp 115–129

Sackett DL, Gent M (1979) Controversy in counting and attributing events in clinical trials. N Engl J Med 301:1410–1412

Sobala GM, Dixon MF, Axon ATR (1989) *C. pylori* is not associated with a distinct dyspeptic syndrome. Gut 30:A733

Talley NJ (1988) *Campylobacter pylori*-associated gastritis. Is antibiotic therapy now justified? J Clin Gastroenterol 10:10–12

Talley NJ, McNeil D, Hayden A, Piper DW (1986) Randomized double-blind, placebo controlled crossover trial of cimetidine and pirenzepine in non-ulcer dyspepsia. Gastroenterology 91:149–156

Talley NJ, McNeil D, Hayden A, Colreavy C, Piper DW (1987) Prognosis of chronic unexplained dyspepsia: a prospective study of potential predictor variables in patients with endoscopically diagnosed non-ulcer dyspepsia. Gastroenterology 92:1060–1066

Talley NJ, Phillips SF (1988) Non-ulcer dyspepsia: Potential causes and pathophysiology. Ann Intern Med 108:865–79

Talley NJ, Phillips SF, Zinsmeister AR, Melton LJ (1990) Prevalence of functional bowel disease: a random community survey (abstract). Gastroenterology 98:A396

Talley NJ, Phillips SF, Melton LJ, Wiltgen C, Zinsmeister AR (1989) A patient questionnaire to identify bowel disease. Ann Intern Med 1989, 111:671–674

Talley NJ, Piper DW (1985) The association between non-ulcer dyspepsia and other gastrointestinal disorders. Scand J Gastroenterol 20:896–900

Thomas LO (1977) Biostatistics in medicine. Science 198:675

Tukey JW (1977) Some thoughts on clinical trials, especially problems of multiplicity. Science 198:679–684

Discussion

Colin-Jones: I think I agree with everything you said with one minor exception and that was in one of your first slides when you listed the criteria that were required. I don't think it is necessarily correct that *H. pylori* is more frequent in the NUD population than in age matched controls.

Talley: I must admit I made that slide a while ago and I agree with you. We can formulate a model which suggests that you need to have a number of different coexistent factors to develop dyspepsia. *H. pylori* may be one of those factors; if *H. pylori* is removed, then you no longer find dyspepsia in the group that is predisposed. However, you must have all the factors together to get dyspepsia. *H. pylori* perhaps, plus possibly genetic factors, perhaps an adequate threshold of acid secretion and so on.

Petersen: I have to disagree with you concerning your advice to exclude those with gastroesophageal reflux symptoms or irritable bowel symptoms. The main reason is that a huge proportion of patients that may be termed nonulcer dyspepsia have such symptoms. If you then exclude such a large proportion you end up with a group of patients that is very artificial, and the external validity of your study is then very limited.

Colin-Jones: If you were to classify your patients very carefully by predetermined criteria and then put them into several groups, would that not give you a better opportunity to find which subgroup benefits from your therapy?

Talley: I think that is true. You would be doing really three or four trials in one, which is an enormous task, but I agree that this could be done.

Tytgat: One of your entry criteria was normal endoscopy or no endoscopic abnormalities, what do you really mean by that, what is a normal endoscopy?

Talley: I think that is a difficult question and you are an expert in that area. I would argue that erosive disease and chronic ulcer disease perhaps comprise part of the same spectrum, *H. pylori* may be the link, although I cannot be sure. Again I would argue for purity. The endoscopist will often see perhaps only erythema or no mucosal abnormality at endoscopy, I would argue that this group *is* a purer group than one which includes erosive disease of any severity. It is debatable, however.

Tytgat: How common is severe gastritis without erosions?

Talley: It is quite common.

Tytgat: I know it is quite common, and I see it too, but I am just wondering. May I have a last question? I mean, this is of course the ideal world and we would love to do such studies, but to be very honest, is it truly possible or will it ever be possible to conduct such a study even on a multinational and multicenter level?

Talley: I would argue it is possible to do these studies. I agree it is very difficult, I agree that the patients do not always like being followed for prolonged periods of time, which is one of the critical issues. However, I believe these studies need to be done if we really want to establish *H. pylori* as a cause of a subgroup of nonulcer dyspeptic patients. I think if we do not do these studies, we will continue to argue about this issue the next international meeting, perhaps many meetings to come.

Colin-Jones: Well that is a good way to end and I can now close the discussion. Thank you all very much indeed. The comment about normal endoscopy reminds me of a London professor of medicine who is reputed to have said there is no such thing as a normal person, a normal person is someone who has been insufficiently investigated.

Optimal Design for Peptic Ulcer Studies

H. PETERSEN

Introduction

The optimal study of peptic ulcer and *Helicobacter pylori* should focus on the most important questions related to the subject which still remain unanswered or to which there are only unsatisfactory answers. In my opinion, the most important question is still whether *H. pylori* plays a significant etiological role in peptic ulcer disease (PUD). In spite of rapidly accumulating evidence strongly favouring such a role, the group of "nonbelievers" among gastroenterologists is still large.

The second main question that needs to be focused on is how *H. pylori* plays a role in PUD. This question, however, can or must be subdivided into a large number of separate questions related to the many possible pathogenetic mechanisms which may operate. Because only a small number of such questions can possibly be solved in a single study, a selection has to be made. In the following, an attempt is made to justify the priority given to certain questions.

A considerable number of abnormalities have been described in patients with PUD [1]. Typical for all of these abnormalities is that there is a great overlap in patients with and without the disease. Well-known examples of this overlap are acid hypersecretion and increased parietal cell sensitivity to pentagastrin in patients with duodenal ulcer [2]. Only a proportion of the patients with duodenal ulcer in fact show true acid hypersecretion. Research on *H. pylori* has, however, identified several more or less new abnormalities in PUD that appear to be present in almost all patients [3, 4].

Gastritis is always found in patients with gastric ulcer, at least if the ulcers due to Zollinger-Ellison syndrome or the use of nonsteroid anti-inflammatory drugs are excluded. The same is true of the presence of *H. pylori* in the stomach: patients with duodenal ulcer nearly always have antral gastritis and associated *H. pylori* infection. The same may also be true of duodenitis, duodenal *H. pylori* infection and at least the superficial type of gastric metaplasia [5]. My guess is that this may also turn out to be true of the heterotopic type of gastric metaplasia if this condition is studied more carefully.

What, then, may happen if humans are exposed to *H. pylori* (Fig. 1)? Probably all will develop some degree of acute gastritis that may heal or progress into chronic active gastritis. It is likely that chronic gastritis will either heal or progress into atrophic gastritis. At some stage in this process, a gastric ulcer may develop. Probably at least partly independent of what happens in the stomach, the overflow of *H. pylori* from the antrum may result in duodenal *H. pylori* infection and duodenitis. A certain degree of gastric metaplasia is the most likely prerequisite for this to happen. The

H. Menge et al. (Eds.)
Helicobacter pylori 1990

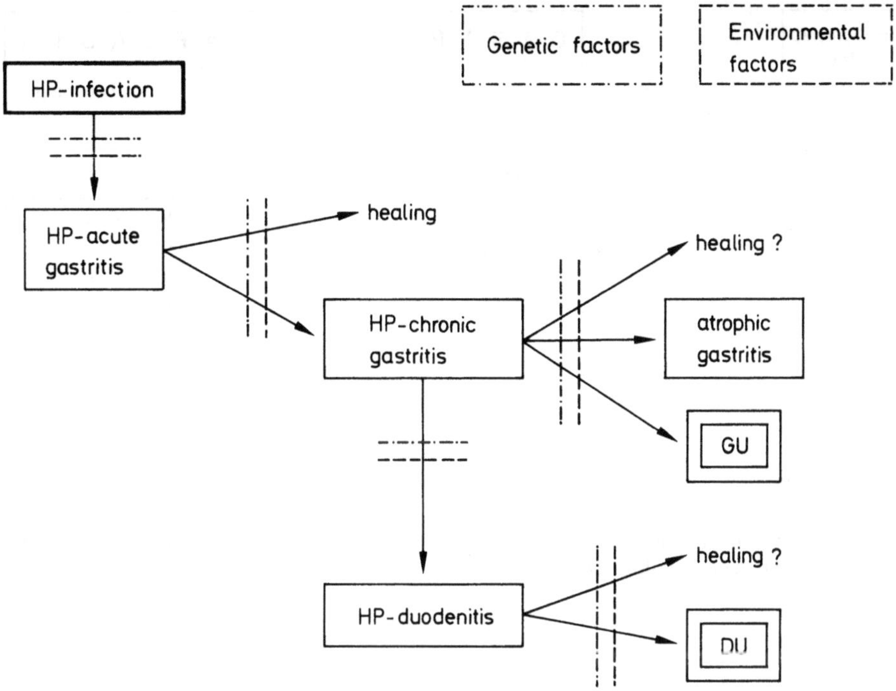

Fig. 1. The possible consequences of infection with *Helicobacter pylori (HP)*

duodenitis is likely to heal or fluctuate between an active and inactive stage. Some of these patients tend to develop a duodenal ulcer.

It is easy to accept that *H. pylori* is the true cause of the gastritis and duodenitis with which it is found to be associated. It is also not difficult to understand that *H. pylori* infection and the inflammation associated with it may weaken the mucosa's general ability to withstand the aggressive forces of acid and pepsin, thereby creating the optimal climate for an ulcer to develop. But still we are left with the question as to which local factor is also in operation.

Let us turn to gastric ulcer first. Parietal cells and G cells do not occur together, parietal cells being found in the mucosa of the corpus and G cells in that of the antrum. There is, however, a variable transitional zone between corpus and antrum where parietal cells and G cells tend to occur together [6]. This border zone is also the border between the site of chronic gastritis and normal corpus mucosa, where gastric ulcers tend to occur [7]. In this transitional zone, where G cells and parietal cells may be close neighbours, local paracrine hyperstimulation of parietal cells and local hypersecretion of acid causing local mucosal damage are feasible.

In the duodenum, there is a close anatomic relationship between *H. pylori* and gastric metaplasia [5]. Superficial gastric metaplasia contains only mucus cells and probably develops in response to damage in general. Damage as a consequence of exposure to too much acid and pepsin is perhaps the most interesting possibility apart

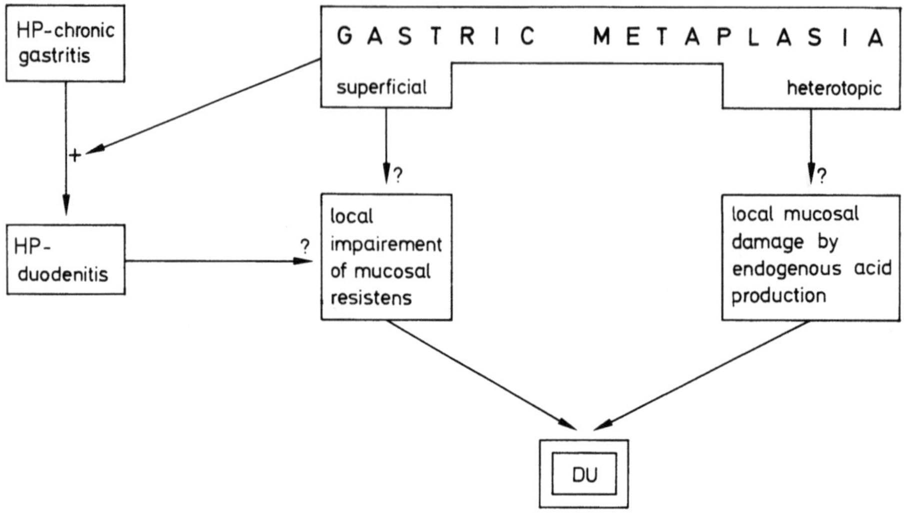

Fig. 2. The possible relationships between *Helicobacter pylori (HP)*, gastritis, duodenitis, gastric metaplasia, and duodenal ulcer *(DU)*

from *H. pylori* infection itself (Fig. 2). The heterotopic type of gastric metaplasia, which may also harbour *H. pylori,* contains functional glands with parietal cells and chief cells. These islets of heterotopic gastric mucosa are therefore capable of producing acid, which may cause local mucosal damage that may ultimately lead to a duodenal ulcer. Using pentagastrin as a stimulant and the Congo red staining method, Carrick et al. [5] recently identified acid-producing gastric metaplasia in close anatomic relationship to duodenal ulcer. The occurrence of superficial and heterotopic gastric metaplasia in the duodenum and its relationship to acid secretion deserves, in my opinion, more attention.

The association between *H. pylori* infection and duodenal ulcer disease actualizes the possibility of gastrin hyperstimulating acid secretion. Hyperstimulation of acid, caused by increased sensitivity of the parietal cells to gastrin [2] or simply due to hypergastrinemia, may not only be important for the development of gastric metaplasia in general, but may also play a role in the degree of local acid production in the duodenum and thus in the risk of local damage. The actuality or importance of gastrin in connection with PUD is supported by a preliminary finding suggesting inappropriate hypergastrinemia in patients infected with *H. pylori* [8]. Gastrin release is inhibited by a low antral pH. By means of its urease activity, *H. pylori* produces large amounts of ammonia and probably protects itself against the low pH in the stomach with a cloud of ammonia. It is possible that the ammonia produced by these microorganisms, particularly in the case of extensive infection, interferes with the antral pH-gastrin feedback mechanism. The effect of *H. pylori* infection and gastritis on serum gastrin urgently needs more attention.

The Optimal Study

The main purpose of the study that I would like to propose would be to examine the effect of eradication of *H. pylori* on the clinical course of PUD, i.e., symptoms, healing, and recurrence. Additional aims would be to examine the effect of this eradication on gastric and duodenal histology, serum gastrin, and gastric secretion. Another goal would be to study the relationship between gastric metaplasia and acid secretion.

An effective drug treatment for *H. pylori* infection does not yet exist. The optimal choice today probably would be a combination of amoxicillin and metronidazole. Bismuth preparations [9] are not regarded as appropriate in an optimal study because of the many possible effects they can have apart from the effects on *H. pylori* and the fact that bismuth is absorbed to a certain degree and kept in the body for a long time [10]. According to a preliminary report, the strong acid inhibition induced by omeprazole may improve the effect of amoxicillin on *H. pylori* [11]. In the light of this finding and because the use of antibiotics for *H. pylori* in the treatment of PUD deserves to be compared with the new gold standard of PUD treatment, a combination and comparison of the treatment of *H. pylori* with antibiotics and omeprazole is suggested. Three treatment groups are proposed (Table 1). The duration of treatment should be standardized; 6 weeks is suggested, but it is possible that even 2 weeks may be sufficient. Pilot studies on the effect of a large dose of omeprazole combined with amoxicillin and metronidazole on the eradication of *H. pylori* are required.

Careful pretreatment characterization of the patients according to history, symptoms, endoscopy, and histology is required (Table 1). Quantitation of symptoms and

Table 1. Pretreatment evaluation and treatment in a suggested optimal peptic ulcer study

Pretreatment Evaluation

Evaluation category	Specific definition
History	with use of nonsteroid anti-inflammatory drugs
Symptoms	graded
Endoscopy	degree of inflammatory changes
	ulcer location
	ulcer size
Histology	grading of duodenitis and gastritis
	grading of superficial and heterotopic gastric metaplasia
Serum gastrin	basal and meal-stimulated
Gastric secretion	basal and pentagastrin-stimulated acid and pepsin secretion

Treatment

Group	Drugs
A	anti-acid
	anti-*H. pylori*
B	anti-acid
	anti-*H. pylori* placebo
C	anti-acid placebo
	anti-*H. pylori*

Proton pump inhibitor; Anti-*H. pylori*, antibiotic(s) effective against *H. pylori*

Table 2. The course of a suggested optimal peptic ulcer study indicating recommended times for specific evaluations *(plus sign)*

	Symptom	Endoscopy	Histology	*H. pylori*-status	Serum gastrin	Gastric secretion
Treatment phase						
Time elapsed (weeks)						
0	+	+	+	+	+	+
2	+	+		+		
4	+	+		+		
6	+	+	+	+	+	+
Observation phase						
Time elapsed (months)						
3	+	+	+	+	+	+
6	+	+		+		
12	+	+	+	+	+	
24	+	+				

histological features, particularly superficial and heterotopic gastric metaplasia, should be attempted. The pretreatment characterization should also include basal and meal-stimulated serum gastrin, or perhaps even a 24-h serum gastrin curve, as well as basal and pentagastrin-stimulated gastric secretion.

During the treatment, symptoms should be recorded daily on a visual analogue scale and endoscopy is required at least every second week (Table 2). At the end of treatment, in addition to repeated symptomatic, endoscopic, and histologic characterization, the serum gastrin and gastric secretory pattern should also be re-evaluated. Serum gastrin and gastric secretion should be examined at least 1 week after stopping treatment and 2 year follow-up is suggested. Endoscopy is advocated every third month during the first half year. Three months and possibly also 12 months after stopping treatment, an evaluation not only including endoscopy and histology, but also serum gastrin and gastric acid secretion may be justified.

Provided it includes a sufficiently large number of patients with gastric, prepyloric, and duodenal ulcer, a study, as suggested, may make an important contribution to our knowledge about the role played by *H. pylori* in PUD, and hopefully also throw some light on the important interrelationships between *H. pylori* infection, duodenitis, gastritis, serum gastrin, and gastric acid secretion.

References

1. Richardson CT (1985) Pathogenetic factors in peptic ulcer disease. Am J Med [Suppl 2C] 79:1–6
2. Petersen H, Myren J (1975) Pentagastrin dose-response in peptic ulcer disease. Scand J Gastroenterol 10:705–714
3. Axon ATR (1988) Campylobacter pylori. In: Pounder RE (ed) Recent advances in gastroenterology, vol 7. Livingstone, Edinburgh, pp 225–244
4. Graham D (1989) Campylobacter pylori and peptic ulcer disease. Gastroenterology 96:615–625

5. Carrick J, Lee A, Hazell S, Ralston M, Daskalopoulos (1989) Campylobacter pylori, duodenal ulcer and gastric metaplasia: possible role of functional heterotopic tissue in ulcerogenesis. Gut 30:790–797
6. Stave R, Brandzaeg P, Nygaard K, Fausa O (1978) The transitional body-antrum zone in resected human stomachs. Anatomical outline and parietal-cell and gastrin-cell characteristics in peptic ulcer disease. Scand J Gastroenterol 13:685–691
7. Stadelman O, Elster K, Stolte M, Miederer SE, Deyle P, Demling L, Siegenthaler W (1971) The peptic gastric ulcerhistopathographie and functional investigations. Scand J Gastroenterol 6:613–623
8. Smith JTL, Pounder RE, Evans DJ, Evans DC, Graham D (1959) Inappropriate 24 hours hypergastrinemia in asymptomatic campylobacter pylori infection. Gastroenterology 96:A479
9. Tytgat CNJ (1987) Colloidal bismuth subcitrate in peptic ulcer a review. Digestion [Suppl 2] 37:31–41
10. Gavey CJ, Szeto ML, Nwokolo CU, Sercombe J, Pounder RE (1989) Bismuth accumulates in the body during treatment with tripotassium dicitrato bismuthate. Aliment Pharmacol Ther 3:21–28
11. Unge P, Olsson J, Gad A, Gnarpe H (1988) Does omeprazole, 40 mg o. m., improve antimicrobial therapy directed towards gastric campylobacter pylori in patients with antral gastritis (Abstr)? International Symposium on Omeprazol, Monte Carlo

Discussion

Colin-Jones: There was a time when I was doing clinical trials when they were fun and the patients thought they were fun too. The criteria we are laying down now, I'm sure this is right, should be very much stricter than they used to be, but I am just concerned about your requirement especially for gastric secretion, Hermod. Could I just question you on that, because that means a lot of extra work for the patients.

Petersen: It has something to do with my background. For a century – half a century at least – we have been extremely interested in gastric acid secretion. I think there is good reason to believe that gastric metaplasia and perhaps also heterotopic gastric metaplasia is due to an increased acid exposure. I think you will agree with me that gastric metaplasia in the duodenum is a very crucial thing and the relationship to acid secretion is, therefore, also very important.

Graham: That study you just described is basically what we are more than half way through. With the exception that we do our follow-up endoscopies every 3 months for 2 years instead of every 6 months, and so I am pleased to see that we designed it properly.

Börsch: I have some difficulties with the aims of your study. The end points are symptoms, healing, and recurrence. You suggest using omeprazole as acid-reducing agent. I do not see any chance that you could speed the healing of ulcers beyond the healing rate induced by omeprazole alone, neither by adding any other further drug, nor by adding *H. pylori* therapy. The other point is that we should distinguish between things which are interesting and those which are essential. I think that it is not the rapidity of healing of ulcers which is essential for the *H. pylori* theory, but just recurrence rates. Once the ulcer, the hole has been generated in the stomach or the duodenum the factors governing the healing are probably different from those factors that have induced the hole. So if you want to do an essential study, you can stick to recurrence rates only.

Petersen: I have a lot of understanding for your objections, but I am not quite so sure as you are that the healing rate achieved with omeprazole cannot be improved. Not all patients are healed with omeprazole. I think that knowledge about if and to what degree *H. pylori* eradication may speed up the healing rate is of enough interest to justify such a design.

Tytgat: Dr. Petersen, you said the majority outside are nonbelievers. I wonder what the arguments are that these people use to support their non-believers' attitude.

Graham: Why don't you try that in Saudi Arabia? I mean it is religion we are talking about.

Petersen: I have a lot of nonbelievers in my surroundings. They are making pleas for more documentation without knowing that there is a fair amount of such documentation. So the most important reason for most nonbelievers is, in my opinion, lack of knowledge.

Tytgat: But can you in all fairness at the present time think of arguments which can explain the findings in a different way as explained now? I am asking the audience that, too. I mean, this is something that puzzles me too and I would like to know.

Petersen: I am not quite happy with the fact that the majority of the studies have involved bismuth preparations, simply because of the many possible other effects that bismuth preparations may have, and the fact that bismuth may accumulate in the body. I know the argument presented yesterday about the difference between *H. pylori* negative and *H. pylori* positive, but that is still a background for being a little sceptical. I do not like the fact that you are trying to force me into the nonbeliever group.

Colin-Jones: I am going to just stay with your comment, if I may. It seems to me the crucial thing here is what is the drug that we are going to use in this trial? I think the trial has been carefully outlined, and with modification and adaptation I think it could give us some very valuable answers. It seems to me the crucial thing is which drug regimen do we use? Should we have bismuth or should we not? That is one question. What does the audience think about this?

Tytgat: If I may answer. The point is if you make the people achlorhydric, you really get bacteriologically contaminated stomachs. And I am not so sure that what you propose is the right combination in the long run. Dr. Rauws followed a group of patients on long-term omeprazole therapy, and month after month you see the breath tests going up. There is no other explanation for this phenomenon than that the bacterial load increases in the stomach. I am not so sure that the combination of total achlorhydria, which is what you aim for to speed up healing, with or without antibiotics, is the best combination to be considered at the present time.

Graham: I can give you another explanation for the breath test going steadily up besides an increase in bacterial load: if you go to your pernicious anemia population and do breath tests, many will be positive and yet have no *H. pylori.* They have other bacteria growing in their stomachs contributing to the urease activity and not just *H. pylori.* You must quantitate the bacteria and look at measurements of surface area that is involved in order to make the assumption that the breath test is actually giving you a measurement of *H. pylori* urease and not just a total global assessment of urease. And you also have to measure CO_2 production, otherwise you do not have values that are really the same. Can I answer Dr. Börsch's question about why it is so critical to measure healing rates? Even though you are right, and it is probably not going to change, you have just designed a study that is going to take 3 or 4 years if you figure it will take 1 year or 18 months to enter patients and then 2 more years until the last patient has finished his follow-up. So, at least, at the first time point, you will get another paper asking does it heal more quickly or not, and that is important to keep the investigators involved.

Marshall: My feeling is that to convince the sceptics and change prescribing practice throughout the world, you must use the gold standard current therapy in your group. For example, treat ulcers with 6 weeks of ranitidine and follow that with 2 years of maintenance therapy at half dose. Then you put a small placebo group in and keep the investigators honest. The aim of the study is to show that the new treatment is better than the gold standard, so we must have a placebo group that receives no maintenance therapy. The other group of course is your active therapy which eradicates *Helicobacter pylori* and is followed by no maintenance therapy at all.

Colin-Jones: And which active therapy would you use, Barry?

Marshall: The ideal study, of course, is to just use an antibiotic or antibiotic combination as the active therapy. Inclusion of a bismuth drug would affect blindness.

Colin-Jones: That's an interesting reply – what does the rest of the audience think? David, are we allowed to ask what you are using in your trial?

Graham: We're comparing ranitidine 300 mg in the evening with ranitidine plus triple therapy. The triple therapy lasts 2 weeks, which is probably longer than necessary. The ranitidine is continued until the ulcer is completely healed, and then there is no therapy of any kind given to the patients. If I have omeprazole, I would probably give 60 mg and do everything just for 2, 3, or 4 weeks and then have one follow-up endoscopy instead of what we do now. We are interested in healing rates and I suspect that we will show a more rapid healing and we will show a larger percentage of patients going to complete healing because we have a percentage that do not completely heal just with one course of ranitidine, even at 16 weeks.

Colin-Jones: Thank you very much.

Tytgat: At the end of this meeting, I would like to say just two words. First of all, I personally enjoyed this meeting very much. I think the standard was very high and I'd like to thank all the speakers and discussants. But above all, I would like to thank the Röhm-Pharma, the board of directors, and Mrs. Klein for the tremendous job they did in bringing us here, and for the way, the frank open way we could discuss all the problems we have in clinical practice.

MIX
Papier aus verantwortungsvollen Quellen
Paper from responsible sources
FSC® C105338

If you have any concerns about our products,
you can contact us on
ProductSafety@springernature.com

In case Publisher is established outside the EU,
the EU authorized representative is:
Springer Nature Customer Service Center GmbH
Europaplatz 3, 69115 Heidelberg, Germany

Printed by Libri Plureos GmbH
in Hamburg, Germany